Equivalents

2 cups ground meat = 1 pound

5 large eggs = 1 cup

8 egg whites = 1 cup

16 egg yolks = 1 cup

1 square butter = 1 tablespoon

2 cups butter = 1 pound

4 cups grated cheese = 1 pound

1 pound fresh peas (shelled) = 1 cup

1 cup uncooked rice = 2 cups cooked

1 cup uncooked macaroni = 2 cups cooked

1 cup uncooked noodles = 1 1/4 cups cooked

1 large lemon = 1/4 cup juice

1 medium orange = 1/2 cup juice

2 cups dates = 1 pound

3 cups dried apricots = 1 pound

2 1/2 cups prunes = 1 pound

2 1/2 cups raisins = 1 pound

1 1/2 pounds apples = 1 quart

3 large bananas = 1 pound

1 cup shortening = 1/2 pound

1 cup molasses = 13 ounces

1 cup nut meats = 5 ounces

1 pound potatoes = 4 medium-sized potatoes

1 pound tomatoes = 3 medium-sized tomatoes

LET'S COOK IT RIGHT

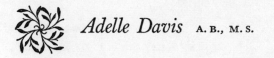

LET'S COOK IT RIGHT

NEW REVISED EDITION

HARCOURT, BRACE & WORLD, INC. New York

Dedicated to my daughter, Barbara,
in the hope that her husband and children
will not have to eat TV dinners

PREFACE

The application of nutritional knowledge in the kitchen has lagged decades behind the progress made in nutritional research. It is in the hope of helping to rectify such a deplorable situation that this book has been written. Only when nutrition is applied in planning and preparing meals day after day can health be attained.

The author wishes to express her thanks to the many friends who have contributed to this book, aided in testing recipes, and offered valuable criticisms. Outstandingly helpful have been Mrs. Helen Moler, Mrs. Glenn Howe, Mrs. Roscoe Wood, Mrs. Gladys Lindberg, and Mrs. Anne Mihaylo.

The author also wishes to thank the following companies for materials used in testing recipes: the Century Metalcraft Corporation for Guardian Service and Presto Pride cooking utensils; Plus Products for powdered milk and tiger's milk; the El Molino Mills for whole-wheat-bread mix and many varieties of flour; and the Lindberg Nutrition Service for organically raised fruits and vegetables, meats from naturally grown animals, fertile eggs, and numerous other supplies.

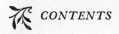

CONTENTS

	PREFACE	vii
1	Let's Cook It Right	3
2	You Need Have No Failures in Cooking Meats	14
3	Make Delicious Gravies or None at All	123
4	Dress Up Your Meats with Dressings	128
5	Sauces to Be Served with Meats, Fish, or Vegetables	134
6	Get Acquainted with Fish	145
7	Meat Substitutes and Extenders for Limited Budgets	171
8	Make Your Leftovers a Treat	203
9	Meats and Meat Substitutes for Hot-Weather Dinners	219
10	Serve Eggs and Cheese Daily	235
11	Appetizers Contribute to Health	251
12	Serve Your Salads First	260
13	Salad Dressings	287
14	Soups Are Fun to Make	293
15	Keep the Flavor and Nutritive Value in Your Vegetables	317
16	If You Want to Bake Bread	403
17	Fortify Your Cereals	434
18	Milk Cannot Be Overemphasized	438
19	Freezing, Canning, and Pickling	452

20   Desserts Can Contribute to Health   467

21   Candies and Candy Substitutes   527

22   Revising and Creating Recipes   539

23   Where to Buy Foods of High Nutritive Value   542

24   Your Reward   544

    NOTES AND OTHER RECIPES   545

    INDEX   555

LET'S COOK IT RIGHT

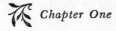 *Chapter One*

Let's Cook It Right

Surely we all agree that our foods should be both delicious and sufficiently health-building to enhance our enjoyment of life; and that dishes which are good for you but almost impossible to eat deserve little praise. Since we spend approximately a thousand hours each year eating our meals, they should be pleasant hours, times of family unity and companionship and, if a blessing is asked, of family worship. Good food is a symbol of love, having psychological value which may even exceed its sensory and physiological contributions. To show how foods can meet these combined needs and retain their delightful flavors as well as their rewarding nutrients is the purpose of this book.

Spiritual and emotional hungers which induce psychosomatic illnesses are undoubtedly as widespread as are vitamin and mineral hungers, and therefore faulty nutrition is by no means the only cause of illness. It has been fully proved, however, that if we are to have the vitality necessary to make our lives richly rewarding, we must obtain some sixty nutrients daily; and that a lack of one or more of these nutrients results first in a below-par drag and eventually in serious illness. Aside from sickness that results directly from nutritional inadequacies, a contributory cause in the onset of infections, allergies, and possibly all illnesses is carelessly chosen food. The degree of health any family enjoys depends to a large extent upon which foods are selected and how they are prepared.

Despite the need to retain maximum value in all food preparation, women are advised by thousands of recipes to extract and discard nutrients or to destroy them by high temperatures, long cooking, or the incorporation of air. The cumulative use of such cooking methods over a period of years can lead to a nightmare of illness and staggering medical bills. It has, therefore, been my purpose in all the following recipes to show the homemaker how to retain the greatest number of nutrients.

Since the values of each nutrient have been fully dealt with elsewhere,* they are referred to only briefly in the succeeding chapters. Nor has space been given to attractive table settings, a subject excellently handled by women's magazines and one of importance; if food is to be well digested and absorbed, one must dine rather than merely eat. Beauty has health value, and its achievement is worth considerable effort.

In this revision I have tried to answer all the questions concerning cooking which have reached me since this book was first written; time does not permit personal correspondence on the subject. Any part which a user found confusing has been rewritten and clarified.

Most of the policies of the original edition have been retained. Preceding each chapter is an introduction which gives the principles of cooking and the fundamentals of nutrition as they apply to the particular group of foods discussed. The recipes are planned for a family of four. All measurements are level, made with standard equipment. Block-style recipes are used to achieve greater clarity and to avoid repetition; the ingredients are listed in the order in which they are to be added. Variations are given for all basic recipes, thus allowing the homemaker to avoid monotony or to substitute another ingredient for one which is not available or which her family does not enjoy. And in every recipe, an attempt has been made to keep dirty dishes to a minimum.

For the most part, recipes are simple and procedures short. Since busy women often prepare sketchy and near-valueless meals because they are convinced cooking is difficult, I have tried to show how easy cooking is. There are actually only four fundamental recipes: those which tell you how to stew, fry, broil, and bake. When you have once learned to cook by these four methods,

* Davis, Adelle: *Let's Eat Right to Keep Fit,* Harcourt, Brace & World, Inc., New York, 1954.

you know the essentials of food preparation. All recipes are variations of these four, the main variation being nothing more than seasonings.

Seasoning brings out flavor. Although it is as impossible to do good cooking without using herbs, seeds, and spices as it is without salt and pepper, the greatest weakness in American cookery is the failure to season food interestingly. Since this phase of cooking is so important, a few fundamental rules should be quickly learned: 1) All seasonings contain aromatic oils, which volatize, or evaporate, easily, and these oils should be kept in the seasonings until they are to be used. Finely ground herbs, like ground pepper, soon have the staleness of a last year's cigar butt, especially if exposed to air. Fresh herbs should therefore be chopped, dried ones crushed, seeds mashed, and whole peppercorns ground immediately before being added to food. 2) The aromatic oils must be treated gently during cooking. The food should be steeped much as is tea, and the oils given time to pass into it. Many old recipes call for hours of cooking, and though the oils gradually pass into the food, nutrients are destroyed: It is preferable to shut off the heat and merely allow the food to stand for a time. 3) If submitted to high temperatures, the aromatic oils take off like a covey of frightened quail. Nothing can be in two places at one time, and the odor of cooking indicates that the food itself is losing flavor. 4) Excessive amounts of any seasoning can quickly ruin a dish; therefore, err on the side of adding too little rather than too much. And garlic, like make-up, should never be obvious. Observation of these four simple rules determines the difference between excellent meals and barely edible ones.

As I see it, a cookbook should not merely teach a beginner how to prepare foods or list proportions of ingredients any housewife may easily forget. One of its chief purposes is to aid in menu planning, bringing to mind, as one flips its pages, foods enjoyed yet infrequently served. Variety lends interest to meals. A woman should be able to prepare thirty or more different entrees without repeating a menu if she wishes to do so; once she has used a recipe it is hers for a lifetime. Housewives who prepare only a few dishes quickly become bored with cooking. And the dinners we plan while gazing at the meat displays in the market, thinking simultaneously of frozen peas, those leftover mashed potatoes, and that tired head of lettuce which needs to be used up are uninteresting both to cook and to eat.

Much of the ease and pleasure in cooking as well as retention of nutritive value depends on the use of proper kitchen equipment. Each housewife must determine what equipment she needs according to the size of her family and the amount of cooking she does. Because many kitchen utensils are used for a lifetime, only those of good quality should be purchased. Certain equipment seems to me to be essential for convenience and efficiency: knives sharp to the point of danger; meat and cooking thermometers; an inexpensive combination shredder, grater, and slicer; measuring cups and spoons; lightweight mixing bowls; a liquefier, or blender; a combination electric mixer and juicer; one or two attractive heat-resistant casseroles in which foods can be both prepared and served; and two or three utensils designed for waterless cooking. These pots and pans should have tight-fitting lids; they should be made of a thick but lightweight material which will not develop hot spots and to which foods will not stick; and they should distribute heat so evenly that food cooks from the sides and top as well as from the bottom.

Unfortunately, no ideal cooking utensils have as yet been made. Enamelware, glassware, ceramic-like plastic cookware, and even copper-clad stainless-steel utensils heat unevenly, causing food to stick or burn. Glassware conducts heat slowly and allows the destruction of vitamin B_2 in foods by exposure to light. Small amounts of aluminum oxide dissolve into foods cooked in aluminum utensils.

Stainless steel was at first welcomed as a metal unlikely to contaminate foods. Investigation, however, has shown that if even the best stainless steel utensils are scoured only once with an abrasive powder, scratch pad, or steel wool, small amounts of chromium, nickel, and other highly toxic metallic compounds dissolve into every food cooked in them thereafter. If stainless steel utensils are always soaked clean and no abrasives are used, they appear to be completely harmless. Unfortunately, food is frequently burned the first time such a utensil is used, and the pan is quickly scoured.

Some authorities believe chromium and nickel are so toxic that none should be ingested; they recommend discarding any utensil which has been scoured even once. Exactly how dangerous these metals are is unknown at present, but they do appear to be considerably more toxic than aluminum. Ingested aluminum combines with phosphorus, a nutrient excessively abundant in the American diet; the resulting aluminum phosphate is excreted from the body.

Since no cooking utensils are perfect, each housewife must reach her own decision as to the kind she wishes to use. I use stainless steel when making soups and preparing foods which cannot stick easily, and aluminum utensils for other cooking.

In this edition dozens of new recipes have been added, old ones rewritten, some little-used ones deleted, and hundreds changed to keep pace with recent findings in nutrition. For example, since radioactive fallout appears to be particularly dangerous to persons whose calcium intake is inadequate, it has become especially important to use calcium-rich ingredients in cooking. To show how this calcium need can be supplied, hundreds of ordinary recipes have been fortified with non-instant powdered milk (the bulkier instant milk is unsatisfactory for fortification; it often causes foods to become gummy or gritty).

A major change throughout the book has been to reduce the use of solid fats to a minimum and to increase that of vegetable oils. Research has shown that excessive intake of solid, or saturated, fats is conducive to a high level of cholesterol in the blood, which may result in coronary disease, strokes, gall-stone formation, and other abnormalities. All hydrogenated cooking fats, hydrogenated peanut butter, processed cheeses, artificially hydrogenated lard, and the ordinary variety of margarines have been omitted from recipes. The use of partially hardened margarines which require constant refrigeration has been suggested, although their content of unsaturated fatty acids varies from as high as 50 per cent to as low as 6 per cent, or little more than occurs naturally in butter. The softer the margarine when it is chilled, the richer it is in the valuable fatty acids. A fat of known unsaturated-fatty-acid content can be obtained by beating a cup of oil, such as soy or safflower, into a pound of butter. The flavor of the butter is retained, yet the cholesterol-increasing action of a highly saturated fat is decreased.

It has been found that the need for vitamin E increases greatly when large amounts of oils, or unsaturated fatty acids, are consumed, particularly if the oils have been heated. Unless 60 to 100 units of this vitamin are taken daily (an amount impossible to obtain from foods), trying to prevent coronary disease by substituting oils for solid fats may lead to other abnormalities.

In the following recipes, an attempt has been made to avoid ingredients which contain possible cancer-producing additives, not an easy task. During the past fifteen years, chemicals by the thousands have been poured into our foods: mold, rancidity, and staleness preventers; a large variety of preservatives and bleaches; artificial sweeteners, flavorings, and dyes; texture modifiers, softeners, agers, and fresheners; emulsifiers, fumigators, anti-foaming and anti-sprouting agents, and paraffin sprays. In addition contaminants get into food from lacquers, enamels, and plastics used in canning, packaging, and shipping; waxed wrapping papers and cartons; and sprays to keep food from sticking to pans. No fewer than 75,000 processing plants are now putting chemical additives into our foods, sometimes as many as a dozen chemicals in a single item.

More than a thousand food additives and contaminants have been shown to produce cancer in experimental animals. Many of these substances—butter yellow, agene flour bleach, mineral oil and paraffin waxes, to mention only a few—had been considered harmless for years. The cancers produced in experimental animals resulted when only *one* additive was fed to them; families using such foods as packaged mixes, brown-and-serve rolls, cold meats, prepared mashed potatoes, and bottled condiments have been found to consume an average of 45 different chemicals daily. Theoretically no food which contains an additive or contaminant in amounts that exceed a specified "safety" level is allowed to be marketed. Studies have revealed, however, that many foods contained twenty to fifty times more DDT than was considered safe; and an analysis of food in certain restaurants showed DDT contamination in everything except black coffee. Yet these studies concern only one out of thousands of food contaminants. Too many "margins of safety" can add to a sum of danger.

The number of additives and contaminants has increased so rapidly that it has been impossible for our government agencies to determine their wholesomeness; it is estimated that seven years are required to investigate a single chemical. Furthermore a number of food additives, apparently safe in themselves, have been found, when combined with others, to produce cancer in animals. Until each additive and every combination of additives have been thoroughly investigated, none can be considered completely safe. Because these chemicals are used to increase attractiveness and retain the appearance of freshness, they are financially advantageous to food processors. Any individual or group which raises a voice against them is quickly declared a "faddist" spreading "scare" propaganda. Yet if we view the situation with apathy, we may well be producing cancer in our children, our husbands, and ourselves in the same way that it is produced in experimental animals.*

The picture would be less grim were there truth in the frequently made statement that we are the best-fed nation in the world. The falsity of this statement is shown by the fact that seven men must now be drafted to obtain two physically and mentally fit for service; and that, although the standards of fitness have been greatly reduced with each war, the number of unfit has steadily increased and is still rapidly increasing.

We have perhaps the greatest *quantity* of food, but quality has been lost. The growth of produce raised on our exhausted soils must be forced with heavy applications of chemical fertilizers. Such foods contain smaller amounts of proteins, vitamins, and minerals than does produce grown on fertile soils. Almost every fresh food in our markets shows signs of plant deficiencies and diseases: uneven ripening, split stalks, rust, spotting, quick spoilage, and an appalling lack of flavor. Plants raised on sick soils quickly become infected with insects; two to three billion pounds

---

* Anyone wishing to learn more about food additives and contaminants is referred to *Stay Young Longer,* by Linda Clark (1961) and *Our Daily Poison,* by Leonard Wickenden (1955), both published by The Devin-Adair Company, New York; and *The Poisons in Your Food,* by William Longgood (1960), published by Simon and Schuster, New York.

of poison sprays and their solvents—many of them already proved to be carcinogenic to animals—are dusted or sprayed annually over our foods. Soils sprayed only once have been found to be still contaminated fifteen years later. Many crops are sprayed a dozen or more times during a single season; these poisons accumulate, and a larger portion seeps into the foods each year. The residues from pesticides and weed killers, even though potentially cancer-producing, cannot be washed off foods. Almost none lie on the surface. They dissolve in the soil solution, are carried throughout the plant, and become imprisoned within each cell of the food itself.

In countries where soils are continuously rebuilt, no insecticides used, and no food additives allowed, the cancer rate, already much lower than ours, is said to be decreasing. Our own sickness and death rate from this dreaded disease increases steadily, the greatest increase now being among our children. That this increase will become even greater in the future can scarcely be doubted.

Nor is that all. Despite the fact that arsenic compounds and such synthetic hormones as stilbestrol are known, from animal experiments, to be potential cancer-producers, the growth of 90 per cent of all chickens and meat animals marketed has been stimulated by these substances. Overheated fats and the smoky residues from burned and blackened meats have long been recognized as carcinogenic, yet charcoal- and ersatz-charcoal-broiled meats have become dangerously popular. Added to this dismal situation is the fact that a large proportion of our foods are highly refined, their nutrients discarded; and, to cut down calories, many foods are now being diluted with indigestible cellulose, which may interfere with absorption and irritate the intestinal tract. It appears that almost any foreign substance introduced into the body is harmful in one way or another.

Only a trickle of the vast amount of money spent on cancer research has been allocated to the study of prevention. A few encouraging results, however, have come to light. Research indicates that adequate protein, vitamins A and E, the many B vitamins, and certain trace elements each play a role in slowing the onset and growth of malignant tumors in rats and mice. In tests involving many hundred food additives and contaminants found to produce cancer in dogs, the nutrient most efficacious in preventing tumor growth was vitamin B_2. Since milk is a rich source of this vitamin, I have over a period of years asked persons previously treated for cancer if they were heavy milk drinkers; none of them were, and most drank no milk at all. In light of the fact that we live in a sea of carcinogens, no one could make the statement that adequate nutrition may prevent cancer, much less correct it. That nutrition plays a role in the time of onset and rate of growth of malignant tumors, however, can no longer be doubted.

We may well ask ourselves what can be done. Our first reaction is usually to say, "Pass more laws," and some are needed. Certainly the spraying of tomatoes, pears, cucumbers, and other foods with carcinogenic waxes should be immediately prohibited. We already have many laws controlling food production, however, and they are difficult to enforce. Furthermore, each food grower has a right to the money value of his crop, which would be quickly ruined, under present farming conditions, if spraying were prohibited.

It seems to me a more positive approach would be to make every effort to obtain foods free from potentially carcinogenic sprays and additives. Many health-food stores already carry not only fruits and vegetables of superb flavor and amazing keeping qualities which have been grown on composted, mulched soils free from chemical fertilizers and insecticides, but also fertile eggs from hens allowed barnyard freedom and meats and fowl from naturally grown animals. The supply of such products can be increased as soon as a demand exists. Enthusiastic "organic" gardeners are to be found from coast to coast, and thousands of former garden plots, now lying fallow, can be put into use any time their owners are convinced the reward is worth the effort.

Although much is still to be learned before blood cholesterol levels can be controlled, an attempt to prevent coronary disease is relatively easy. If we wish to, we can use oils for home cooking; avoid bakery products and packaged mixes loaded with saturated shortening; and forego doughnuts, potato chips, French fries, and restaurant-prepared seafoods cooked in hydrogenated fats, often at dangerously high temperatures. We can also increase our intake of the B vitamins (particularly cholin), which help the saturated fats to be used normally in the body.

Trying to protect ourselves against dangerous potential carcinogens imposes a much more serious problem. Some, such as air contaminants, we cannot control. Many others we may not wish to give up: cigarettes, for example, or hair dyes, lipsticks with their pigments and paraffin base, mineral-oil cold creams, and almost an endless list of foods containing dyes, synthetic flavorings, and other additives. But if we choose to do so, we can avoid most foods loaded with chemicals, control the temperature of fats when cooking, and take care that no hot food touches wax paper or paraffin-coated cartons.

Since melted fat from meats broiled or barbecued above charcoal drips into the fire, causes flames to flare up and produces possible carcinogenic substances not only in the charred surface of the meat but also in the fatty residues deposited on it by the smoke, this dangerous method should be discarded. Instead we can broil or barbecue our meats at low temperatures with the heat above or beside them. We can sear our other meats slowly at moderate temperatures, if at all. Certainly each of us should form the habit of reading the fine print on the labels on everything we buy. Yet we must keep in mind that many additives are not mentioned on labels, and that dozens of foods containing them, such as candies and products one buys from a bakery, are not labeled at all.

Most of the additives are to be found in packaged and already prepared foods; therefore, the housewife who does her own cooking has relatively few to worry about. She must, however, decide whether or not to use synthetic coloring and flavorings, hot dogs to which both dye and preservatives are added, potatoes sprayed to prevent sprouting, yams which have been colored red, and commercial butter, margarines, and Cheddar-type cheeses to which yellow dyes have been added. When the popularity of foods like butter or margarine demands, or the nutritive value, as in yellow cheese, is high, I have included them in the recipes, although I am not sure of the wisdom of the decision.

The stresses of modern life have made the need for adequate

nutrition probably greater than it has ever been before. The more numerous the processed foods in our markets, the greater becomes the desirability of a return to home cooking. Although we live in an era of vitamin capsules and mineral tablets, good health must still come essentially from good food which has been properly cooked. This cookbook, therefore, is not intended merely to show how delicious foods may be prepared. Its purpose is to aid the housewife in building in her family that degree of health which is a basis for a full and rewarding life.

You, the homemaker, are the guardian of the health of your family. If you accept this responsibility, you cannot view yourself as a kitchen drudge, doing work formerly assigned to servants and slaves. Yours is a role of tremendous importance. Your goal is to see that the food you serve daily supplies the ideal amounts of each vitamin, mineral, and the many other body requirements in so far as possible. The nutritive needs of the body are many, and several of its requirements are most difficult to obtain from the American diet. If nutrition is to be successfully applied, therefore, good cooking becomes a necessity.

It is my hope that these recipes, designed to build health, may help you reach this goal.

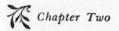

Chapter Two

You Need Have No Failures in Cooking Meats

Since meat is the most expensive item on the food budget and since protein deficiencies are widespread, it is more important to know how to cook meat than any other food. Menus are planned around meats or meat substitutes. Should a housewife learn nothing more about cooking than how to prepare meats well, she would know enough to be a passable cook.

The secret of cooking meats successfully is to remember that a high temperature makes protein tough. This statement explains a thousand cooking failures and is the basis of dozens of household rules. It explains why a milk bottle rinsed first in hot water is difficult to wash; why a blood-stained handkerchief remains stained if put into boiling water; why baking in a hot oven makes a soufflé shrink and toughens an angel-food cake. It explains why eggs fried in smoking fat might be used for vulcanizing tires and why cheese browned under the broiler usually resembles chewing gum. Thousands of dollars' worth of tender, delicious meats have been ruined, many a guileless steer blamed, and many an innocent butcher cursed because housewives have not realized that high temperatures make proteins tough. Meats need not be ruined if one merely glances at a thermometer and controls the heat.

Research in meat cookery has been carried on by the National Live Stock and Meat Board, the United States Department of Agriculture, and the Departments of Home Economics of many state universities. More than 20,000 cuts of meat have been cooked under experimental conditions. Meats have been measured before and after being cooked by different methods, and the percentage of shrinkage has been computed. The escaped juices have been collected and weighed, and the amounts compared. The toughness or tenderness of the cooked meats has been tested by the pounds of force needed to tear the meat fibers. The meats have been tasted by thousands of people whose opinions as to the best flavor and the tenderest and juiciest meat have been pooled and analyzed statistically. The findings of this tremendous amount of research can be summarized in a single sentence: *Meats should be cooked at low temperatures.*

Actually every piece of meat successfully cooked since the legendary shack burned down with a pig in it has been cooked at low temperature. Often, however, the heat has been kept high, and effort, money, and fuel have been wasted to achieve the low temperature. A housewife may fry or broil meat with high heat, but by turning the meat frequently she may allow one side to cool before it has time to heat through. Broiling is often done with high heat and the meat put many inches from it, as wasteful a process as if a furnace were turned on full tilt and the windows opened. Since cold fat conducts heat slowly, people pay high prices for meats streaked with fat which will cook at a low internal temperature even when the cooking temperature is high.

There are many advantages in cooking meats at low temperatures. The least tender cuts may be roasted and served rare, an accomplishment formerly thought to be impossible. There is no danger of meat burning or becoming tough. Meats cook evenly throughout with the same degree of rareness or doneness from surface to center; when high temperatures are used, the outside may be burned while the inside is raw. At low temperatures meats shrink little and are more attractive; they are juicier and more delicious. Studies have shown that the fuel consumption is less during several hours of low-temperature cooking than during an hour of cooking at high temperature; thus money is saved. The meats need little watching when cooked at low temperatures, and almost no work is involved; the method, therefore, also has social advantages.

The principles of meat cookery are clear when you understand that lean meat is muscle tissue. Muscles are made of long fibers such as those seen in the stringy meat of overcooked stew. In raw meat, the protein in the fibers is delicate and soft, like the proteins in a raw egg. Since muscles must be strong, the soft fibers are given strength, held together, and bound into bundles by a tough yet elastic substance known as connective tissue from which gelatin is made. Although the sheets of connective tissue are thin in tender cuts of meat, in meats sold for soup they are so thick that they look like strips of tough gelatin, or gristle. The meat juices, containing flavor, vitamins, and minerals, are held in and around the muscle fibers by these sheets of connective tissue. A bundle of muscle fibers, therefore, is somewhat like fresh, moist stems of a corsage of violets held together by Scotch Tape.

When meat is cooked at low temperatures, the proteins of the muscle fibers, like those of a gently cooked egg, merely become firm. The sheets of connective tissue, which keep the meat from being tender, gradually soften. The softening is brought about because some of the connective tissue when heated changes to gelatin. Tender meats contain little connective tissue; therefore, they need to be cooked only a short time. The less tender cuts, which contain much connective tissue, must be cooked slowly for a long time so that the connective tissue will have time to soften. When meat has been cooked to doneness at low temperature, the softened connective tissue continues to hold the meat fibers together so that the meat slices evenly without tearing apart; it continues to hold the juices, flavor, and nutritive value in the meat; the meat is therefore juicy and its flavor delicious.

When meats are cooked at high temperatures, the heat causes the proteins to contract, shrivel, and become hard, dry, and tough. The effect of heat is usually seen in bacon fried until crisp. The protein, or lean part, may contract until the fat is gathered into a ruffle; the lean meat is so hard and dry that if it were thick, it would not be edible. The high temperature causes the connective tissue surrounding the meat fibers to break down and split; part of it changes completely to liquid gelatin. The contracting proteins act like a hand squeezing water from a sponge; they squeeze the delicious meat juices through the holes split by the heat in the sheets of connective tissue. If you have ever attempted to brown ground meat, you have probably noticed this squeezing process. Heat penetrates such tiny pieces of meat almost immediately. You found that the more you tried to brown the meat, or the higher the temperature you used, the more the juices poured out, the tougher the meat became, and the more stubbornly it refused to brown.

These processes are less noticeable when you cook large cuts of meat, because heat penetrates them gradually. The same changes nevertheless take place whenever meat is heated to high temperature. As the proteins contract and juices are squeezed out, the meat shrinks. A large attractive cut which you thought would be enough to serve six or eight people may become small, shriveled, ugly, and may be scarcely enough to serve four persons. When meats are broiled or roasted, telltale juices in the dripping pan show the unnecessary dryness of the meat and the loss of flavor and nutritive value. If meats are fried, the temperature is often so high that spilled juices evaporate immediately and cannot be noticed.

Everyone agrees that well-cooked meat should be delightfully tender. It is equally important, however, that the connective tissue should remain firm. Only then are juices and flavor held in the meat. Whenever connective tissue is allowed to break, the meat becomes less delicious and will not slice evenly without pulling apart.

In cooking meats, you must keep two temperatures clearly in mind: the temperature inside the meat, or the internal temperature; and the temperature outside the meat used for cooking it. The inside temperature can be known only by using a meat thermometer. The outside temperature, or the cooking temperature, usually ranges between 185° F., or that of simmering water used for stewing and steaming, to 350° F., sometimes used for broiling and roasting. How long it takes the inside of the meat to heat depends on how high the cooking temperature is, how large the cut is, and what kind of heat is used. The moist heat of water or steam penetrates meat twice as quickly as the dry heat of the oven or broiler at the same temperature.

Think of the connective tissue throughout meat as being tough gelatin, and of cooking meat as a process of softening such gelatin. If you put a set gelatin into a warm oven, it becomes softer. How quickly it becomes soft depends on how large and tough it is and how warm the oven is. If left in a warm oven for a certain time, it will become soft throughout without becoming liquid. If put into a hot oven, it will become liquid quickly. The "gelatin" must be softened without being allowed to change to liquid.

Like a gelatin, the connective tissue throughout meat softens as heat penetrates the inside of the cut. Little softening occurs until the internal temperature reaches 120° F. The longer meat cooks, the more tender it becomes even at this low internal temperature. If the heat outside the meat is increased, tenderness can be developed more rapidly. The catch in heating meat quickly is that the connective tissue near the surface heats first and breaks down before that in the center has had time to become tender. The change to gelatin is slow at first, but juices are lost rapidly after the temperature reaches 170° F., the point at which proteins start to become tough. If you want meats to be juicy, tender, and delicious, to shrink as little as possible, and to slice as well as commercially cooked ham, you must give the connective tissue sufficient time to become tender largely between the internal temperatures of 120 and 160° F. The entire trick of roasting, broiling, pan-broiling, and sautéing, or the so-called dry-heat methods of cooking meats, lies in maintaining this range of temperature inside the meat until it becomes tender.

When meats are ground, the cut connective tissue does not need to be softened by heat. If it is not to become tough and dried out, such meat should be allowed to heat only to 170° F. or less. Unless ground meat is packed into a firm loaf, as in meat loaf, heat penetrates it especially rapidly. Ground meat added to boiling soup, for example, is cooked well done in less than a minute. Pounding meat breaks down part of the connective tissue and softens the remaining part. A well-pounded but less tender cut should be cooked as if it were a tender one containing little connective tissue. Such meats, therefore, should be cooked for a relatively short time even at low temperature.

If the external and internal temperatures at which meats are cooked are known and controlled so that the meats can become delightfully tender without reaching the point where connective tissue breaks down and proteins become tough, one need have no failures in cooking meat. These temperatures, therefore, should be carefully checked with thermometers whenever possible. During one's lifetime, inexpensive thermometers can save hundreds of dollars' worth of meats. The use of thermometers changes hit-and-miss methods into exact ones; it puts the amateur on a par with the experienced cook. To prepare meats by methods handed down from one's great-great-grandmother is comparable to cooking as she did on an open hearth.

Keep the Juices in the Meat

Even if meats are cooked carefully at low temperatures, juices may be drawn out in other ways. Just as salt in a shaker attracts water during rainy weather, salt sprinkled on the surface of meat draws out juices. All meat juices, moreover, are salty because the animal from which meat came had to eat salt to live, so if juices are drawn out, the meat is robbed not only of moisture and flavor but also of salt. It tastes so flat that much salt must be added to make it palatable. Several days after meat is salted, the salt has not penetrated it more than half an inch. In making stew or a meat soup, however, salt is added to draw out juices which give flavor to the gravy or stock.

Seasonings other than salt do not bring out juices, but their aromatic oils are largely lost if the meat is to be cooked a long time. Seasonings cannot penetrate meat any more than can salt. The flavor of garlic slipped into meat is not distributed, and someone invariably gets the garlic in his mouth. Onion, peppers, and celery quickly overcook and their flavor becomes stale. When seasonings are added shortly before serving, the freshness of a spring garden is served with the gravy or sauce. If thin cuts of meat, to be cooked only a short time, are allowed to stand with the seasonings until the aromatic oils penetrate the meat, they may be seasoned before cooking without loss of flavor.

To prevent the loss of juices through evaporation in broiled and roasted meats, brush the lean meat carefully with oil. Moisture cannot penetrate a layer of fat. Meat streaked with fat stays juicy after it is cooked, because melted fat coats the meat fibers and prevents evaporation. Unless carefully brushed with oil, a flat roast loses more moisture through evaporation than does a cube-shaped one, because much surface is exposed to heat. Tying a roast compactly decreases evaporation. A roast should be set with the fat side up so that melted fat will drip over it as the meat cooks.

Contrary to public opinion, basting dries out meat; it increases evaporation by washing off the fat. If you like to hover lovingly over meat as it cooks, baste it with a pastry brush dipped in oil.

The old belief was that juices could be held in by searing, or browning, meat at high temperature. Far from being held in, juices are spilled as the proteins contract, but they evaporate too quickly to be noticed. When meat is submitted to high tempera-ture, part of the protein breaks down chemically and develops the delightful "browned-meat" flavor and appetizing color. Al-though searing has long been used as a means of developing flavor, it may cause carcinogenic substances to be produced; brown meats only with the aid of flour, crumbs, molasses, paprika, or sweetened fruit juices which brown easily. Red meat, such as roast beef or broiled steak, does not need to be seared but will brown by the time it is ready to serve.

If you want juices drawn out for soup or gravy, salt the meat before cooking it. If you want the meat to be juicy, salt it just before it is to be eaten.

Cook Your Meats to Retain Maximum Nutritive Value

The principal contribution meat makes to health is the pro-tein of lean meats. The human body is built of protein supplied by foods. The health of the muscles, internal organs, hair, nails, blood cells, antibodies, and hormones, each made of protein, is limited by the kind and amount of protein eaten. An extensive survey made by the United States Department of Agriculture indicates that nine out of every ten Americans suffer from pro-tein deficiencies.

Proteins are not harmed when meats are cooked at low tem-peratures; at high temperatures, some of the essential amino acids are broken apart by heat, and their health-promoting value is decreased. Overcooking can also harm the proteins. Try not to cook any meat longer than is necessary to make it tender. With the exception of pork, meats served rare are nutritionally superior to well-done meats.

Every movement of a muscle, whether animal or human, requires the aid of many and perhaps all of the B vitamins. Since meats are muscles, they are therefore rich sources of these vitamins. With the possible exception of folic acid, an anti-anemia vitamin, the B vitamins are not harmed even by long cooking at low temperature except at the surface of the meat. Above the boiling point, the destruction of several B vitamins increases in proportion to the temperature.

All the B vitamins and the minerals supplied by meat, iron, copper, and phosphorus, dissolve in water and can be lost if meats are soaked or boiled and the cooking water not used. Juices which seep from frozen meats during thawing and those which are lost in the broiling pan should be used in gravy or added to soup stock. Try to make only the amount of gravy which will probably be eaten at a meal; use leftover gravy in sauces, soups, dressings, and meat loaf.

You can increase the nutritive value of meats containing bone by soaking or cooking them with a little acid, as tomatoes, vinegar, or sour cream. The acid dissolves some of the calcium from the bones into the gravy or sauce. If the cut does not contain bones, purchase bone to cook with any meat to be braised or stewed. A single serving of pickled pigs' feet has been found to supply as much calcium as 3 quarts of milk.

When uncooked meat and bones are soaked with a small amount of vinegar for 48 hours, the cooking time is often decreased by a third to a half. The meat, however, must be no thicker than 1 inch, so that the acid can penetrate it. Acid softens connective tissue. Tomatoes, sauerkraut juice, sour cream, dark molasses, and cooking wines may be used, but the acids they contain are less concentrated than is the acetic acid of vinegar. If any trace of vinegar remains, it can be evaporated off before the gravy is made.

The high temperatures used when meats are fried, boiled, or cooked in a pressure cooker are particularly destructive to the health-promoting value of the protein. Moreover, the proteins are toughened before the connective tissue has time to soften. The meat must be overcooked until the proteins change chemically and again become soft; by this time much connective tissue has broken down, juices have been squeezed out, and the meat is usually hard, dry, or stringy. When meats are boiled, so much water is used that both the meat and the gravy lack flavor. If any of the cooking water is discarded, as it often is after ham or tongue is boiled, much of the vitamin and mineral content of the meat is lost.

To fry meat means to cook it in the heat of fat, which can soar quickly to extremely high temperatures. What housewife has not fried bacon which seemed to be progressing well one minute and burned the next? The heat under the frying pan did not suddenly become hotter and burn it. When meats are protected by flour or batter, the high temperatures of hot fat are excellent for browning, but such a method requires continuous attention. Hot fat does not sputter unless moisture is added to it; the inevitable sputtering of frying meat tells that juiciness and flavor are being lost.

A 10-Minute Method for Learning the Cuts of Beef

Innumerable housewives buy meat year after year, often spending hundreds of dollars, without any conception of why one roast or steak is delicious and another a failure. When they learn the cuts of meat and can tell the approximate age of the animal, such hit-and-miss results can be eliminated.

If you are willing to make yourself utterly ridiculous, you can learn the cuts of meat in a few minutes and forever afterward have a basis for buying and preparing each cut. The trick is more fun when done with others but is usually interrupted by everyone's rolling on the floor with laughter. Get down on all fours, imagine you are a steer, try to imitate the movements a steer would make, and notice which muscles you use. The lean meat of the frequently used muscles will have the most flavor; the least used will be most tender. (For example, chickens raised on wire can take so little exercise that their meat, though tender, lacks flavor.)

By now you should be chewing cud, a peaceful exercise but one you persist in. The large muscles in your cheeks may be used for soup meat, hamburgers, or chicken-fried steak. If you wiggle your ears, you find there are muscles attached to them and to the skin of your scalp, used for head cheese. Your brain is little valued but is nevertheless excellent food. Your tongue is a much-used muscle without bone or fat.

You are a curious animal, often turning, lowering, and raising your head; the muscles of your neck will be rich in flavor. Your legs and arms get much use; the muscles of your fore quarters are smaller and cut into less attractive steaks and roasts than those of your hind quarters. You occasionally wiggle the muscles on either side of your backbone to frighten away a fly; certainly they will be tender. The muscles around the rump are used in walking and swishing the tail; they will be flavorsome. In general, the muscles across your back are the most tender, and flavor increases in the order of shoulders, hind legs, front legs, neck, and jaw muscles.

You may now lie down in a shady spot and ponder morbidly over how you will be butchered. You will first be quartered by being cut lengthwise along your backbone and breastbone and crosswise around your waist, the cut slanting in front to well below your ribs. The sections from your hands to elbows and from feet to knees are sold as soup bones. Your elbows and knees, including some of the muscles and bone above them, are your fore and hind shanks. The upper part of your arms, your shoulders, shoulder blades, the first six ribs, and the back of your neck are collectively called the *chuck,* usually sold for pot roasts. The large muscle over your shoulder blade is the *clod.*

Between your shoulder blades and your waist, the large muscles and ribs are usually cut into *roasts.* The ribs may be cut off, leaving a boned *rib roast,* or the meat rolled into a rolled rib roast. If the ribs are tied into a circle giving the appearance of a crown, it becomes a *crown roast,* but if nothing is done to the roast, it is called a *standing rib roast.* The muscles over the last rib at your waist are the most tender; a roast including this rib is spoken of as a *prime rib roast.* The ribs and muscles may be cut into *rib steaks;* if the bones are removed, rib steaks become *Spencer steaks.*

The front of your chest, from your neck to just above your waist and from the cut along your breastbone to your shoulders, is the *brisket.* This cut includes the upper chest bones, the muscles which move your chest in breathing, and other muscles which pull your head grassward; such muscles are rich in connective tissue and flavor. The wall of your upper abdomen and lower chest is a flat, platelike cut known as the *plate.* The ribs under your arms, between the plates and rib roasts, are cut only 5 to 7 inches long and are called *short ribs,* delicious when barbecued.

In the hind quarters, the lower part of your back below your waist is the *loin* section, usually cut into steaks which become larger and slightly less tender as they near the rump. Uppermost are the small *club steaks.* Next are the *T-bones,* which contain short bones protruding from the backbone in semblance to a T. Following the T-bones are the still larger *porterhouse steaks,* named for a certain Mr. Porter who served them frequently years ago in his hotel, or "house," in England. Finally come the large *sirloin steaks,* which include the muscles to the side of the hips. The sirloin steaks nearest the porterhouse steaks are spoken of as the *top sirloin.* The sirloin may be left uncut and cooked as a roast.

The large, frequently used muscles of the buttocks are cut as a *rump roast,* usually boned and rolled. The tail, sold as *oxtail* regardless of the sex of the animal, contains flavorful muscles and much cartilage; it surpasses other cuts for making delicious soup.

The muscular wall of the abdomen is the *flank.* It is a thin layer of flavorful muscles with fibers running lengthwise. The flank may be cut into steaks or rolled as a roast.

Surrounding the thigh bones are round clumps of muscles customarily cut into steaks known as the *upper,* or *top, rounds,* the *middle round,* and the *bottom rounds.* These well-exercised muscles are usually prepared as Swiss steaks or chicken-fried steaks. Between the bottom round and the hind shank is the heel of the round which contains so much connective tissue that it is customarily used for stews. The round steaks become progressively smaller and less tender as they near the shank.

A muscle which must contract before you can lean forward runs along the inside of the backbone. Since steers infrequently bend their backs into semicircles, this muscle is tender regardless of the animal's age. It may be sliced directly across the grain into a small steak known as a *filet mignon;* filet means boneless and mignon means delicate, lovable, and pleasing. In case this delicate, lovable, boneless pleasure is cut diagonally, larger steaks result known as *New York cuts.* The term New York cut, however, is sometimes used to refer to a top sirloin or a boned porterhouse steak.

You have now learned the cuts of beef. Has it taken 10 minutes?

If you cannot remember the name of a cut, look at the size and shape of the muscles and bones. Where in your body are bones and muscles of comparable shape? A cut with a small round bone must be a leg. A rib you readily recognize. Large chunks of muscles and flat bones must be shoulder or rump. It is easy, once you think about it.

When the cuts of beef are known, cuts of other meat are easily learned. Veal is cut into *fore shank, breast, shoulder, rib, loin,* and *round.* The shoulder may be sold as *roasts* or *blade* and *arm steaks;* the rib section, as *roasts* or *rib steaks.* The loin is cut into *kidney chops,* followed by *loin chops,* and lastly *sirloin steaks. Veal cutlets* are sliced from the thighs and are comparable to the round steaks of beef. The breast includes the entire under part of the body, the chest bones and muscles and the abdominal wall; it may be rolled as a roast or cut into riblets, stew meat including the riblets, or ground meat for veal patties. In other respects the cuts are similar to those of beef.

Lamb is cut in the same manner as veal. The rib section along the backbone, comparable to the rib roasts of beef, is known as the *rack.* Both the rack and loin may be sold as roasts or cut into chops. The thigh, or *leg of lamb,* includes the rump; although it is usually left whole, it may be cut as small roasts and steaks. Mutton cuts are similar to those of lamb and veal.

People in general are familiar with the cuts of pork. The shoulder and fore leg may be cut together and sold as a *fresh pork roast* or cured as a *picnic ham.* The ribs and loin section are sold as *fresh pork roasts* or *pork chops.* The *spareribs* include all the chest bones of the under part of the body. The abdominal walls are cured as *bacon* or *salt pork*. The muscle along the inside of the backbone, comparable to the filet mignon of beef, is the *tenderloin;* when cured, it becomes *Canadian bacon. Ham* includes muscles of the rump and the pelvic bones at the larger, or butt, end; the smaller, or shank, end includes the large bones and cartilage of the knee joint.

How to Determine the Tenderness, Flavor, and Juiciness of Meat before Buying It

When you buy meat, you have a definite flavor in mind which you want it to have after it is cooked. Certainly you want it to be tender and juicy. You can easily learn to tell the tenderness, flavor, and juiciness of meat merely by looking at it provided you have some idea of the age of the animal from which it came.

In general, tender meats are muscles which have been used little because life was short or used little during a long life. Tenderness is also determined by the amount of fat throughout the meat. Fat is deposited in the connective tissue and divides it into thin sheets as it is in tender meats. Meats streaked with fat can be depended upon to be tender. The lack of fat allows very lean veal and other meats to be quite tough, even though the muscle has been little used during a short life.

Little-used muscles or meat from young animals have a more delicate flavor than frequently used muscles or meat from older animals. Tender beef from a young steer, for example, may resemble veal rather than stew meat. The more a muscle is used and the older the animal becomes, the more pronounced is the flavor of the lean meat.

It is the fat which gives the characteristic flavor to the meat of each species. Just as you can disguise tuna as creamed chicken if you wash off the oil and cook it with chicken fat, so you can change the flavor of any meat by removing the fat and preparing the meat with fat of another species. This principle is used in preparing liver with bacon and in cooking mutton chops, trimmed free of fat, with butter or oil. Aside from the flavor of the lean meat, the amount of flavor in any cut of meat is in proportion to the quantity of fat throughout the meat fibers.

When meats are served hot, much of the so-called juice is actually melted fat. Fat also makes for juiciness by preventing evaporation. The juiciest meats are those from mature young animals and from less frequently used muscles; such meat has high moisture as well as high fat content, hence is the most expensive.

Just as veal differs in color from stew meat, so does all meat vary in color in proportion to age. The meat of a young steer is a light or cherry red; that of an old animal is dark red or purplish red.

Meat fibers become larger with use. The small fibers of young animals cause a cut surface to have the velvety appearance seen in veal chops. Because of the large fibers of older animals, a cut surface is somewhat rough like that of beef cut for stew.

If you compare veal bones with soup bones, you will notice that they are different in appearance. Relatively few minerals are deposited in the bones of young animals. Such bones contain a large proportion of connective tissue which is white and shiny. Since growing bones must be well supplied with blood, a cut surface of these bones has a pinkish cast and a smooth, glossy appearance. The bones of older animals contain much larger amounts of minerals, and no blood vessels can be seen; such bones have a yellowish-gray color, and a sawed surface is rough and grainy.

Young animals, such as calves, are so active that they store little fat. As the animal becomes well developed, fat is usually stored throughout the little-used muscles. The meat of a young, fattened steer will show much fat throughout such a muscle and around it. Since streaks of fat through the dark lean give the appearance of marble, such meat is spoken of as "well marbled." When older animals are fattened, the meat may show no marbling but be surrounded by fat an inch thick or more.

The color of fat depends largely on the presence or absence of carotene, the yellow pigment which is changed into vitamin A in the body. The fat of a young animal is white because there was little time to store carotene, and requirements for vitamin A are high during growth. If the animal's diet is adequate, carotene is stored in proportion to the length of time it lives; the older the animal, the more carotene stored in the fat and the deeper yellow the color. Jersey and Guernsey cattle, however, store carotene more efficiently than do other breeds; certain feeds cause the fat to be yellow; and an animal of any age, when fed dry feed, quickly uses up stored carotene, and its fat becomes white. The color of the fat, therefore, can serve as only a rough guide, but in general the more yellow the fat, the older the animal, and the more nutritious and flavorful but less tender the meat.

If a cut is cherry-red, has a velvety surface, contains pink and white bones, and is marbled with white fat, you may be sure that it comes from a young animal, will be tender and juicy, and will have much flavor of fat. If the cut is rough and dark red, the sawed bone is grainy and yellowish-gray, and the meat shows no marbling but is surrounded by a thick layer of yellow fat, it comes from an older animal. Between these extremes lie all degrees of variations.

When you know the cut of meat and the approximate age of the animal, not only can you buy the cut with the flavor you desire but also you know, by looking at the meat, how to cook it. If the meat is a less tender cut from an older animal, you know that you can make it tender by grinding, pounding, or cooking it a long time at low temperature. The less fat and more connective tissue it contains, the longer it must be cooked and the lower the cooking temperature must be. If the meat comes from a young animal and has a mild flavor, you can add flavor by browning it in flour or crumbs or serving it with a highly seasoned sauce. If the meat is lean and you enjoy the flavor of fat, you can add this flavor by grinding the meat with fat, by browning it in fat, or by cutting it into small pieces and serving it in a gravy. If the meat is well marbled and comes from a mature animal, you know that it has a delicious flavor of both fat and protein and can be broiled or roasted without any seasonings added to it. If the meat comes from a much-used muscle of an old animal, you know it will make delicious stew or soup.

Prepare your meat to have the flavor you most enjoy. Add flavor, leave it alone, or divide the flavor with the gravy.

Cook Pork Carefully

You have been repeatedly cautioned to cook pork thoroughly in order to destroy any possible trichinae. You have probably been told not to broil pork for fear that it may be eaten undercooked. As a result, women who are aware of trichinosis usually overcook pork until it loses much flavor, juiciness, and nutritive value. Trichinae are destroyed when pork is cooked for an hour at 122° F. (50° C.) or a few minutes at 131° F. (55° C.).* Even rare beef is customarily not served under an internal temperature of 140° F.

Pork is richer in B vitamins than is any other meat. Unnecessary overcooking of pork causes destruction of considerable amounts of many of these vitamins.

Just as overcooking should be avoided, so should undercooking be avoided because of the possibility that trichinae are present. Trichinosis is caused by a parasite which is transmitted from pork to humans. Almost all pork is infected with it. The trichinae hatch in the human body and burrow into the muscles and tendons. The body forms capsules of calcium around the parasites, making itself the oyster in which they are the pearls. These walled capsules eventually cause pain whenever the infected person moves about. When the diet is inadequate in calcium or in vitamins C or D, the capsules break, the trichinae migrate elsewhere, multiply rapidly, and burrow into other muscles and tendons. Although trichinosis is difficult to diagnose, autopsies indicate that 20 per cent of all persons are infected with it; that millions of people spend years of their lives feeling below par from this one cause alone.

This infection is the result of carelessness and ignorance. Women sometimes taste uncooked pork sausage when seasoning it. Tenderized hams are frequently undercooked because housewives confuse them with precooked hams. Restaurants where "short order" cooking is done have long been considered the worst offenders in spreading trichinosis.

* Ransom, B. H., and B. Schwartz, "Effects of Heat on Trichinae," *Journal of Agricultural Research*, 17:201–221 (1919).

Whenever possible, pork should be cooked with a meat thermometer which can show the temperature at which trichinae will have been destroyed and can also prevent overcooking to the extent that flavor and nutrients are lost. Since pork has changed from pink to light gray by the time the internal temperature is 150° F., the absence of pink can serve as a guide when the thermometer cannot be used.

Broiling Captures the Campfire Flavor

There are only three basic methods of, or recipes for, cooking meats: broiling, roasting, and braising, or steaming. Other methods are only variations of these three. The easiest method, and the one many people enjoy most, is broiling.

The authors of recipe books often confuse broiling, or cooking by direct heat, with roasting, or cooking by dry heat surrounding the meat. Recipes often advise you to heat the broiler before using it, to keep the temperature high during broiling, and to have the broiler door closed. Naturally the meat dries out, shrivels, curls, and toughens; juices pour from the contracting protein and burn on the broiler pan; the kitchen often resembles a smoke barrage. Unless you are as agile as a monkey and grab the meat at the instant it is done, it is ruined.

When you go camping or perhaps deer hunting and broil steaks, you do not cook them with the high temperatures of the flames but with the low heat of glowing coals. Only the side of the meat exposed to the coals is cooked at one time. The other surface is possibly bathed with wind or snow; no heat surrounds the meat which could dry it out. The steaks to be served to persons wishing them well done are cooked longer than those for persons who enjoy rare steaks; well-done and rare steaks alike are cooked by low temperature. To duplicate this method in the kitchen is simplicity itself.

You can broil meat perfectly 100 per cent of the time if you do not preheat the broiler compartment, if you keep the heat low, if you leave the broiler door open, and if you watch the internal temperature with a meat thermometer. The "wind and snow" are essential in preventing the meat from being dried out. If you are using a gas range in which the heat can be easily controlled, set the broiler rack on the top ledge. The tiny flames, intensely hot at the tips, slowly brown the meat, yet give off too little heat to toughen it. Once you adjust the heat, you need not glance at the meat until you turn it, or until half the calculated cooking time has expired. A few glances at the thermometer tell you exactly when the meat is ready to serve. It is juicy, beautifully browned, and delicious; the broiler pan is not burned; no wisp of smoke and almost no juices have escaped; and you, as a cook, rank with the experts.

Since the thermostat on a broiling compartment controls the temperature only when the door is closed, disregard the thermostat and adjust the heat by hand. If you have a strange broiler door which snaps shut when the rack is pushed inside, find a mechanically talented child to tear it apart. If you use an electric range, your only choice is to place the meat 5 or 6 inches from the heat. When the temperature becomes high, use stored heat for a short time.

Just as broiling over a campfire is the same whether you broil fish, venison, or beef, so is broiling at home the same regardless of whether you cook chicken, steak, or ham. It is particularly important for you who are amateurs at cooking to realize that if you can broil one steak successfully, you can broil any meat successfully.

Cooking Times and Temperatures for Broiling, Pan-broiling, and Sautéing Meats

Refer to the following table each time before broiling, pan-broiling, or sautéing meat; the information is not repeated in each recipe.

Adjust estimated cooking time to characteristics of meat. Use figures for shorter cooking time when meat shows little marbling, contains bone, or has been frozen. Use figures for longer cooking time when meat is well marbled or contains no bone.

Cooking Times and Temperatures for Broiling, Pan-broiling, and Sautéing Meats

TYPE OF MEAT	THE CUT, OR THICK- NESS OF SLICE	BROILING TEMPERA- TURE AT SURFACE OF MEAT	INTERNAL TEMPERATURE AT WHICH TO BE SERVED	APPROXI- MATE COOKING TIME IN MINUTES
Bacon		Very low		12–15
Beefsteaks, less tender	1 inch	Very low	Rare, 135° F. Medium, 150° F. Well done, 160°F.	35–40 45–50 50–55
Beefsteaks, tender	1 inch	Low	Rare, 140° F. Medium, 155° F. Well done, 165° F.	25–30 35–40 40–45
Brains	¾ inch	Low	175–185° F.	15–20
Chicken, fryer or young broiler	Quartered or halved	Low	165–170° F.	45–50
Ham or shoulder, tenderized	1 inch 1½ inches	Low Low	150–155° F. 150–155° F.	20–30 35–40
Ham or shoulder, not tenderized	1 inch 1½ inches	Low Low	165–170° F. 165–170° F.	40–45 55–60
Kidneys	½ inch	Very low	140–155° F.	12–16
Lamb chops, patties, or steaks	1 inch 2 inches	Low Low	140–160° F. 140–160° F.	20–30 40–45
Liver, beef, veal, or lamb	¾ inch	Low	140–155° F.	12–18
Liver, pork	¾ inch	Low	155–160° F.	18–22
Milt	Uncut	Low	140–155° F.	15–18
Pork chops or steaks	1 inch 1½ inches	Low Low	165–170° F. 165–170° F.	30–35 40–45
Rabbit, young fryer, 2 pounds, dressed	Quartered	Low	165–170° F.	45–50
Veal cutlets	1 inch	Low	175–180° F.	30–35
Wieners		Very low	130–140° F.	8–10

BROILED BEEFSTEAK

Select steaks cut approximately 1 inch thick; they may be club, T-bone, Spencer, rib, sirloin, porterhouse, or filet mignon.

If steaks are well marbled, use the cooking time and temperature for tender steaks; if a flank steak or one which contains little fat, use the cooking time and temperature for less tender steaks.

Set meat on broiler rack and allow it to heat to room temperature, or remove from refrigerator about ½ hour before cooking. Trim off fat, leaving ⅛ inch to prevent evaporation. If drippings are not to be used for gravy, cover dripping pan with aluminum foil.

Carefully insert punch for meat thermometer, holding it parallel to the surfaces of the meat, and making a hole in the center of the thickest portion, avoiding bone or fat; withdraw punch and insert thermometer. Brush all surfaces of the meat lightly with oil.

Estimate cooking time. At the calculated number of minutes before time to serve the meat, put it under the broiler with the reading of the meat thermometer down.

If heat can be controlled, put broiler rack on upper ledge about 2 inches from heat; turn heat on low; if using an electric range, set rack 5 or 6 inches from heat. See that the part of the steak holding meat thermometer gets no more heat than any other.

When half the estimated cooking time has passed, turn the meat; the thermometer should now be facing up.

Check reading of the meat thermometer frequently; remove meat when reading is 135 or 140° F. for rare, 150 or 155° F. for medium, 160 or 165° F. for well done.

Sprinkle steaks with **freshly ground peppercorns. Salt at the table.**

VARIATIONS:

Just before serving, rub surface of meat lightly with mashed garlic. If broiling only 1 steak, broil on cake rack set over a pie pan.

In broiling each of the meats listed in the table on page 32 giving cooking times and temperatures and in the following variations, the procedure is identical with that outlined in the recipe for broiling beefsteak, referred to as the basic recipe. When preparing other meats, mentally substitute for steak the name of the meat you plan to cook; follow this basic recipe in broiling all meats.

Before cooking, sprinkle paprika generously over such meats as brains, liver, chicken, rabbit, and pork chops to give a delightfully brown appearance.

Bacon: If no more than 5 strips of bacon are to be broiled, place on a cake rack set over a pie pan; omit oiling and thermometer. If bacon curls, the heat has been allowed to become too high. Cooking bacon on a rack in a slow oven is a satisfactory substitute for broiling it.

Brains: Use 1 pound of uncooked beef, lamb, pork, or veal brains; remove membranes under running water; dry on paper towels, slice, and place on oiled baking sheet; oil and sprinkle generously with paprika; proceed as in basic recipe.

Chicken: Cut broilers (1½ to 2 pounds) into halves along backbone and breastbone; insert thermometer in center of breast muscle, making sure it does not touch bone. Brush all surfaces well with **vegetable oil** and sprinkle generously with **paprika** before broiling. If a young chicken weighs 3 to 4 pounds, cut each half into quarters, one piece including leg, thigh, and lower back, and the other including breast and wing. It is regrettable that only occasionally does a housewife broil chickens; they can be delicious.

Hamburger steaks: Use 1½ pounds of ground stew meat, flank, or round steak; season with **freshly ground black peppercorns, sautéed onions, and/or pinch of savory, basil, or marjoram;** *do not salt;* form into firm cakes 1¼ inches thick or pack firmly into cardboard milk carton; slice meat through cardboard before removing it; broil as a tender beefsteak; insert thermometer when turning.

Meat patties: Prepare meat patties (p. 111) and broil as hamburgers.

Kidney: Use 1 to 1½ pounds of beef, lamb, or veal kidneys; slice beef or veal kidneys into ½-inch slices; cut lamb kidneys in half lengthwise; remove all white tissue; lay on baking sheet and brush both sides lightly with **vinegar**, then with **vegetable oil**. Before serving, rub well with **garlic**; serve with tart mint sauce (p. 143).

Pork kidney: Broil to internal temperature of 155° F.; after removing from heat, rub with **mashed garlic** and sprinkle with **ground mustard, freshly ground peppercorns,** and **chopped parsley.**

Lamb chops, steaks, or patties: Mix 1 teaspoon **dill seeds** with 1 pound ground lamb for patties; broil as in basic recipe.

Liver: Use baby beef, veal, or lamb liver sliced ¾ inch thick; brush with **vegetable oil**; before serving, rub with **mashed garlic** and sprinkle with **freshly ground peppercorns.**

Pork liver: Before oiling sprinkle with **caraway seeds** and press into surface; broil slowly to internal temperature of 155° F.; if slices are too thin to hold thermometer, test temperature by inserting thermometer for a moment diagonally to surface. This is a delicious recipe.

Pork chops or steaks: Do not broil without a meat thermometer; trim off fat; sprinkle both sides generously with **paprika** before broiling.

Stuffed pork chops: Buy chops 2 inches or more thick; cut pocket by inserting knife into side and rotating to edge of lean meat. Fill with **1 cup of crumb, fruit, or vegetable stuffing** (pp. 129–133); broil as in basic recipe.

Pounded steaks: Choose a Swiss steak about 1 to 1½ inches thick, cut from young animal; pound well and cut into serving sizes; broil as tender steak; brush with **vegetable oil** before broiling and when steaks are turned.

Tenderized steaks: choose moderately tender steaks; rub with **garlic** or sprinkle with **minced garlic**; cut into individual servings, put in refrigerator dish and pour **1 tablespoon lemon juice or French dressing** over each serving; let stand in refrigerator 24 hours. Broil as a less tender steak.

Sweetbreads: Clip off elastic tissue with kitchen scissors; cut into serving sizes; broil as brains.

Veal cutlets: Brush with **vegetable oil** before broiling and when turned; broil on an oiled baking sheet; after broiling rub with **mashed garlic** and sprinkle with **ground white peppercorns**.

Wieners: Need not be oiled; broil as in basic recipe.

Pan-broiling

Pan-broiling is a variation of broiling, or of cooking by direct heat. The utensil used to hold the meat is not greased; it serves only as a rack and dripping pan. The ideal utensil for pan-broiling is a grill surrounded by a groove into which the fat drains as it is rendered out. The method is confined to cooking well-marbled steaks and meats having a sufficiently high fat content so that they will not stick to the pan during cooking; the meats must also have flat surfaces. At the beginning of cooking, pork chops, bacon, sausage, and ham are customarily pan-broiled. As the fat is rendered out, the meat fries, or is cooked by the heat of the fat, which almost invariably becomes so hot that flavor and juices are lost. If the fat drains off or is poured off as it is rendered out, the cooking temperature can easily be kept low; the meat does not dry out, shrivel, curl, burn, or need careful watching.

Pan-broiling, like broiling, is similar to cooking over glowing coals: the temperature is low; unless searing is desired, the utensil used should be cold; the meat is not covered at any time. If the meat is covered, the temperature becomes too high, juices seep out and heat quickly to boiling temperature; the meat curls, shrivels, and becomes tough. Any fat rendered from the meat should be poured off before it has time to soar to a high temperature. When you understand the procedure of pan-broiling, you can cook meat by this method without failure.

Since many people do not have good equipment for pan-broiling and since heat cannot always be kept low, it is sometimes difficult to brown meat satisfactorily without searing it first. In this case, the grill or pan is heated until extremely hot before the meat is put on it. The meat is then allowed to sear so short a time that the high temperature does not penetrate the interior of the cut. Immediately after searing, the heat should be turned off or, if electricity is used, the utensil moved and the meat allowed to cook only from the heat of the utensil until it has cooled to moderate temperature. The meat should then be put over extremely low heat until it reaches the internal temperature desired.

A meat thermometer should be used in pan-broiling all meats which are thick enough to hold it. To make room for the thermometer, pan-broiling should be done on a flat grill such as is used for cooking pancakes, Many women who would not broil meat without a thermometer believe that a thermometer is not necessary for pan-broiling. If gravy is to be prepared from the meat juices, a frying pan must be used and the thermometer inserted and removed once or twice before the meat is taken up. The cooking times and internal temperatures for pan-broiling are the same as for broiling (p. 32).

PAN-BROILED PORK CHOPS

Choose pork chops 1 to 1½ inches thick; allow 30 to 35 minutes for cooking 1-inch chops; 40 to 45 for 1½-inch chops.

Trim fat, leaving ⅛ inch. Carefully pierce hole for thermometer, holding punch parallel to the surface of the meat and driving it into the center of the thickest portion. Insert thermometer. Sprinkle chops generously on both sides with **paprika**.

Put chops on extremely hot pan or grill; sear 2 or 3 minutes on each side; immediately turn off heat or move utensil until cooled; then continue cooking over extremely low heat. *Do not salt the meat or cover the grill.*

In 15 to 20 minutes turn the chops; drain off any rendered fat; continue to keep heat low. Take reading of meat thermometer frequently.

Take up when the thermometer reading is 165 to 170° F. Sprinkle chops with **freshly ground white peppercorns**.

Heat on hot grill:

½ cup vegetable-cooking water   pinch each of savory and sage
1 tablespoon chopped chives

Pour sauce over meat.

VARIATIONS:

A minute before taking up, sprinkle with dry mustard and/or horse-radish.

Buy pork chops at least 2 inches thick; cut a pocket in one side and stuff with sautéed onions, or any crumb, fruit, or vegetable dressing (pp. 129–133).

Steam sauerkraut or cabbage in a heat-resistant casserole; season with 1 teaspoon caraway seeds; put pork chops on top and serve.

In the following variations the procedure, unless otherwise stated, is exactly the same as outlined in the recipe for pan-broiling pork chops, referred to as the basic recipe. When preparing other meats, follow the basic recipe, merely substituting for pork chops the name of the meat.

Bacon: If time permits, allow 15 minutes for bacon to cook; do not sear; put on cold grill and keep heat low throughout cooking; pour off fat as it accumulates. Bacon cooked by this method is flat, evenly browned, and extremely delicious. If oven is in use and temperature low, cook there.

Beefsteak: Choose any tender steak, such as club, T-bone, porterhouse, sirloin, or filet mignon; steak may be stuffed with **spiced fruit or lightly sautéed onions or leeks**; pan-broil as in basic recipe.

Ham: Trim fat from ham slices, preferably ½ inch thick; pan-broil slices without searing and put on serving platter; dice ham fat into ½-inch cubes and quickly brown until crisp; drain and add **1 teaspoon each dry mustard and brown sugar**: stir well and serve over ham. Don't miss this recipe; it's delicious. Vary by mixing **chives, chopped green onions, or minced fresh herbs** with browned ham fat.

Ham and veal with sage: Cut matched servings of ham and veal sliced ½ inch thick; put **2 leaves minced fresh sage or ¼ teaspoon dried sage** on ham, and fasten veal on top with toothpicks; sear veal surface only; take temperature by piercing diagonally with thermometer; remove meat and add **½ cup white wine** to drippings; mix well, heat, pour over meat. This is an Italian recipe worthy of its fame.

Ham steaks: Cut slices from cured or tenderized ham or shoulder, preferably 1 inch thick; proceed as in basic recipe; before serving sprinkle surface with **ground mustard** if desired. Increase heat and sear slices of **canned pineapple**.

Hamburger steaks: Form ground meat into firm cakes; insert a thermometer when meat is nearly done. Mix **caraway seeds, minced garlic, or lightly sautéed onions** with meat before forming cakes, but *do not salt*.

Pork steaks: Use steaks cut from a fresh pork leg or shoulder; cook in frying pan, inserting thermometer once or twice before taking up.

Lamb chops, steaks, or patties: Pan-broil as in basic recipe; insert thermometer in patties when nearly done.

Mutton chops: Select 2-inch chops; trim off fat; cut pocket in side and stuff with **sautéed onions**; pan-broil, allowing 50 minutes for cooking.

Pork sausage: Mold sausages into firm cakes; do not sear; remove fat as it is rendered out; insert meat thermometer when sausage is nearly done.

Link sausage: Pierce casings of 1 pound of link sausages in several places with fork so that steam can escape; omit thermometer; pan-broil for 12 to 15 minutes.

Venison, elk, or bear steaks, or steaks from other big game: Choose rib or loin steaks; proceed as in basic recipe. If strong game flavor is not enjoyed, marinate overnight (pp. 100–101).

Sautéed Meats

Although sautéing is frequently confused with frying, it is a variation of broiling; the food is cooked by direct heat, not by the heat of fat. The utensil is merely brushed with fat to prevent the food from sticking to it; otherwise the method is identical with pan-broiling. The advantages of sautéing over frying are that the heat can be easily controlled, the meat requires little watching, and there need be no danger of the temperature becoming so high as to dry out the meat or rob it of flavor.

The meats which are sautéed rather than pan-broiled are those which are low in fat. Since they lack the prominent flavor of fat, flavor is added by dredging them in wheat germ, flour, or crumbs.

As in pan-broiling, the temperature should be kept low except for a few minutes of searing. A flat grill surrounded by a ½-inch rim is best for sautéing. Such a utensil allows room for the meat thermometer to be inserted into one serving. The cooking times and temperatures are the same as those used for broiling (p. 32).

Unless the taste of fat meat is actually enjoyed, meats to be dipped in wheat germ, flour, crumbs, or batter should be carefully trimmed.

Meats to be sautéed may be salted before cooking; the juices are caught and held in the flour, crumbs, or batter, and thus add flavor to the crust.

SAUTEED VEAL CUTLETS

Trim cutlets; dredge in wheat germ; insert thermometer into thickest portion, and brown on each side on grill brushed with vegetable oil; cook slowly, taking 25 to 30 minutes; *do not cover at any time.*

When internal temperature reaches 175 to 180° F., salt veal and put on serving platter; heat in drippings:

½ cup vegetable-cooking water	dash of salt
2 tablespoons minced chives	freshly ground peppercorns

Pour sauce over veal.

VARIATIONS:

Dredge veal with wheat germ or flour and pound well with meat tenderer; cook at moderate temperature 10 minutes on each side.

Dip cutlets in egg stirred with 2 tablespoons milk, 1 teaspoon salt, a generous pinch of savory; dredge in wheat germ or sifted whole-wheat-bread crumbs; after removing cutlets heat 1 cup tomato sauce (p. 140) and serve over meat.

Dip veal in batter (p. 158) and sauté; insert thermometer before dipping in batter.

In the following variations, the procedure is the same as that outlined in the recipe for sautéing veal cutlets, referred to as the basic recipe. Follow this recipe when preparing other meats, merely substituting the name of the meat for veal cutlets. Refer to table (p. 32) for cooking times and temperatures.

Beef Stroganoff: Buy 1 or 1½ pounds round steak cut ½ inch thick; dredge in **whole-wheat flour,** pound well, and cut with scissors into strips ½ inch wide and 3 or 4 inches long; dredge again, brown 5 minutes, and sauté slowly until tender, or about 10 to 20 more minutes; add **1 cup sour cream;** salt and sprinkle with **freshly ground black peppercorns;** serve as soon as heated through. Vary by sautéing **mushrooms** with beef; or omit salt and instead of sour cream add **1 can condensed mushroom soup, 1 tablespoon lemon juice or vinegar, ¼ cup milk.**

Beef paprika: Prepare beef as in preceding recipe; sauté with beef **1 finely chopped onion;** when tender, put beef in serving dish and prepare **2 cups country gravy** (p. 125); add **1 to 3 teaspoons paprika;** stir beef and onions into gravy to reheat before serving.

Brains with chives: Remove membranes from uncooked lamb, veal, or beef brains while holding under running water; cut into ½-inch slices; dredge, sprinkle with **paprika** and **salt,** and sauté; before serving sprinkle generously with **chives.** When time permits, pack brains firmly into ice tray, freeze. Remove and slice before sautéing.

Chicken-fried steak: Trim, dredge, pound, and brown ½-inch slices of round steak in rendered suet, allowing 25 to 30 minutes for total cooking time. Serve with country gravy seasoned with sage.

Chicken-fried venison, elk, or bear meat: Dredge and pound thoroughly; sauté as in basic recipe. Serve with country gravy seasoned with a pinch each of savory, marjoram, sage.

Lamb steaks: Sauté as in basic recipe or dip in **egg or milk and crumbs.** Serve with dill or caper sauce (pp. 136–137).

Liver: Use lamb, baby beef, veal, or pork liver cut into ½-inch slices; brown no longer than 2 minutes on each side, and reduce heat, cooking slowly 5 to 8 minutes longer; sprinkle generously with freshly **ground black peppercorns.** Serve with raw creole sauce (p. 141).

With bacon: Cut strips of bacon in half and pan-broil before sautéing liver; drain on paper; pour off drippings; after liver is browned, put bacon above liver to reheat; serve at once.

With onions: Chop fine **2 cups sweet onions;** sauté in **vegetable oil** 8 to 10 minutes before sautéing liver, using same utensil; put on serving dish; just before serving, add onions to liver and reheat.

Pork: Use pork chops, tenderloin, or steaks; trim off fat and sauté as in basic recipe or dip in **egg** mixed with **2 tablespoons milk** and then in crumbs. Serve with country gravy (p. 125) seasoned with sage.

Quick Swiss steak: Since Swiss steak is pounded, it should be cooked as a tender cut of meat; the *utensil should not be covered* at any time. Purchase a Swiss steak about 1 to 1½ inches thick; dredge and pound thoroughly; sauté with **3 tablespoons vegetable oil;** cook slowly to an internal temperature of 140 to 165° F., or about 30 minutes. Meanwhile steam together in another utensil **1 or 2 each quartered onions, un-peeled potatoes, carrots, turnips;** when vegetables start to be tender, add **1 cup fresh or frozen peas.** When steak is done, put on serving platter and prepare brown or tomato gravy (pp. 125–127). Season gravy with **salt, crushed black peppercorns, basil, savory;** combine vegetables and gravy and pour over meat. This type of Swiss steak in my opinion is far more delicious than the overcooked variety.

The Person Who Works at Roasting Ruins the Meat

To roast meat means to cook it with dry heat. Meat to be roasted is set on a rack above a dripping pan, brushed with oil to prevent evaporation, and allowed to cook until the meat thermometer indicates the degree of doneness most enjoyed. What else can you do without ruining the meat? If you salt it, sear it in a preheated oven, or baste it, juices are drawn out or lost by evaporation, and the meat is left drier. If you cover the meat with a lid, it is steamed instead of roasted. If you set it on a pan instead of a rack, the lower surface is first steamed, eventually rests in melted fat, fries, and becomes tough. If you want delightfully roasted meat, let it alone and honor its privacy.

Meats cooked in a covered "roaster" are not roasted but steamed, even though they are cooked in an oven. A so-called pot roast is really a "pot steam." If a "roaster" is not used for cooking on top of the range, it should be planted with herbs.

When roasting meat, set an upright oven thermometer on the rack beside the roast. A thermostat, or heat control, can give nothing more than a general indication of the oven temperature. Every woman knows that heat rises and causes a cake to brown more quickly at the top of an oven that at the bottom. The temperature in one part of an oven is often 360° F. and in another part, 275° F. Moreover, thermostats are rarely accurate. I have checked oven temperatures of ranges of perhaps two dozen of my friends and have yet to find a thermostat which, when turned to 300° F., for example, is not 25 to 50 degrees too high

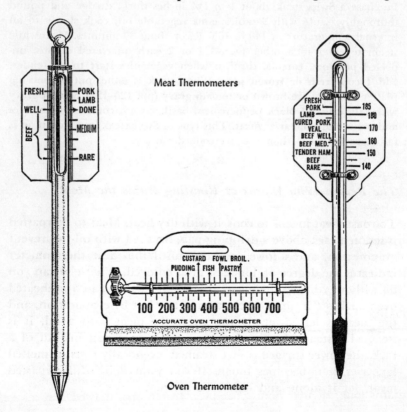

Meat Thermometers

Oven Thermometer

or too low. Unless the cooking temperature is known, there is no way of determining whether the meat will be done an hour before dinnertime or 2 hours later.

The tables giving the estimated cooking times and temperatures should be referred to before roasting any meat. Although these tables are worked out to help you know when to put the meat on to cook, they can be nothing more than a rough guide. Unless you carefully consider the characteristics of each individual roast, you may have eggs for dinner.

Roasts with certain characteristics cook slowly: those which contain no bones or only short, compact bones; cube-shaped or rolled roasts which have relatively little surface through which heat can penetrate; and a well-marbled roast, since fat is a poor conductor of heat. On the other hand, meats which show no marbling heat through rapidly. Long, slender bones conduct heat readily; a crown roast often cooks in half the time needed for the same amount and cut of meat made into a rolled roast. Meats which have been frozen and thawed cook more quickly than fresh meats. A large flat roast, cut like a pot roast, may cook in half the time required for a thicker roast which weighs less. In terms of minutes per pound, a large roast cooks much more quickly than does a small one. Putting a preheated stuffing into a roast also shortens the cooking period. Consider all of these factors and allow yourself plenty of time. If the roast gets done before time to serve, take it from the oven when it is 5 degrees below that of desired doneness; it will continue cooking from its own heat for an hour or more.

As in broiling, if you have successfully roasted one meat, you can roast any meat. The only variations lie in the cooking times and temperatures and the preparation of the meat before it is put into the oven.

Cooking Times and Temperatures for Roasting or Barbecuing Meats with Moderate Heat

In calculating time when meat is to be put on to cook, use figures for shorter cooking time if the roast shows little marbling, contains long, slender bones, has been frozen and thawed, has a relatively large surface area, is flat, weighs 4 pounds or more, or is stuffed with preheated dressing. Use the figures for longer cooking time when meat is well marbled, contains no bones or has short, compact bones, is rolled or cube shaped, or weighs less than 4 pounds.

TYPE OF MEAT	APPROXIMATE COOKING TIME IN MINUTES PER POUND	EXTERNAL TEMPERATURE OF UPRIGHT OVEN THERMOMETER	DEGREE OF DONENESS	INTERNAL TEMPERATURE AT WHICH MEAT IS SERVED
Beef,	45–50	225–250° F.	Rare	135° F.
less tender cuts	55–60		Medium	150° F.
	60–70		Well done	160° F.
Beef, tender cuts	18–20	300° F.	Rare	140° F.
	20–25		Medium	155° F.
	27–30		Well done	165° F.
Chicken, roasting	35–45	300° F.		185° F.
stewing	60–70	225–250° F.		185° F.
Duck, young	25–30	300° F.		185° F.
Goose, young	25–30	300° F.		185° F.
Ham, home cured	25–30	300° F.		165–170° F.
tenderized	20–25	300° F.		150–155° F.
Lamb, leg	25–30	300° F.		155–160° F.
shoulder	40–45	275° F.		155–160° F.
Liver, uncut	15–20	300° F.		145–160° F.
Mutton,	60–70	225–250° F.		180–185° F.
leg or shoulder				
Pork roast	35–40	300° F.		165–170° F.
Rabbit	30–35	300° F.		180° F.
Spareribs	30–35	300° F.		180–185° F.
Turkey, large	15–18	300° F.		180–185° F.
small	20–25	300° F.		180–185° F.
Veal, standing	40–45	275° F.		180–185° F.
roast rolled	45–50	275° F.		180–185° F.

ROAST BEEF, LESS TENDER CUTS

Select roast weighing 3 pounds or more cut from chuck, clod, round muscles, or rump of prime or choice grade or from rib or loin section of good, commercial, utility, or canner grade. My favorite of all roasts is a standing clod.

Allow meat to reach room temperature, or allow about ½ hour per pound if taken from refrigerator. If it is frozen, put over dripping pan to thaw.

Estimate cooking time, considering characteristics of meat (p. 44).

Trim off fat, leaving ½ inch for self-basting.

If desired, use **vegetable, fruit, or crumb stuffing** (pp. 129–133); if roast is not compact, tie with heavy strings 1 inch apart to prevent evaporation.

Carefully pierce hole for meat thermometer, inserting punch into center of thickest part of roast and being careful not to touch fat, bone, or dressing; insert meat thermometer.

Put meat on broiler rack above broiler pan or on similar rack above dripping pan; brush all lean surfaces with **vegetable oil**; set roast with fat side up and put into oven preheated to 225 or 250° F.; *do not salt or season in any way.*

Set oven thermometer on rack beside meat. After 15 minutes read oven thermometer and adjust thermostat accordingly; if adjustment is necessary, check reading and readjust heat again in 15 minutes.

As end of calculated cooking time approaches, take reading of meat thermometer.

Make gravy when meat is 5 degrees below the temperature desired for serving. Season gravy with savory and marjoram.

Serve meat when internal temperature, shown by meat thermometer, is 135° F. for rare, 150° F. for medium done, and 160° F. for well done.

VARIATIONS:

If meat is to be served cold, subtract 10 degrees from desired temperature of doneness; turn off heat and let meat cool in oven.

In the following variations, the meats are roasted in the same manner outlined in the recipe for less tender beef roast, referred to as the basic recipe. Regardless of the type of meat you wish to roast, follow the basic recipe, merely substituting for beef the name of the meat.

Beef, tender cut: Roast as in basic recipe except at higher temperature and shorter cooking time (p. 44).

Chicken: Salt chicken inside if desired; fill with stuffing (p. 130).

Brush with **vegetable oil** and proceed as in basic recipe, inserting thermometer into dressing at tail end. Set chicken on special rack with breast down.

Duck and goose, domestic: Stuff duck with **apple, onion, or buck-wheat stuffing** (pp. 131–133); goose with **apples, celery, and/or onions** to be discarded before serving. Insert thermometer into thigh muscle next to body; roast as in basic recipe. Note location of fat deposits on goose before cooking. Each hour during cooking, barely prick the skin over fat deposits with a sharp-tined fork to allow melted fat to escape; remove fat from dripping pan with basting syringe to prevent discoloration. The French consider goose fat a great delicacy for use in general cooking.

Ham, whole or half, home-cured or tenderized: Wash well if home-cured; trim, leaving ½ inch of fat; save trimmings for seasoning; leave skin over shank, or more pointed end, cutting skin with kitchen shears into star-shaped or semicircular border; score fat into diamonds by cutting diagonally across surface; brush with **dark molasses** and put **clove** in center of each diamond; roast as in basic recipe. Serve with sauce made of dry mustard and fresh horseradish.

Lamb: Select leg, shoulder, loin, rack, or breast; have butcher remove oil gland from leg; bone and stuff leg if desired; or bone, stuff, and roll breast; or make pocket between bones and meat in breast or shoulder roast for stuffing. Do not remove thin membrane covering leg or shoulder. Proceed as in basic recipe; garnish platter with **sprigs of fresh mint.**

Liver: Buy 2 pounds or more of unsliced baby beef, veal, lamb, or pork liver; make pocket in center of liver, stuff with **onion dressing** (p. 131), or roast without stuffing; cut 2 or 3 slices of bacon in half and put over top, holding them securely with toothpicks; roast as in basic recipe.

Mutton: Buy leg, shoulder, rack, or loin roast; ask butcher to remove oil gland from leg. Cut off all mutton fat and cover with **slices of bacon** held in place with toothpicks. Roast as in basic recipe. Garnish roast and platter with **fresh mint.**

Pork: Select fresh shoulder, leg, loin, or tenderloin; bone and stuff shoulder or leg (p. 128) if desired; proceed as in basic recipe.

Rabbit: Select a mature rabbit; stuff with **rice and tomato dressing** (p. 131); insert meat thermometer into thigh muscle next to body; roast as in basic recipe. Garnish platter with **sprigs of parsley.**

Roast suckling pig: Should weigh 9 to 12 pounds; clean thoroughly, wipe with cloth, fill half the pig with **rice or buckwheat stuffing** (p. 132), and half with **onion dressing** (p. 131); tie front legs together and pull backward; tie hind legs together and bring forward, as if the pig were lying down; then tie all four legs together securely. Prop mouth open with small raw potato. Insert thermometer in top of hip muscles; set with back up. Roast as in basic recipe at 350° F. for 5 hours or more, or until internal temperature is 165 to 170° F. Put on serving platter, place a small red apple in pig's mouth, fresh cranberries in eyesockets, and a wreath of parsley around neck.

Spareribs: Select 2 or 3 pounds of meaty spareribs; cut pocket between meat and bones and stuff with onion dressing or fill with sauerkraut seasoned with caraway seeds; or put dressing between two matching sections. Insert thermometer in dressing.

Barbecued or glazed spareribs: Use meaty, farmers' style ribs without stuffing. When ribs are half cooked, brush with sauce of ½ cup catsup, ¼ cup each vinegar and dark molasses, 1 grated onion, ½ teaspoon each chili powder, freshly ground peppercorns, and salt. Bake 30 minutes longer, applying remaining sauce every 10 minutes.

Turkey: Stuff with giblet dressing (p. 130); insert thermometer into dressing; roast as in basic recipe, preferably on rack with breast down.

Veal: Select breast, leg, loin, rib, or shoulder roast; bone, stuff, and roll if desired; cover with ¼-inch layer of kidney fat if there is no fat on meat. Proceed as in basic recipe.

Venison, elk, moose, buffalo, bear, or other big game: Roast as a less tender cut of beef, cooking to medium or well done.

Wild duck, grouse, pheasant, wild turkey, prairie chicken, or squab: Stuff with buckwheat, wild rice, or apple stuffing (pp. 132, 133). Insert meat thermometer into dressing or into thigh next to body. Roast duck to 140° F., other wild fowl to 185° F. Follow cooking time for chicken, depending on age and probable tenderness of meat. Roast as in basic recipe.

Slow Roasting

In experiments where identical roasts were cooked at different oven temperatures to the same degree of doneness, roasts cooked for 20 to 24 hours were preferred in 100 per cent of the taste tests to roasts cooked in 3 hours or less. Although the cooking time seems startling at first, the meat is so amazingly delicious, juicy, and tender, slices so beautifully, and shrinks so little that meats cooked at higher temperatures no longer taste good to you.

In slow roasting, the oven temperature is set approximately at the temperature you want the meat when it is done. Just as meat taken from a refrigerator will warm to room temperature, so will meat put into such an oven heat to oven temperature. It cannot burn; it needs no watching; vitamins and proteins cannot be harmed at such low heat; almost no fuel is needed to cook it. One might say that it cooks itself. Many warming ovens are adjusted so that a pilot light maintains a constant temperature of 165° F., ideal for this type of roasting.

Probably you often buy a roast the day before you plan to cook it. If you wish to use this method, instead of putting the meat in the refrigerator, simply brush it with oil, insert the meat thermometer, set the meat in a preheated oven at 300° F. for 1 hour to destroy bacteria on the surface. Then adjust the heat to the internal temperature desired, and forget about it. The longer the meat cooks, the more tender it becomes.

After the period of preheating, which should assure complete sterilization of all surfaces, the cooking time is approximately three times that of moderate-temperature roasting, although there is considerable variation between different roasts. In using the method, estimate the time needed to cook the roast at moderate temperature (p. 44), multiply by three, and add the hour of preheating.

Slow roasting is an ideal method if persons must be away throughout the day and have warming ovens, adjustable oven pilot lights which can reach slow-roasting temperatures, or well-insulated ovens which can maintain low temperatures at almost no cost. The chief advantage of a knowledge of slow roasting is that you can cook your meat at a temperature which most suits your convenience. Combine moderate-temperature roasting with slow roasting or use any cooking temperature between 140° F. and the temperature recommended in the table on page 44 for the type of meat you wish to cook. Within this range, the lower the temperature used in cooking, the more delicious the meat will be, particularly if the cut is a less tender one. Since the lower temperature requires longer cooking, its use must depend on when you wish to serve the meat. You might have a roast which could be cooked at moderate temperature in 3 hours; yet you wish to be away from home for 6 hours. You could cook the roast at moderate temperature for a short time while you are at home, decrease the temperature to that of desired doneness when you must be away, and if the meat is not done when you get home, increase the temperature again. Thus your roasting can be adjusted entirely to your convenience.

At first the objection to using variation of temperatures appears to be that you cannot tell when the meat will be done. If you cook it at a temperature of desired doneness, or 160° F. or below, the connective tissue softens but breaks down little or none, even if the meat is cooked longer than necessary; hence the exact cooking time is less important than when higher temperatures are used. Remember only that the lower the cooking temperature, the longer the meat must be cooked. Allow yourself plenty of time when using low temperatures and let your meat thermometer be your guide to the degree of doneness you desire.

Barbecuing in the Kitchen

When meat is barbecued over an open fire or charcoal flames, a revolving spit allows it to broil on one surface while the other surfaces cool; the flames some distance away cause the meat to be surrounded by dry heat as if it were in a slow oven; thus barbecuing is a combination of broiling and roasting. Barbecuing at home can be done by cooking meat in a broiler compartment with the door closed. If carefully cooked, the meat is delicious indeed. Since the temperature of both the direct and accumulated dry heat can be controlled, turning the meat more than once is unnecessary.

An advantage of barbecuing rather than roasting is that the surface becomes beautifully browned; yet the low direct heat cannot penetrate far into the meat. The meat therefore shrinks much less than if it were browned to the same degree in an ordinary oven. The method is especially well adapted for cooking meat with flat surfaces, as a chuck roast cut as a thick pot roast, although the size of the meat to be barbecued is limited only by the size of the broiling compartment.

The procedure of barbecuing differs from roasting in that the meat is turned when half the estimated cooking time has passed. The fat side of the meat should be placed down during the first half of barbecuing, and turned to the direct heat for the remainder of the cooking time. Fowl, tied so that their legs and wings are held close to the body, are laid breast side up during the first half of the cooking period. The surface of the fowl or meat should be brushed with oil at the beginning of cooking and again at the time it is turned. If barbecue sauce is to be poured over the meat, it should not be applied until 15 minutes before the meat is served.

Since the procedure for barbecuing meat is so nearly the same as that for roasting, only one basic recipe is given. Any meat which can be roasted may be barbecued by following this basic procedure. The cooking times and temperatures to be used are the same as those used for roasting (p. 44).

Still lower temperatures may also be used, and the meat will be even more delicious. If the meat is barbecued in a gas range, it may be placed so that the top surface is 3 inches from the flames; if electricity is used, the top surface should not be nearer than 5 inches. Persons with electric ranges seem particularly enthusiastic about this method of cooking meat.

Do not try to barbecue meat without using thermometers; the chances are ten to one that you will ruin the meat.

BARBECUED LEG OF LAMB

Select leg of lamb of desired weight; ask butcher to remove oil gland. Estimate cooking time at 25 to 30 minutes per pound.

Wash thoroughly and dry; trim off undesired fat, leaving ¼ to ½ inch; *do not remove membrane over lean meat.*

Put on broiler rack, lean side up, and brush lean surface with **vegetable oil.** Press punch into thickest part of lean meat, withdraw, and insert thermometer.

Place in broiling compartment so that top of surface is 3 inches below gas heat or 5 inches below electric heat. Set oven thermometer on rack beside meat; turn on heat and adjust thermostat to 300° F.

After 15 minutes read oven thermometer; adjust heat if necessary.

Turn meat fat side up after it has been cooked for half the estimated cooking time; brush surfaces with **vegetable oil.**

Cook until meat thermometer shows internal temperature of 155 to 160° F.

Serve with caper sauce (p. 136) or gravy seasoned with dill (p. 127).

VARIATIONS:

Bone leg of lamb and stuff with **onion dressing** (p. 131).

Barbecue beef, chicken, duck, ham, fresh pork, or other meat by same procedure. For preparing meats, follow directions given under roasting.

The Moist-Heat Methods of Cooking Meat

The methods of meat cookery discussed thus far, broiling, roasting, and their variations, are known as the dry-heat methods. Since dry heat penetrates meat slowly and is easy to control, meats properly cooked by these methods lose so little flavor and are so delicious that no seasonings are needed. When meats are cooked by moist heat, or by hot water or steam, the internal temperature reaches 185° to 212° F. within a few minutes, a temperature so high that much flavor is lost; therefore such meats are usually served well seasoned.

A myriad of recipes exists for cooking meats with moist heat. They may be called braised, smothered, potted, fricasseed, baked (in a covered utensil), or half a dozen other terms. They run the gamut of all the less tender cuts of meat of all sizes and from all the animals commonly used as food. These recipes include almost every known vegetable and seasoning and combinations of vegetables and seasonings. As a result they are so confusing and their number so appalling as to convince an amateur that she will never learn to cook.

Meat cookery becomes simplified when you understand why thousands of so-called separate recipes exist. In past centuries, when few vegetables and fruits were known, meat was the chief food. It spoiled easily, yet had to be eaten to prevent starvation. The spoiled meats were highly seasoned with spices and herbs to make them palatable. Thousands of lives were lost in the search for trade routes to obtain spices; and America was discovered because of spoiled meat. Through generation after generation, thousands of ideas for seasoning meats have been written down into what are now considered to be different recipes. The person who originated each idea was probably no more intelligent than you; his ideas are probably no better than yours.

Aside from seasonings, there are really only four variations in recipes for cooking meat by the moist-heat methods: the method of browning; the vegetables cooked with the meat; the amount of moisture used in cooking; and the type of gravy prepared. The meat may be browned by frying, sautéing, pan-broiling, or roasting; it may be seared or dipped in wheat germ, flour, crumbs, or batter. The vegetables used, like the seasonings, will depend on what your family happens to enjoy and which ones you have on hand. The gravy may be clear, brown, or made with milk or tomatoes. Stripped of their excess baggage, the thousands of recipes may be reduced to two recipes, or methods—braising and stewing.

If you are aware of these variations and can cook one meat successfully by a moist-heat method, you can cook all meats with equal success. Moreover, you can throw away all recipes (including mine) and make up your own. When the principles of cookery are known, the only value of recipes is to suggest ideas which you may not think of at the moment.

Braise Meats to Retain Their Flavor

According to schools of cookery, to braise meat means to cover it during cooking. The covering may be hot coals or stones, the lid of a utensil, or a browned crust. Regardless of its type, the covering holds steam around the meat so that it is cooked by steam.

When meat is cooked in water, much of the meat flavor passes into the liquid. If meat from a young animal or a muscle which has been little used is stewed, almost no flavor is left in the meat, and the gravy is unworthy of the name. If the meat is steamed, or cooked on a rack standing ¾ inch above the bottom of the pan, this unnecessary loss of flavor is largely prevented. When little or no gravy is to be made, meat should be braised, or steamed, rather than stewed. Since the rack allows steam to surround all surfaces of the meat, they are evenly heated and the cooking time is shortened by a third or more.

Steam held in a utensil stays at exactly the same temperature as the water below it. It is extremely important that the water used not be allowed to go above simmering temperature, or 185° F. Even this temperature quickly toughens the protein. Although connective tissue starts to break down below 185° F., the less tender cuts used for braising contain thick sheets of connective tissue which soften and break down slowly. If the water (hence the steam) does reach boiling temperature, the connective tissue breaks down more rapidly, but the proteins become so tough that much flavor is lost and the cooking time must be prolonged an hour or more before the proteins become tender again. When braising meat, turn the heat as low as you can get it; check the temperature of the water with the cooking thermometer. If the heat is still above 185° F. and cannot be turned lower, set the utensil to one side so that it covers only half or a third of the heating unit. Since steam heat penetrates rapidly, the meat cooks at an internal temperature of 185° F. and a meat thermometer is rarely needed.

Such meats as pot roast and Swiss steak are often cooked by steam formed only from meat juices, no water being added. Since most cooking utensils allow some steam to escape, the meat shrinks more and is less moist than if water is added at the beginning of cooking. As the meat nears doneness, however, the water may be allowed to evaporate off to ensure rich, luscious gravy.

Unless rolled in flour or crumbs, most meats to be braised should not be salted until ready to serve because salt draws moisture from the meat; these are less tender cuts already low in moisture. They are usually served with a sauce, which may be generously salted.

Since vinegar and other acids tenderize meat and shorten the cooking time, use them in all braising. If the meat does not contain bone, buy a small amount of bone and cook it in the water and acid used for steaming; thus calcium and a delightful flavor are added to the gravy or sauce.

Braised meats are frequently overcooked. The test of a well-cooked meat is that it will slice evenly without pulling apart. If it is stringy, flavor has been lost which cannot be recaptured

The simplest form of braising is that which serves as a substitute for boiling, a criminal means of cooking meat. Not only is flavor lost in boiling, but valuable nutrients are discarded when the liquid left from cooking such meats as tongue or ham is thrown away.

BRAISED, OR STEAMED, CHICKEN

Select stewing chicken; wash outside thoroughly; disjoint or leave whole. If disjointed, put neck and wing tips in the bottom of the utensil. Set a rack standing ¾ inch high over bones; place chicken on rack and add:

½ to 1 cup water   1 tablespoon white vinegar or white wine
                               for each pound of chicken

Cover utensil and set over simmer burner or extremely low heat; after 10 minutes check temperature of water with cooking thermometer; if it is greater than 185° F., adjust heat or set utensil to one side of burner. No bubbles should burst on the surface of the water.

Cook until tender when pierced with a fork, or about 2 to 2½ hours. Use chicken in making soufflé (p. 195), chicken loaf (p. 226), chicken salad (p. 232), or creamed chicken (p. 211).

VARIATIONS:

Although the types of meat in the following variations differ widely, they are steamed in the same manner outlined in the recipe for steamed chicken, referred to as the basic recipe. Merely substitute for chicken in the basic recipe the name of the meat you wish to prepare.

Corned beef: Prepare as in basic recipe, using vinegar and steaming 3⅓ to 4 hours; 10 minutes before serving, set meat on platter, skim off excess fat from drippings, and steam sauerkraut or shredded cabbage in same utensil; add 1 to 4 teaspoons caraway seeds.

Ham: Steam as in basic recipe, allowing 20 minutes per pound for large ham, 30 for small, half, or picnic ham; save drippings for seasoning.

Heart: Use half a beef heart, 1 veal or pork heart, or 4 lamb hearts; wash well and clip out tough membranes; score (p. 62); steam as in basic recipe, allowing 3½ hours for beef heart, 2½ hours for pork, veal, or lamb hearts. Slice meat while hot, serving beef heart with celery or curry sauce, pork with caraway or horseradish sauce, lamb with caper or dill sauce (pp. 136–137); or slice and serve cold with chilled sauces (pp. 141, 143).

Stuffed heart: Select whole heart which has not been cut; steam as above; prepare 1½ cups fruit, celery or crumb stuffing for beef or veal heart; cornbread stuffing for pork heart; rice stuffing seasoned with 1

STANDARD LAMB CUTS

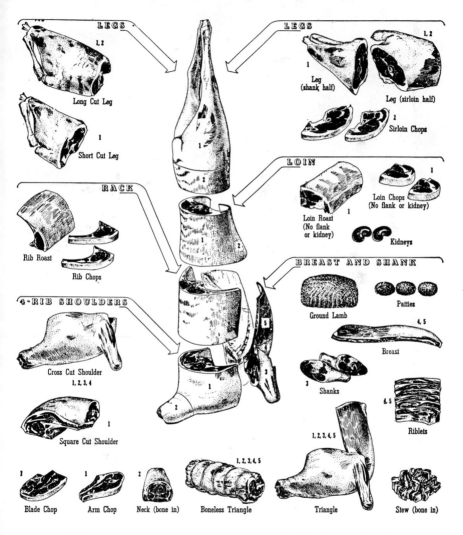

LEGS

Long Cut Leg

1

Short Cut Leg

RACK

Rib Roast

Rib Chops

4-RIB SHOULDERS

Cross Cut Shoulder
1, 2, 3, 4

1

Square Cut Shoulder

Blade Chop

Arm Chop

Neck (bone in)

1, 2, 3, 4, 5

Boneless Triangle

Triangle

Stew (bone in)

LEGS

Leg
(shank half)

Leg (sirloin half)

Sirloin Chops

LOIN

Loin Roast
(No flank
or kidney)

Loin Chops
(No flank or kidney)

Kidneys

BREAST AND SHANK

Ground Lamb

Patties

Breast

Shanks

Riblets

PRIMAL (WHOLESALE) LAMB CUTS AND THE RETAIL CUTS MADE FROM EACH

STANDARD VEAL CUTS

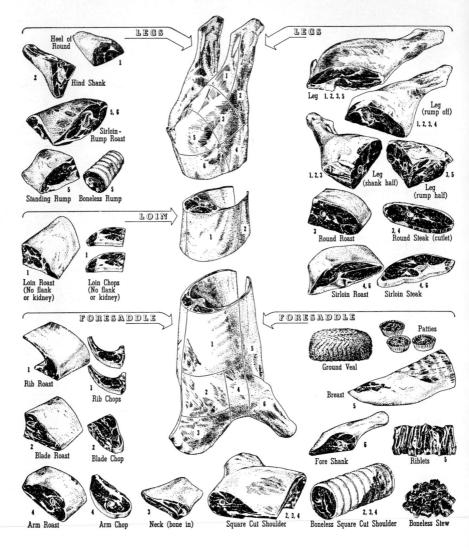

PRIMAL (WHOLESALE) VEAL CUTS AND THE RETAIL CUTS MADE FROM EACH

STANDARD BEEF CUTS

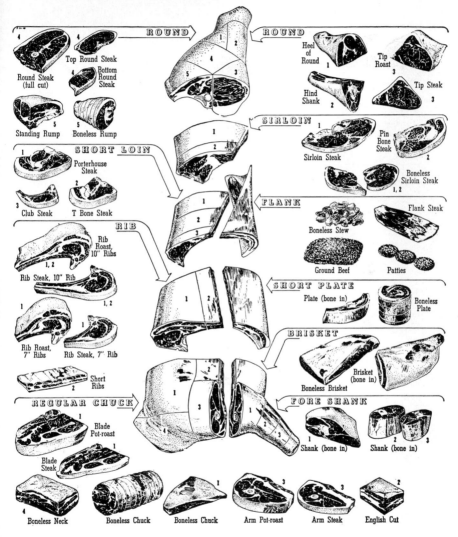

ROUND

Top Round Steak

Round Steak (full cut)

Bottom Round Steak

Standing Rump

Boneless Rump

ROUND

Heel of Round

Tip Roast

Hind Shank

Tip Steak

SIRLOIN

Sirloin Steak

Pin Bone Steak

Boneless Sirloin Steak

SHORT LOIN

Porterhouse Steak

Club Steak

T Bone Steak

FLANK

Boneless Stew

Flank Steak

Ground Beef

Patties

RIB

Rib Roast, 10" Ribs

Rib Steak, 10" Rib

Rib Roast, 7" Ribs

Rib Steak, 7" Rib

Short Ribs

SHORT PLATE

Plate (bone in)

Boneless Plate

BRISKET

Boneless Brisket

Brisket (bone in)

REGULAR CHUCK

Blade Pot-roast

Blade Steak

FORE SHANK

Shank (bone in)

Shank (bone in)

Boneless Neck

Boneless Chuck

Boneless Chuck

Arm Pot-roast

Arm Steak

English Cut

PRIMAL (WHOLESALE) BEEF CUTS AND THE RETAIL CUTS MADE FROM EACH

STANDARD PORK CUTS

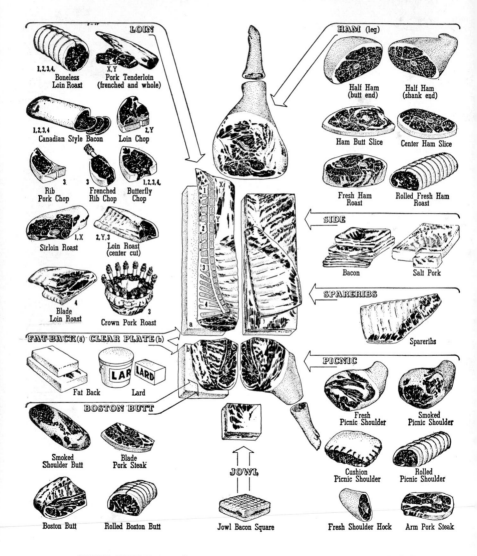

LOIN

1,2,3,4
Boneless
Loin Roast

X,Y
Pork Tenderloin
(frenched and whole)

1,2,3,4
Canadian Style Bacon

2,Y
Loin Chop

3
Rib
Pork Chop

3
Frenched
Rib Chop

1,2,3,4,
Butterfly
Chop

1,X
Sirloin Roast

2,Y,3
Loin Roast
(center cut)

4
Blade
Loin Roast

3
Crown Pork Roast

FAT BACK (a)   CLEAR PLATE (b)

Fat Back

LARD   LARD

Lard

BOSTON BUTT

Smoked
Shoulder Butt

Blade
Pork Steak

Boston Butt

Rolled Boston Butt

JOWL

Jowl Bacon Square

HAM (leg)

Half Ham
(butt end)

Half Ham
(shank end)

Ham Butt Slice

Center Ham Slice

Fresh Ham
Roast

Rolled Fresh Ham
Roast

SIDE

Bacon

Salt Pork

SPARERIBS

Spareribs

PICNIC

Fresh
Picnic Shoulder

Smoked
Picnic Shoulder

Cushion
Picnic Shoulder

Rolled
Picnic Shoulder

Fresh Shoulder Hock

Arm Pork Steak

PRIMAL (WHOLESALE) PORK CUTS AND THE RETAIL CUTS MADE FROM EACH teaspoon dill seeds for lamb hearts. As soon as meat is tender, heat stuffing thoroughly in drippings; pack into heart, sprinkle dressing generously with **paprika,** and brown under broiler. Don't miss this recipe; it makes an excellent inexpensive entree.

Liver: Use unsliced lamb, pork, or baby beef liver; insert meat thermometer and steam about 8 minutes for each inch of thickness; take up when internal temperature is 155° F.; slice and serve hot or cold with creole sauce (pp. 140, 141). Prepare liver in this way for persons who must use a reducing or low-fat diet.

Tongue: Use 1 fresh, pickled, or smoked beef, veal, or pork tongue or 6 to 8 lamb tongues; wash thoroughly and steam 1 hour per pound; remove skin while hot; slice diagonally. Serve beef, veal, or pork tongue hot or cold with horseradish sauce (p. 137), lamb tongues with caper sauce (p. 136).

Creamed lamb tongues: Steam 1 pound of lamb tongues as above; prepare 2 cups caper or dill sauce; cut tongues into fingers and add to sauce 5 minutes before serving.

Braised Meats Browned by Frying

Strange though it may seem, fried chicken and other meats which are dipped in flour or batter and browned in fat are cooked by the heat of steam, or are actually braised. The browned crust serves the same purpose as does the lid of a utensil, holding in steam formed from meat juices. If chicken were fried without the protective coating, the meat would be so dry and tough you could not eat it.

The chief purpose of frying is to utilize the heat of fat not merely to brown the crust but to carry heat into curves and contours of meat which cannot lie flat on the surface of a utensil. The only meats which should be browned by frying are those which have irregular surfaces. In braising tender meats which cook in a relatively short time, it is important that the utensil not be tightly covered. If steam is held in even for a few minutes, it is quickly heated by the hot fat to boiling temperature; the meat becomes tough, is less juicy, and much delightful flavor is lost.

Before refrigeration for farm homes was heard of, I lived on a farm where we ate delicious fried chicken at almost every breakfast, dinner, and supper from the time spring chickens were large enough to eat until it was cold enough to butcher hogs without danger of the meat spoiling. Being an optimist, I have persistently ordered fried chicken in restaurants over a period of twenty years and in almost every state, but like a homesick New Englander who orders Boston baked beans and finds them cooked with tomatoes, I leave the restaurant a sadder person. The way you can depend on getting delicious fried chicken is to ask a genuine farmer's wife to fry one for you; these women are gracious and wholehearted and will not let you down. If you are lucky enough to find one like Mrs. Johnson, who lived on our farm near Lizton, Indiana, along with the fried chicken and country gravy you will be served creamed peas, new potatoes, sliced tomatoes, corn on the cob, homemade cottage cheese golden with rich cream, a pitcher of milk, home-canned peaches, and fresh berry pie; and your hostess will apologize because she did not get around to baking a cake.

Although everyone who enjoys fried chicken has his own standards as to the way it should be cooked, most people would probably agree that every bit of surface should be an even and golden brown, that the crust should be crisp but tender, and that the meat should not be dried out. These standards we met quite accidentally years ago. It was difficult to urge the old wood stove to produce efficient heat; hence the surface of the meat was browned at moderate temperature, flour which dropped from the meat was not burned, and the meat was not dried out. Since there were usually huge jars of lard in the cellar, we used a generous amount in browning the chicken; curved surfaces which could not touch the bottom of the skillet were thus browned as golden as the flat surfaces. We did not own a lid which fitted the frying pan; hence steam could not be held in to make the crust soggy or to reach a temperature which could overcook or toughen the meat. To prepare delicious fried chicken, these conditions should be duplicated.

The chief problem now lies in finding chickens worth buying or even safe to eat. Chickens raised on wire get neither enough good food nor enough exercise to develop flavorful meat. Caponized fowl are usually tasteless, and according to some health authorities, lack nutritive value because of lack of hormones. Some of the brands of frozen chicken breasts, thighs, and other pieces come from fowl raised on the ground and have more flavor than chickens purchased fresh.

The type of fat used in frying chicken must be determined by the flavor you wish in the gravy and by the degree of health you want your family to enjoy.

CRISP FRIED CHICKEN, INDIANA STYLE

Allow approximately ¾ hour for frying a 3-pound chicken and 1 hour for a 4-pound chicken.

If you dress the chicken, disjoint so that each piece will be as flat as possible; cut lower back into 2 pieces; crack and flatten ribs along upper spine; wash quickly and dry immediately.

Before frying, mix in a paper bag:

3 or 4 tablespoons whole-wheat flour   ½ teaspoon freshly ground peppercorns
1 teaspoon salt

Dredge chicken by shaking 2 or 3 pieces at a time; lay on wax paper and allow 10 minutes for the flour to be dried on the surfaces; dredge a second time if a thick crust is desired.

Meanwhile heat in a frying pan:

½ cup lard, butter, partially hardened
margarine, or vegetable oil

When fat is moderately hot, carefully shake off any excess flour as chicken is put into pan; place larger pieces in center of pan over source of heat; put smaller pieces around edge, or brown them later. Keep out liver and brown it 10 minutes before serving.

See that fat is sufficiently deep to reach into all curves of the lower surfaces of the meat; add more fat if needed. Leave frying pan uncovered, or set lid to one side, allowing steam to escape. Maintain heat at moderate temperature and allow crust to brown slowly; there should be no smoking fat or sputtering.

As soon as lower surfaces are deep golden brown, turn and brown other surfaces; when all surfaces of a piece are completely browned, pile it on top of those browning so that it can cook at low temperature; continue browning slowly until all surfaces are golden.

When browning is complete, lower heat and cook until meat is tender, keeping lid to one side; pour off excess fat, leaving 2 tablespoons for each cup of gravy desired; make country gravy (p. 125) seasoned with a pinch of sage.

VARIATIONS:

If several chickens are to be browned at one time, use deeper fat; when each piece is well browned, set chicken in a moderate oven at 300° F. on a flat pan or broiler rack. Do not cover pan. Roast until tender, or for 15 to 30 minutes.

Chicken fried in batter: Make a batter by beating together ½ cup each milk and whole-wheat flour, 1 teaspoon salt, 1 egg, ¼ teaspoon freshly ground white peppercorns, pinch of sage, dash of cayenne; dip the chicken in batter and fry as in basic recipe, or in deep fat at 300° F.

Chicken fried in crumbs: Beat 1 egg slightly with 3 tablespoons milk, 1 teaspoon salt, ⅛ teaspoon each paprika and freshly ground black peppercorns; dip chicken in egg, then in sifted whole-wheat-bread crumbs; fry as in basic recipe. Or use wheat germ instead of crumbs.

Chicken paprika: Brown chicken as in basic recipe; drain fat, leaving about 4 tablespoons; add 2 or 3 chopped onions or leeks and sauté as chicken continues to cook; pile chicken to one side and stir in 2 tablespoons whole-wheat flour; cook slowly 10 minutes; put chicken on serving tray; add to flour and onions ½ teaspoon salt, 1 to 2 teaspoons paprika, 2 cups sour cream or yogurt; stir well and heat through. Pour the sauce over the chicken.

Chicken, Spanish style: When chicken is browned, add 1 minced clove garlic, ½ cup each chopped onions, celery, green peppers and/or pimentos; set chicken on top of vegetables; keep heat low and simmer 15 minutes; put chicken on serving platter; add to vegetables and heat quickly 2 cups tomatoes, 1 teaspoon salt, dash of cayenne; pour sauce over chicken.

Fried duck, goose, guinea hen, and other fowl: Choose a young fowl and fry as in basic recipe, allowing ¾ to 1 hour for cooking time. Serve with country gravy seasoned with a pinch of sage.

Fried rabbit: Choose a young rabbit weighing 3 to 4 pounds. Prepare as in basic recipe or any variation of fried chicken, cooking about 45 minutes.

Fried roasting chicken: Choose a young roasting chicken and disjoint; brown at moderate temperature as in basic recipe; set on rack above dripping pan and roast in moderate oven at 300° F. until tender, or about ½ hour. Serve with country gravy.

Fried turkey: Select a young turkey, preferably weighing between 8 and 10 pounds; disjoint and cut into pieces approximately the size of those of chicken prepared for frying; split thighs into 2 parts along bone; cut breast into 6 or 8 pieces, upper back into 3 or 5, and lower back into 4. Proceed as if frying several chickens at one time, setting browned pieces on a rack in a moderate oven at 300° F. and cooking until tender, or from 25 to 40 minutes; or pile browned turkey in large baking dish, add 1 cup cream, and finish cooking in oven.

When mature rabbits, stewing chickens, and other less tender meats with irregular surfaces are browned by frying and then braised, the procedure is identical with that of frying chicken except that the cooking time is longer, the utensil is tightly covered, the meat is preferably placed on a rack above water, and usually a highly seasoned gravy or sauce is prepared. Since these meats are lean, the purpose of browning is to add the flavor of fat as well as that of browned flour or crumbs. These meats, which are low in moisture, should not be salted until ready to serve.

Many cookbooks advise that meats to be braised be "baked" in a covered utensil in the oven for several hours. Since the cover holds in steam and baking means to cook with dry heat surrounding the food, to follow such advice is impossible. Steaming in the oven is recommended because oven heat penetrates slowly and can easily be controlled; there is less danger of the steam reaching boiling temperature than when meat is carelessly cooked on top of the range. Such a procedure, however, is extravagant; you use 10 to 15 times more fuel and obtain less heat when you braise meats in an oven rather than over a surface burner.

BRAISED CHICKEN BROWNED BY FRYING

Select a stewing chicken weighing 4 to 5 pounds; singe, wash, disjoint, and dredge in **wheat germ or whole-wheat-pastry flour**; follow procedure for frying chicken (p. 57), allowing 30 minutes to brown all surfaces to a deep golden. Pour off fat not needed for gravy; *do not salt.*

Set all chicken except wing tips and neck on rack standing ¾ inch above bottom of utensil; add:

½ **cup water**	1 **tablespoon white vinegar for**
¼ **cup dry white wine or**	**each 2 pounds of chicken**

Cover utensil; put over simmer burner or extremely low heat; steam chicken until starting to be tender, or about 2 to 2½ hours.

Lift rack holding chicken to serving platter; increase heat, boil a few minutes if any odor of vinegar remains, and add:

1 cup vegetable-cooking water	3 or 4 diced unpeeled carrots
pinch of thyme or sage and basil	2 to 4 diced green onions with
¼ teaspoon crushed white pepper-	tops
corns	1 teaspoon salt

Stir or shake until smooth:

4 tablespoons whole-wheat flour	½ cup vegetable-cooking water

Add thickening slowly to sauce, stirring well; boil 2 or 3 minutes; put tray of chicken over sauce; cover utensil and simmer until chicken and vegetables are tender.

Before serving add 2 tablespoons chopped parsley.

Taste for seasonings; put chicken on platter, sprinkle with salt, and pour sauce over it.

VARIATIONS:

Before browning dip chicken in 1 egg stirred with 3 tablespoons milk; roll in wheat germ or whole-wheat-bread crumbs.

Instead of carrots and onions cook in sauce any of the following combinations of vegetables: 1 cup fresh or frozen peas, 3 or 4 fresh or canned pimentos; celery, carrots, zucchini; 1 cup each mushrooms, diced carrots, leeks; cauliflower and string beans seasoned with basil; green peppers, chopped onions, carrots.

Braised chicken with fruit: Omit vegetables and herbs; make gravy with cup of fruit juice and add dash of allspice and cinnamon, 1 cup chunk pineapple or pitted red or black cherries. Serve chicken on bed of rice with fruit sauce over it; serve remaining sauce separately.

Braised chicken with spinach: Omit vegetables, seasoning, and thickening of basic recipe; when chicken is tender, set aside on rack; add 1 minced clove garlic, 1 bunch shredded spinach and cook greens until tender; stir in 1 slightly beaten egg and let stand about 6 minutes; salt; put greens on serving platter with chicken in center; sprinkle chicken well with salt. Prepare any other greens in the same way.

Braised chicken with sour cream: Omit seasoning, thickening, and vegetables of basic recipe; when chicken is tender, evaporate broth to ¼ cup and add salt, peppercorns, 2 tablespoons each chives and parsley, 2 cups sour cream or yogurt. Vary by adding 1 cup mushrooms, dash of cayenne or Tabasco.

Braised chicken with cream sauce: Instead of sauce in basic recipe prepare 2 or 3 cups caper, celery, dill, mushroom, mock Hollandaise, or olive sauce (pp. 136–137), using **chicken broth** instead of part of the fresh milk. Place chicken on serving platter, pour sauce over it; garnish with parsley and paprika.

Braised chicken with tomato sauce: Instead of sauce in basic recipe prepare 2 or 3 cups tomato sauce (p. 140); pour over chicken.

Braised duck: Prepare as in basic recipe or any variation for braised chicken, steaming 3 to 3½ hours.

Braised duck with sauerkraut: Braise as directed; set tray of duck aside when tender; add to broth **1 or 2 teaspoons caraway seeds, 3 or 4 cups sauerkraut;** steam 10 minutes; put sauerkraut on serving platter with duck in center; sprinkle meat well with **salt and paprika.** Duck prepared in this way is delicious.

Braised goose, guinea hen, and other tame fowl: Braise like chicken, steaming 2½ to 3 hours; season sauce with **sage, tarragon,** or **basil.** Prick skin of goose several times during cooking to allow melted fat to escape. Remove goose fat from meat juices with a basting syringe. Vary by making sauce of **2 cups orange juice;** salt and thicken as in basic recipe, mixing flour with orange juice; add **2 teaspoons grated orange rind.** Omit other seasonings.

Braised squab: Cut in half along breastbone and backbone 2 or more squabs; flatten pieces and brown as in basic recipe; set aside on rack; bring to boiling **2 cups vegetable-cooking water,** add slowly **1 cup brown** or **wild rice, ¼ to ½ teaspoon crushed black peppercorns;** set tray of squab over rice and steam 40 minutes; season rice with **1 teaspoon salt, 2 chopped pimentos.**

Braised rabbit: Use a 3- to 5-pound stewing rabbit; braise as in basic recipe or any variation for chicken. Or after browning put into casserole with **4 to 6 sliced onions, 1½ teaspoons salt, ¼ teaspoon each sage** or **thyme** and freshly ground **peppercorns;** add **1 cup fresh** or **reconstituted milk.** Simmer on top of range or bake for 45 minutes at 325° F., or until meat is tender. Sprinkle with **paprika** and serve.

Curried chicken: See page 74.

Braised Meats Browned by Sautéing

Meats which have flat surfaces, such as Swiss steaks and pot roasts, should be browned by sautéing rather than frying. The heat can be easily controlled, and there is far less danger of toughening or drying out the meat. When meat contains fat, as does a pot roast, the fat melts during cooking and the gravy becomes greasy if additional fat has been used for browning. Meats browned by sautéing may be browned with or without being dredged in wheat germ, flour, or crumbs, depending on the flavor you desire. Since, however, the high temperatures often used for searing may cause carcinogenic substances to be formed in overheated fat, it is preferable to brown meats slowly and with the aid of wheat germ, crumbs, or flour.

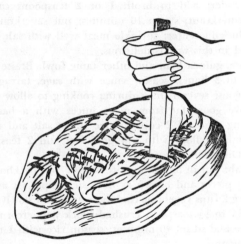

Whenever meat to be braised contains so little bone that a knife can penetrate it readily, the meat should be scored thoroughly. Scoring shortens the cooking, thus allowing a more delightful flavor to be retained. The modern method of scoring is to use a sharp-pointed knife and push it through the meat at ½-inch intervals, being particularly careful that the blade is at a right angle to the meat fibers. If the knife is ½ inch wide, a ½-inch cut alternates with ½ inch which is not cut. Although stabbed full of holes, the meat itself remains intact; the cut holes quickly seal over during cooking so that juices are not lost.

This type of scoring is extremely easy, takes only a moment, and works like a charm. The usual method of scoring, or cutting the surface of the meat diagonally to the fibers to the depth of ¼ to ½ inch does not cut the connective tissue in the center of the meat. Hence tenderness is increased but little, especially when the cut is thick. Moreover, so much surface is exposd that many juices are lost and the meat becomes dry and lacks flavor.

POT ROAST OF BEEF

Select pot roast weighing 3 pounds or more; purchase bone if it contains none. Score meat by pushing knife through it at a right angle to meat fibers and at intervals of ½ inch in rows 1 inch apart; turn and score the other side, making slits between those already made.

Put on wax paper and dredge meat well with:

4 to 5 tablespoons whole-wheat flour (optional)

Put meat into dry pan containing no fat. The floured surface will brown as readily without fat as with it. Brown meat well on both sides; keep heat moderate, taking 15 to 20 minutes. Lift meat and set rack under it, leaving bone in bottom of utensil; add:

½ cup vegetable-cooking water	1 tablespoon white vinegar for
¼ cup dry red wine or	each 2 pounds of meat

Cover utensil, put over simmer burner or extremely low heat. Simmer until almost tender, or about 3 hours.

When meat is tender, set lid of utensil to one side; let any excess moisture evaporate; set rack of meat over serving platter and make 2 cups brown gravy or tomato gravy (pp. 125–127); add and cook in gravy:

2 or 3 unpeeled carrots cut into quarters lengthwise	1 diced bell pepper or fresh pimento or paprika
2 or 3 unpeeled turnips cut into quarters	1 minced clove garlic
1 or 2 potatoes, preferably unpeeled, cut into quarters	1 or 2 sliced onions, leeks, or green onions with tops
¼ to ½ teaspoon crushed black peppercorns	½ crushed bay leaf
	pinch of basil or savory
	1½ teaspoons salt

Cover utensil and boil 5 to 6 minutes until vegetables are heated through; lower heat to simmering; return tray holding meat, cover utensil, and simmer 10 to 15 minutes, or until vegetables are tender; sprinkle meat with **salt**. Taste gravy for seasonings.

VARIATIONS:

Omit vegetables suggested and add fresh or frozen peas, cauliflower, string beans, zucchini, kohlrabi, or other vegetables, adding them at such a time that none will be overcooked.

Instead of basil or savory, add turmeric, marjoram, rosemary, thyme, tarragon, or other herbs.

Make gravy with milk; cook in gravy diced carrots, green peas, 2 or 3 diced pimentos; season with a pinch of thyme.

Omit vegetables, bay, and basil; prepare brown gravy; 5 minutes before serving spread meat with dry or prepared mustard or freshly ground horseradish; or simmer 3 tablespoons finely diced preserved ginger in gravy.

Unless otherwise stated, the meats in the following variations are prepared as in the recipe for pot roast, referred to as the basic recipe. Follow this recipe, merely substituting for pot roast the name of the meat you wish to cook.

Braised beef brisket: Select 3 or 4 pounds of fresh brisket; remove bone to cook under rack; score meat, brown, cook, and season as in basic recipe or any variation, steaming 2½ to 3 hours. Vary by cooking in gravy ½ cup each diced **onion, carrots, celery, green peppers.**

Braised brisket with wheat: Omit vinegar; score and brown brisket and set aside on rack; heat 2½ cups vegetable-cooking water to boiling and add 1 cup unground wheat or dry lima beans; place rack of meat on top and simmer until tender; season with ½ teaspoon **crushed black peppercorns**, 1½ teaspoons salt, omitting gravy, vegetables, and seasonings of basic recipe. Beef brisket with wheat is an Argentine recipe and is delicious.

Braised flank: Select 2 pounds or more of beef flank; score; prepare 1 cup **bread, vegetable, or fruit stuffing** (pp. 129, 133) and spread on flank; fold ends over and pin edges together with skewers, making a roll so that meat can be sliced across the fibers; lace securely with string. Dredge and brown surface of roll; steam as in basic recipe 1½ to 2 hours. This recipe is one of my favorites; it is especially delicious with apple or prune stuffing.

Braised pork roast: Select fresh pork roast weighing 3 pounds or more; if shoulder roast is used, stuff with **prune or apple dressing** (p. 133); trim off excess fat; braise as in basic recipe 2½ to 3 hours. Serve with brown gravy.

Braised lamb or mutton: Select shoulder roast weighing 3 pounds or more; score and braise as in basic recipe, allowing 1½ hours for lamb, 2½ to 3 hours for mutton. Add or omit vegetables or use vegetables suggested under variations.

Braised rump roast: Select boned and rolled rump roast; score, cook, and season as in basic recipe or any variation.

Braised veal roast: Select shoulder or rump roast weighing 3 pounds or more; braise as in basic recipe or any variation, steaming 1½ to 2 hours.

Heart pot roast: Select beef heart and bone from shank sawed into 1-inch pieces; wash heart, trim tough membranes, and cut as stew meat so that each piece lies flat; score, cook, and season as in basic recipe or any variation, simmering 3½ hours.

Pot roast with cherries: Omit vegetables and seasonings except salt. Prepare brown gravy, using 1 cup each water and juice from black cherries; add 1 cup cherries to gravy. Slice meat and serve with cherries and sauce over it.

Pot roast with sour cream: Cook pot roast as in basic recipe; instead of gravy, vegetables, and seasonings, add 2 cups chopped onions, ½ cup chopped celery, ½ teaspoon paprika, 1 teaspoon salt, 1 or 2 cups sour cream or yogurt; simmer 5 minutes and serve with sauce poured over meat; the onions and celery should still be crisp.

Stuffed breast of lamb or veal: Select veal or lamb breast weighing 3 or 4 pounds; make pocket between meat and ribs for **crumb, vegetable, cereal, or fruit stuffing** (pp. 129–133); omit scoring; prepare as in basic recipe, steaming 1½ to 2 hours. Add vegetables suggested in basic recipe or variations, or cook in gravy ½ cup each **chopped celery, onions, pimentos, 1 teaspoon dill seeds.**

Swiss steak: Score or pound Swiss steak well after dredging; prepare and season as in basic recipe, simmering 2 to 2½ hours.

The following braised meats, which are browned by sautéing, are prepared in exactly the same manner as are Swiss steaks and pot roasts. The only essential difference is that the cuts are smaller.

BRAISED LAMB OR VEAL SHANKS

Select 4 lamb or veal shanks; ask butcher to saw 1 inch of bone from smaller ends; score meat from all sides by jabbing a knife into it at intervals of ½ inch in rows ½ inch apart.

Without adding fat of any kind, sear meat slowly in preheated utensil until brown on flat surfaces, first dredging in whole-wheat pastry flour; set shanks on rack, leaving bones in bottom of utensil; add:

2 tablespoons vinegar or cooking   ½ cup vegetable-cooking water
wine

Cover utensil, put over simmer burner or extremely low heat. Simmer 1½ to 2 hours.

When meat is almost tender, set lid of utensil to one side; let excess moisture evaporate. Set rack of meat over serving platter and make 2 cups brown gravy or tomato gravy (pp. 125–127); season gravy with:

1 clove garlic   1¼ teaspoons salt
¼ crushed bay leaf   pinch each of marjoram, basil,
¼ to ½ teaspoon crushed black   and/or savory
   peppercorns

Simmer 10 minutes. Serve shanks in gravy or in separate dish.

VARIATIONS:

Cook in gravy of basic recipe or any variation 2 or more of the following: onions, bell pepper, pimento, paprika, celery, carrots, potatoes, turnips, kohlrabi, string beans, cauliflower, zucchini, fresh lima beans, or other vegetables. Be particularly careful to add vegetables only in time for them to become tender when the meat is ready to serve. Leave vegetables whole or halve, quarter, dice, or cut into fingers.

Omit herbs; add 1 teaspoon dill or caraway seeds; or add whole or powdered turmeric, fresh tarragon, or other herbs.

Prepare the meats in the following variations as outlined in the recipe for braised lamb shanks. Merely substitute for lamb shanks in the basic recipe the name of the meat you wish to cook. Achieve variety by using different herbs in seasoning gravy.

Braised beef brisket: Select 2 pounds or more of brisket, cut into serving sizes; braise 2½ to 3 hours as in basic recipe, removing part of the bone to cook under rack; or cook diced carrots, celery, and onions in gravy.

Braised lamb or mutton breast: Select 2 pounds or more of lamb or mutton breast, cut into serving sizes; have butcher cut off 2 or 3 bones to cook under rack; braise as in basic recipe, steaming lamb 1½ hours, mutton 2½ to 3. If taste of mutton is undesirable, remove as much fat as possible, marinate in ¼ cup French dressing for 24 hours before cooking.

Braised oxtail: Select 2 pounds of oxtail; let 1 or 2 smaller pieces cook under rack; braise and season as in basic recipe, cooking 2½ hours; or cook in gravy 2 each chopped onions and diced carrots, 1 cup tomatoes, ½ cup chopped celery, 3 cloves; add bay, garlic, salt, and peppercorns.

Braised short ribs of beef: Select 2 pounds or more of meaty short ribs cut into serving sizes; remove 2 or 3 bones to cook under rack; braise as in basic recipe but without searing or dredging with flour, steaming 2½ to 3 hours.

Braised veal or lamb riblets: Select 2 pounds or more of meaty veal or lamb riblets; remove 1 or 2 bones to cook under rack; braise as in basic recipe, steaming 1½ to 2 hours.

Curried lamb, beef, or veal: See page 75.

Lamb or veal stew: Select 2 pounds or more of lamb or veal stew meat cut into 2-inch pieces; purchase bone or remove bone to cook under rack; braise 1½ hours and season as in basic recipe; cut carrots, potatoes, onions, green peppers, and celery in 1-inch chunks and cook in brown or tomato gravy, adding each vegetable only in time to become tender. Immediately before serving combine lamb or veal with gravy and vegetables. Do not cook these meats in water. Lamb or veal stew is especially delicious with fresh or frozen peas or fresh lima beans, but any vegetables suggested under variations may be used.

Slow Braising

Probably every person with a discriminating taste would agree that meats which are broiled or roasted, or cooked at low internal temperatures, are more delicious than braised meats which are cooked at the internal temperature of 185° F. or above. Since meats which are braised are the more flavorful cuts, the reverse should be true. Simmering temperature, however, is so high that proteins toughen and much flavor is lost. Commercially "boiled" ham, certainly one of the most delicious of all meats cooked with moist heat, is usually cooked at a temperature of 160 to 165° F. The water used for steaming it is not allowed to go above this temperature at any time. The proteins do not toughen; the connective tissue does not break down; the delicious flavor is retained, and the meat, although delightfully tender, slices beautifully without tearing apart. There is no reason why meats which you braise at home cannot be equally delicious.

If you are fortunate enough to have a low simmer burner, a vigorous pilot light, a burner known as a coffee warmer, a warming oven, or an oven pilot light, set a pan of lukewarm water over the source of heat, let it heat for an hour or more, and check the temperature with the cooking thermometer. If a temperature of 160 to 165° F. can be maintained, you can prepare delicious meats without effort and almost without fuel cost by braising them slowly. Actually, lower temperatures can also be used. I have cooked many large pot roasts over a pilot light which maintained the water under the rack at 140° F. Although it took 24 hours, I have rarely tasted more delicious meat.

Meats to be braised slowly are browned and seasoned in the same manner as when braised at simmering temperature. If browning is not desired, they should be simmered for ½ hour to kill all surface bacteria before being transferred to a pilot light or other extremely low heat. Then you simply forget about them. Hours later you return to find them tender and delicious indeed. The cooking time varies widely with the particular cut of meat, but is roughly three times that required for braising at simmering temperature, or from 8 to 12 hours. This method, which I recommend heartily, is ideal for the person who must be away from home during the day. As in slow roasting, one of its principal advantages lies in being able to combine ordinary braising with slow braising to suit your activities.

Since the purpose of stewing meat is to extract flavor, there is no point in preparing stews at low temperature.

Only the Most Flavorful Cuts Should Be Stewed

Stewing is a variation of braising. The only difference is that enough water is added to make the amount of gravy desired and the meat is cooked in the liquid rather than on a rack. The purpose of stewing meat, aside from developing tenderness, is to prepare delicious gravy and to add the flavor of fat. Only the well-exercised muscles of mature animals have sufficient flavor to share with the gravy. Shank, brisket, neck, or oxtail of cutter or canner grade is preferable to other cuts and grades of beef.

Stew meats may be slowly seared without being dredged in flour, or dredged and seared, or not seared at all, depending on what flavor you prefer. Salt should be added at the beginning of cooking to bring out juices desired for the gravy. One or more bones should be cooked with the meat to supply calcium and additional flavor. Be particularly careful not to overcook stew; although the meat should be tender enough to cut with a fork, it should not fall apart.

Recipes for stewed lamb and veal are purposely omitted. Such meats are much more delicious when braised.

BEEF STEW

Select 2 or 3 pounds stew meat cut into 2-inch cubes, and ½ pound of bone cut from shank; ask butcher to saw bone into 1-inch pieces.

If time permits, put bones and meat into a refrigerator dish; add and stir well:

2 to 3 tablespoons vinegar, lemon juice, or red cooking wine
2 teaspoons salt

1 to 3 teaspoons dark molasses (optional)

Set in refrigerator for 12 to 36 hours; if meat has soaked 36 hours, put on to cook 1½ hours before serving; if soaked 12 hours, put on 2¼ hours before serving; if not soaked, allow 3 hours for cooking.

Shake moisture from meat, dredge with flour, and without adding fat sear meat and bone; keep heat moderate, searing 10 to 15 minutes; lift marrow from bones and mash with a fork; add:

liquid left from tenderizing meat
3 cups vegetable-cooking water or tomato juice

¼ to ½ teaspoon crushed black peppercorns

Cover utensil and simmer until meat is almost tender; discard bones; add the following chilled vegetables:

2 or 3 unpeeled carrots, cut into halves lengthwise
1 quartered potato
2 quartered turnips, rutabagas, or kohlrabi

2 onions or leeks cut into quarters
1 minced clove garlic
pinch each of savory and marjoram

Cover utensil, heat vegetables quickly, and simmer 10 minutes; blend to a smooth paste and add slowly:

½ cup vegetable-cooking water
4 tablespoons whole-wheat flour

more water or tomato juice if needed

Stir well and simmer 10 minutes. Taste for salt. Stir in 3 tablespoons parsley.

VARIATIONS:

Vary stews by adding one or more of the following vegetables only in time to become tender before serving: fresh asparagus, cauliflower, zucchini, string beans, green onions, celery, broccoli, green or red bell peppers, pimentos, fresh lima beans, cabbage, fresh or frozen peas, mushrooms, tomatoes, summer squash, celery root.

Season with Worcestershire, lemon juice, paprika, 1 or 2 chili tepines, 1 whole cayenne, whole turmeric, or 3 to 6 whole cloves; or use any herbs or seeds. If sweet meat is enjoyed, omit vegetables and herbs, and cook any one of the following in the gravy: prunes; wedges of firm, unpeeled apple; raisins; cling peaches; sliced pineapple; black cherries; preserved ginger; or an assortment of fruits.

Beef and kidney pie: Use a heat-resistant casserole and prepare stew as in basic recipe with 1 pound beef. Omit turnips; dice other vegetables and add **1 cup fresh or frozen peas;** season with **thyme and basil;** prepare **wheat-germ biscuit** dough (p. 424) and bake on a pie pan the size of casserole or cut into biscuits. Remove white tissue from **1 beef kidney, 2 veal kidneys, or 3 lamb kidneys;** dice; 5 minutes before serving, add kidneys and **1 tablespoon Worcestershire** to stew; put crust or biscuits on top.

Beef paprika: Prepare beef as in basic recipe, dredging in flour and simmering with ½ cup **vegetable-cooking water** until tender; add **1 cup sour cream, 1 teaspoon paprika;** omit vegetables and other seasonings.

Beef stew with wheat: Prepare as in basic recipe, using **4 cups vegetable-cooking water;** omit vinegar or wine; add and cook with meat **1 cup unground wheat;** 15 minutes before serving add ¼ cup each chopped **onions, celery, green peppers;** add **herbs, parsley, garlic;** omit vegetables.

Heart stew: Select a beef heart, wash, trim, and cut into cubes; tenderize, stew, and season as in basic recipe.

Hungarian goulash: Prepare stew as in basic recipe; omit turnips and herbs; add **carrots, onions, garlic, potatoes, 1 cup canned or fresh tomatoes, 3 chopped fresh or canned pimentos, 1 or 2 teaspoons powdered paprika.**

New England boiled dinner: Cut into cubes and stew 3 hours without tenderizing or searing **2 pounds corned beef or 3 pounds fresh brisket;** about 20 minutes before time to serve, add **small whole carrots, turnips, potatoes cut in half, small cabbage cut into sixths;** add vegetables in order of size and time required for cooking, being careful that none overcooks; thicken gravy, season with **salt and white peppercorns.**

Stewed beef with dumplings: Sear meat and bones thoroughly to develop flavor; add 1½ quarts vegetable-cooking water; when meat is almost tender, prepare dumplings (p. 73); omit potatoes and turnips. Bring liquid to boiling; add carrots, onions, garlic, herbs; drop in dumplings, cover utensil, and cook 15 minutes without removing lid.

STEWED CHICKEN

Select a stewing chicken, dress, disjoint; put into utensil with:

2 cups vegetable-cooking water   2 teaspoons salt
2 tablespoons white vinegar

Simmer for 2½ to 3 hours, or until nearly tender; if odor of vinegar can be detected, remove the lid of the utensil during the last ½ hour of cooking; skim off excess fat.

Combine and shake or beat until smooth:

½ cup vegetable-cooking water   4 tablespoons whole-wheat flour

Stir thickening into sauce and add:

½ teaspoon crushed peppercorns
⅛ teaspoon dry sage

Simmer 10 minutes before serving.

VARIATIONS:

Add 10 minutes before serving, fresh peas, diced carrots, potatoes, asparagus, leeks, lima beans, celery, or onions.

Instead of sage season with fresh or dried savory, tarragon, thyme, or basil.

Shake flour for thickening with 1 cup fresh milk, ½ cup powdered milk.

Spanish chicken: Prepare as in basic recipe; when nearly tender, add 1 cup tomatoes, ½ cup each chopped onions, carrots, celery, 2 diced pimentos, 1 minced clove garlic, pinch of basil or orégano, thickening; garnish with chopped parsley.

Chicken pie: Stew chicken as in basic recipe in heat-resistant casserole; cook 1 cup each fresh or frozen peas and diced carrots in thickened gravy. Prepare wheat-germ biscuits (p. 424), roll out dough, spread over casserole, and bake at 400° F. for 10 minutes.

Chicken with dumplings: Stew chicken in 1½ quarts vegetable-cooking water; when tender, make dumplings of 1 cup whole-wheat flour, ⅓ cup powdered milk, ½ teaspoon salt, 2½ teaspoons baking powder, 1 beaten egg, ⅓ cup cooled chicken broth; put chicken on serving platter; drop dumplings from teaspoon into slowly boiling broth; cover tightly and cook 15 minutes without removing lid.

Chicken with noodles: Stew chicken in 5 cups vegetable-cooking water; make noodles by stirring together 2 eggs, ⅓ cup powdered milk, 1 teaspoon salt, enough whole-wheat-pastry flour to make a stiff dough; knead and roll 1/16 inch thick; let dry 30 minutes and cut into strips ¼ inch wide; put chicken on serving platter, increase broth to a rolling boil, drop in noodles so slowly that boiling does not stop; reduce heat and add sage; cover utensil and simmer 10 minutes.

Chicken with paprika: Prepare as in basic recipe; omit sage, add thickening and 2 or 3 chopped fresh paprika peppers or canned pimentos and 1 or 2 teaspoons ground paprika.

Chicken stew with vegetables: 15 minutes before chicken is ready to serve, add ½ cup each baby lima beans, diced carrots, chopped onions or leeks, celery, bell pepper or pimento. Season with pinch each of sage, basil, thyme.

Chicken with mushrooms and olives: Follow basic recipe; add 1 small can button mushrooms and ¼ cup sliced stuffed olives.

Chicken with pineapple: Omit sage; just before serving add 1 cup well-drained chunk pineapple, 2 tablespoons each soy sauce and diced preserved ginger. Reduce salt to 1 teaspoon.

Chicken with rice: Stew chicken as in basic recipe, using 4 cups vegetable-cooking water; 15 minutes before serving, add 2 cups cooked brown rice or 1 cup uncooked converted rice, ¾ cup diced carrots. Five minutes before serving, add 1 cup fresh or frozen peas. Omit thickening.

Stewed rabbit: Use an old rabbit; disjoint and prepare as in basic recipe or any variation for chicken.

The two following recipes are nothing more than stewed chicken exotically seasoned. They meet the requirements for guest dinners where you wish to have your meal prepared in advance yet serve something rather special.

The curry recipe was given me by an East Indian woman. Perhaps it was the beautiful white sari she wore which made me believe that this curry is superior to any other I have ever tasted.

The coriander seeds give the curry its professional touch. If you wish your curry to be dynamic, add the cayenne rather than the curry powder with a heavy hand. The only change I have made in the original recipe is to shorten the simmering time from several hours to a few minutes. The recipe, however, must be prepared several hours in advance to allow the aromatic oils time to pass from the seasonings into the food. When I plan to serve either curry or Hawaiian chicken, I cook it in the morning, simmer the rice until it is half done, assemble the salad ready for tossing (then cover it and keep it in the refrigerator)—and find getting the guest dinner easier than preparing a meal for my family. Pineapple halves filled with assorted fresh fruits (p. 476) make an excellent dessert to accompany either of these dishes.

CHICKEN CURRY

Mix thoroughly in a large frying pan:

3 tablespoons vegetable oil	1 or 2 tablespoons well-mashed
2 or 3 teaspoons curry powder	coriander seeds
generous sprinkling of cayenne	

Heat oil and seasonings and add:

5 large chopped onions	1 teaspoon salt

Cover pan and cook over low heat for 10 minutes; add:

stewed meat from large hen or	2 cups broth left from stewing
2 pounds breasts and thighs	

Turn off heat; let curry stand at room temperature 4 hours or longer. Allow 10 minutes for reheating. Taste for **salt**.

Serve nested in a bed of rice on a large platter; sprinkle with paprika.

At the table pass dishes of small salted peanuts, shredded coconut, chutney, and seedless raisins to be sprinkled over curry.

VARIATIONS:

Add any of the following seasonings: 1 minced clove garlic; 1 small chili pepper; 1 teaspoon powdered turmeric; dash of nutmeg, cinnamon, or ground ginger; 1 teaspoon cumin, mustard, or cardamon seeds; ¼ teaspoon anise seeds.

Vary accompaniments by serving chopped hard-boiled eggs, white seedless raisins, pickle relish, roasted coconut flakes, or chopped bell pepper or green onions with tops.

Curried beef, lamb, turkey, and other meat: Instead of chicken use **2 or 3 cups leftover diced roast beef, lamb, veal, turkey, or other meat; or use part chicken and part canned tuna.** Let stand or serve at once; do not allow curry to boil after meat has been added.

Curried lobster: Use **1 fresh or frozen lobster tail** for 2 servings; cut into 1-inch hunks; add to onions no sooner than 5 minutes before serving.

Curried shrimp: Shell and remove veins from **2 pounds uncooked shrimp;** add to onions no sooner than 5 minutes before serving. Or use **2 cans shrimp and broth;** let stand with seasonings.

Curry with lentils or split peas: Omit rice; cook **1 cup lentils or split peas in 3 cups water or broth** until consistency of purée; add oil, onions, seasonings, **1 or 2 cups any diced leftover meat, 1 minced clove garlic.** Serve as soon as onions have simmered 10 minutes or let stand.

Imitation chutney: Prepare by mixing **1 cup canned mincemeat, 2 finely chopped raw apples, 2 tablespoons each vinegar and chopped green pepper and onion, dash of cayenne.** Serve without heating.

HAWAIIAN CHICKEN

Combine in cooking utensil:

1 or 2 disjointed stewing chickens or 1 or 2 packages each frozen breasts and thighs	½ cup soy sauce juice from 1 can chunk pineapple 1 cup water or more

Simmer until meat is just tender, being careful not to overcook; add:

2 or 3 tablespoons finely chopped preserved ginger	1 cup chunk pineapple

Taste for salt. If time permits, let stand 2 hours or longer; or serve at once in a bed of rice. Simmer no more than a few minutes after preserved ginger has been added.

At the table pass dishes of sliced almonds and roasted coconut flakes to be sprinkled over chicken.

VARIATIONS:

Instead of preserved ginger cook 1 or 2 small pieces of fresh ginger root with chicken.

Marinate chicken overnight in soy sauce and pineapple juice; lift chicken from marinade, place on broiler rack over aluminum foil, brush with vegetable oil, and sprinkle with paprika; broil under low heat until tender and golden brown. Heat pineapple and ginger in marinade; sprinkle pineapple over chicken and serve hot in marinade as sauce. Or transfer broiled chicken to heat-resistant casserole, cover with marinade, add pineapple and ginger, and simmer for 10 minutes or bake at 300° F. for 20 minutes.

Instead of chicken heat diced leftover turkey, lamb, or veal with ginger, pineapple and juice, and ¼ cup soy sauce.

Chicken with currant jelly: Combine and heat ½ cup water, 1 glass or ¾ cup currant jelly, 1 tablespoon each Worcestershire and lemon juice, 1 teaspoon salt, ½ teaspoon allspice; add thickening of 2 tablespoons whole-wheat-pastry flour mixed with water; bring to a boil and drop in 1 or 2 packages frozen chicken breasts. Transfer to low baking dish, sprinkle with paprika and ground black peppercorns, and cook in oven at 375° F. for 1 hour, or until tender. Baste once or twice.

Eat the Superior Meats Most Often

The meats most important nutritionally are liver, kidney, brain, thymus (sweetbreads), and heart. The liver is the storage place, or the "savings bank," of the body. If there is an excess of protein, sugar, vitamins, and any mineral except calcium and phosphorus, part of the excess is held in the liver until it is needed. Vitamin C, the bioflavinoids, and the many B vitamins dissolve in water; since water is not stored in the body, they cannot be stored. If an excess is available, however, they are held in greater concentration in the liver juices than in other body fluids. Liver is, therefore, nutritionally the most outstanding meat which can be purchased.

Brain, which is one of the richest sources of the B vitamin cholin, and kidney rank close to liver in nutritive value. Pancreas, used in the production of insulin, is not sold on the retail market, but if obtainable after home slaughtering, it should be prepared by recipes given for liver or sweetbreads. The thymus, or sweetbread, is a gland in the chest of young animals.

The function of these meats in the living animal is to carry on vital life processes; therefore, they contain proteins of the most superior quality and larger quantities of many vitamins and minerals than do muscle meats. Although brain and kidney are not glands, these meats are collectively spoken of as glandular meats in contrast to muscle meats, which are cut from muscles into chops, steaks, and roasts.

The heart is a group of muscles and in flavor resembles other muscle meats. Since it must work continuously from the animal's birth to its death, the heart has an abundance of excellent protein and the B vitamins necessary to produce energy. Animals, like people, die quickly when their heart muscles are undersupplied with these nutrients. Heart is not a glandular meat, but it is grouped with these meats because of its nutritive value.

Since these superior meats are especially rich in the B vitamins, they should not be touched unnecessarily with water. If these meats are washed slowly or soaked, they also lose iron, copper, and other minerals.

The housewife who wishes to maintain maximum health in her family is wise to serve glandular meats at least once or twice a week. These meats are more economical than any other because they contain no bones or waste.

Although brains contain more cholesterol than does any other food, they are also extremely rich in lecithin, which aids the body in using cholesterol normally; for this reason, they have not been proved to be detrimental to persons suffering from coronary disease. Since brains are so frequently disliked, I have tried to work out recipes especially for those persons who sincerely wish to develop an enjoyment of them. If time permits, first freeze them in an ice tray, then slice or dice them; most women find them pleasanter to handle this way. They should be neither boiled nor parboiled unless the cooking water is to be used. The secret of making brains enjoyable to the uninitiated is to cook them to the internal temperature at which proteins become quite firm.

BRAINS IN SPANISH SAUCE

Pack 1 pound brains in ice tray and freeze; remove and dice into 1-inch cubes.

Blend well together:

2 tablespoons vegetable oil or partially hardened margarine

3 tablespoons whole-wheat-pastry flour

Add and stir well:

1 cup water and 2 or 3 beef bouillon cubes or
1 cup beef consommé
¼ cup each chopped onions and bell pepper or chili pepper

½ cup tomato purée or diced raw tomato
¼ teaspoon each basil, orégano, and cumin seeds
diced brains

Simmer 15 to 20 minutes, stirring occasionally. Salt to taste.

VARIATIONS:

Add ½ cup celery or 1 cup cooked or canned kidney beans or garbanzo beans.

Substitute 1 teaspoon chili powder for other seasonings or add with herbs.

BAKED BRAINS IN BACON RINGS

Select 1 pound veal, pork, lamb, or beef brains; remove membranes while holding under running water; dry on paper towels.

Make 6 bacon rings, overlapping ends of bacon strips and fastening each with a toothpick; place rings on oiled baking sheet; cut brains into 6 portions and drop into rings; brush with vegetable oil and sprinkle generously with paprika.

Bake in moderate oven at 350° F. for 20 minutes, or until bacon is crisp and brains are firm. Garnish with parsley or chopped chives.

VARIATION:

Broil under moderate heat about 15 minutes on each side.

CREAMED BRAINS

Select **1 pound veal, pork, lamb, or beef brains;** remove membranes while holding under running water; pack in ice tray, freeze, and cube later, or dry on paper towels and dice immediately into ¾-inch cubes. Prepare **2 cups medium cream sauce** (p. 135); when sauce is boiling, drop in brains; simmer until meat is firm, or about 15 minutes. Stir in:

2 tablespoons lemon juice or   **3 tablespoons chopped parsley**
sherry   **1 teaspoon salt**

Serve over whole-wheat toast.

VARIATIONS:

Use ½ pound cubed brains; add to creamed sweetbreads, creamed ham, tuna, chicken, shrimp, fish, or other creamed meats. If it is desirable to disguise brains, this is a way to do it.

Prepare brains as in basic recipe, using any cream sauce (pp. 135–138), such as cheese, caraway, curry, dill, egg, mock Hollandaise, mushroom, olive, or pimento.

Cook brains as in basic recipe, using any brown sauce (p. 136), well-seasoned leftover gravy, or tomato sauce (p. 140).

SAUTÉED BRAINS WITH LEMON SAUCE

Select **1 pound veal, pork, lamb, or beef brains;** remove membranes while holding under running water; dry on paper towels. If time permits, freeze in ice tray, remove and slice; or cut fresh brains into serving sizes. Dip in:

1 egg stirred with   **1 teaspoon salt**
2 tablespoons milk and

Roll in **wheat germ** or dredge with **sifted whole-wheat-bread crumbs** and sauté in a small amount of **vegetable oil** until golden brown on both sides, or about 20 minutes over moderate heat.

Put brains on platter and heat in same utensil **2 tablespoons each partially hardened margarine and capers** (optional); **¼ cup each lemon juice and chopped parsley.** Pour sauce over meat.

VARIATIONS:

Dip in batter (p. 158) and sauté as in basic recipe; or cut into half-size servings, dip in batter, and fry in deep fat at 260° F. until crust is a deep golden.

Mock oysters: Prepare brains as directed and cut into 1-inch cubes; dip in egg and crumbs or in batter (p. 158); sauté as in basic recipe or fry in deep fat at 300° F. Serve with tartar sauce.

With scrambled eggs: Cut brains into 1-inch cubes; sauté with or without wheat germ or crumbs until firm; add eggs and scramble.

With sour cream or yogurt: Dice brains into ¾-inch cubes and prepare as in basic recipe; when golden and well done, add 1 cup sour cream or yogurt, 1 teaspoon salt, 2 tablespoons each diced pimentos and chopped chives. If yogurt is used, do not heat above simmering.

With sautéed tomatoes: Prepare brains as in basic recipe, cutting into slices ½ inch thick; dip firm slices of tomatoes in egg and crumbs and sauté; serve brains over or between tomato slices. Vary by sautéing with eggplant slices (p. 341).

With vegetables: Cut brains in 1-inch cubes and sauté as in basic recipe; sauté with brains 1 each finely chopped onion, pimento, stalk celery; sprinkle with salt and freshly ground peppercorns.

BRAINS IN CASSEROLE

Select 1 pound veal, pork, lamb, or beef brains; remove all membranes while holding under running water; drain and cut into ½-inch cubes. Mix with brains:

2 cups medium cream sauce or leftover gravy	1 teaspoon salt
1 grated onion	¼ teaspoon freshly ground peppercorns
2 tablespoons ground parsley	1 cup cubed Cheddar cheese
¼ cup wheat germ	

Put brains and vegetables in a flat baking dish brushed with oil; sprinkle with wheat germ or whole-wheat-bread crumbs; bake at 350° F. for 35 minutes, or until the surface is golden brown.

VARIATIONS:

Add any diced leftover meat, such as chicken, ham, liver, lamb, tuna, shrimps, or fish.

Omit cheese; add 2 tablespoons lemon juice and 1 teaspoon grated lemon rind.

Brain croquettes: Instead of medium sauce use 1 cup thick cream sauce; add 1 teaspoon dill or caraway seeds; include cheese; combine all ingredients, form into croquettes, roll in sifted whole-wheat-bread crumbs, and sauté in vegetable oil or fry in deep oil at 260° F. until golden.

Brain loaf: Omit wheat-germ cream sauce; add 1 egg, ½ cup each fresh milk and whole-wheat cracker crumbs, ⅓ cup powdered milk, pinch of basil and thyme; chop onion and sauté lightly with 1 stalk chopped celery, 1 diced bell pepper or pimento; combine ingredients with salt, peppercorns, and parsley; use or omit cheese; form into loaf in flat baking dish; sprinkle generously with paprika. Bake as in basic recipe for 1 hour.

Peppers stuffed with brains: Prepare as brain loaf, omitting bell pepper from stuffing; use nippy Cheddar; fill peppers, sprinkle with paprika, and bake as in basic recipe for 45 minutes. Use brains prepared in this way for stuffing cucumbers, zucchini, tomatoes, or onion shells.

BRAIN SALAD

Select 1 pound veal, pork, lamb, or beef brains; remove all membranes while holding under running water; put into utensil with tight-fitting lid and add:

2 to 4 tablespoons water	1 tablespoon vinegar

Simmer 20 minutes, or until texture is firm. Chill, dice fine, and add:

¼ to ¾ cup French dressing	¾ teaspoon salt
4 tablespoons chopped parsley	

Stir well; retain any moisture left from steaming; let brains chill in moisture and French dressing ½ hour or longer. Add:

1 or 2 diced hard-cooked eggs	2 diced pimentos
1½ cups diced celery	2 tablespoons or more mayonnaise

Combine and serve on lettuce or watercress. Brains prepared in this manner are usually assumed to be hard-cooked eggs.

VARIATIONS:

Cut steamed brains into fingers like shoestring potatoes; after marinating in French dressing, add to tossed salad or any vegetable salad.

Add with parsley one or more of the following: 1 grated onion or chopped leek; 1 finely diced pimento or green pepper; 1 or 2 teaspoons dill or caraway seeds or dill sauce; ¼ to 1 teaspoon curry powder; freshly ground horseradish or dry or prepared mustard; 2 tablespoons chives; 1 minced clove garlic. Use these seasonings when it is desirable to disguise flavor of brains.

Brain sandwich spread: Use ½ pound brains; steam and dice fine; decrease celery to 3 tablespoons finely diced; use mayonnaise or French dressing; add any seasonings suggested under variations; use for sandwich spread on rye bread.

Brain sausage: Steam as in basic recipe; pass through meat grinder; omit seasonings except salt; add **fresh or dried sage, freshly ground black peppercorns, ¼ cup each wheat germ and powdered milk**; mold into patties, dredge with **whole-wheat flour**, and fry until golden brown. Add brains prepared in this manner to meat loaf, hamburgers, pork sausage, or other foods.

Brains with sour cream or yogurt: Prepare and season as in basic recipe; stir into **1 or 2 cups sour cream or thick yogurt**; garnish with **parsley and paprika;** serve chilled for buffet. Vary by omitting seasonings of basic recipe and fold into any sour-cream or yogurt sauce (pp. 143–144), such as dill, caper, onion, or curry.

Kidneys Can Be Delicious

Few recipes need revising as much as do the old recipes for preparing kidneys. Generally the recipes were written without a knowledge of anatomy or physiology. Around the outer layer, or cortex, of a kidney are several million tiny knots of capillaries. The walls of these capillaries in a single kidney, if laid flat, are estimated to cover more than a square mile. Through this tremendous surface the force of the blood pressure pushes blood plasma chemically identical to the juices of meats universally considered delicious. The blood plasma flows through tiny tubes surrounding the knots of capillaries into connective tissue, which is white. It is only when the plasma reaches this white tissue that it takes on the composition of urine. In preparing kidneys, therefore, let no water touch them until the white tissue is snipped away with the kitchen scissors.

When kidneys are cooked at too high temperature or over-cooked, the odor of ammonia can be detected. Since ammonia occurs in urine, an untrained person assumes that the odor of improperly cooked kidney proves that the meat is saturated with urine. All proteins and the products into which used proteins are changed contain nitrogen. Much nitrogen is converted by enzymes in the kidney into ammonia, which readily dissolves in water; in this way nitrogen no longer needed by the body can be thrown off. Heat accelerates enzyme action, or the production of ammonia, and also causes ammonia to evaporate. Although this odor does not indicate that urine is in the kidney tissues, a little vinegar should be added to neutralize the ammonia. When kidneys are cooked only a short time, no odor of ammonia can be detected. If a delightful flavor free from all ammonia is to be achieved, kidneys should be cooked so quickly that the internal temperature of even tiny pieces of meat does not exceed 150° F. The main reason powdered milk is used in the following recipes is because it speeds browning.

In preparing any recipe in which kidneys are to be cooked in a sauce, it is important that the sauce be sufficiently thick to take up the juices squeezed from the meat as it cooks. If more thickening must be added, the meat either overcooks or a raw-flour taste lingers in the sauce.

SAUTÉED KIDNEYS

Cut 1 beef or 2 veal or pork kidneys into ½-inch slices; snip out all white tissue with scissors; brush surfaces with **vinegar;** fasten together into serving-size rings with toothpicks; dredge with **wheat germ or whole-wheat-pastry flour** and sear in **vegetable oil** 2 or 3 minutes on each side. Season with **salt and freshly ground peppercorns.**

Serve plain or with herb butter (p. 142) or creole sauce (pp. 140, 141).

VARIATIONS:

Marinate sliced kidneys in French dressing or vinegar and soy sauce for several hours before sautéing.

Mix together 1 egg, 2 tablespoons each powdered milk and fresh milk, 1 teaspoon salt, and 2 teaspoons minced fresh dill or dill seeds; dip kidney slices in egg mixture and then in wheat germ or sifted whole-wheat-bread crumbs; sauté as in basic recipe.

KIDNEY CREOLE

Cut lengthwise 1 beef kidney, 2 pork or veal kidneys, or 4 lamb kidneys; remove all white tissue; dice into ¾-inch cubes and mix well with 2 teaspoons vinegar; put into a paper bag and shake with:

3 tablespoons wheat germ or   2 tablespoons powdered milk
whole-wheat-pastry flour

Sear kidneys about 3 minutes in vegetable oil; turn onto paper towel. Sauté 5 minutes in same utensil:

1 chopped onion   1 minced clove garlic
1 diced pimento or green pepper   1 chopped stalk celery with leaves

Add:

1 cup tomato purée or canned   ¼ teaspoon freshly ground pep-
tomatoes   percorns
1 teaspoon salt   pinch each of basil, savory, thyme

Simmer 10 minutes; add kidneys and reheat. Serve over steamed brown or converted rice.

VARIATIONS:

Season with ⅛ teaspoon each orégano and cumin seeds.

Kidney hash: Sauté with vegetables of basic recipe 1 finely diced carrot; omit tomatoes; prepare kidneys as directed and cut into ¼-inch cubes; when vegetables are tender, add kidneys, salt, pepper, 3 drops Tabasco; stir, heat 3 minutes, and serve.

KIDNEY PATTIES

Slice lengthwise 1 beef kidney, 2 pork or veal kidneys, or 4 lamb kidneys; remove all white tissue, chop in a chopping bowl until fine; add and mix well:

2 teaspoons vinegar

Sauté lightly in vegetable oil:

1 chopped onion or leek   1 minced clove garlic

Meanwhile add to kidneys:

¼ cup powdered milk	1 teaspoon salt
¼ cup wheat germ	1 egg
¼ cup fresh milk	4 drops Tabasco

Stir in sautéed onion and garlic. Drop onto hot grill brushed with vegetable oil, shaping with spoon into patties; brown quickly on both sides and serve.

VARIATIONS:

Instead of kidneys use chopped raw liver or brain.

Shred 1 potato and brown with high heat before adding onions and garlic; add to other ingredients with 2 teaspoons chopped fresh dill, dill seeds, or dill sauce; mix together thoroughly. Vary by omitting garlic and cooking 1 or 2 teaspoons caraway seeds with potato.

Omit onion and garlic and add 3 chopped fresh or canned pimentos or ½ cup lightly sautéed sliced mushrooms.

KIDNEYS WITH SOUR CREAM

Remove all white membrane from 1 beef, 2 veal or pork, or 4 lamb kidneys; cut into fingers ½ inch thick and mix with:

1 tablespoon vinegar

Shake kidney in paper bag with:

3 tablespoons whole-wheat-pastry flour or wheat germ	½ teaspoon paprika
	¼ teaspoon freshly ground black
2 tablespoons powdered milk	peppercorns
1 teaspoon salt	

Brown quickly in vegetable oil.
Stir in:

1 cup sour cream	1 small can mushrooms (optional)

Serve as soon as heated through.

VARIATIONS:

Omit sour cream and mushrooms; pour 1 cup cream sauce over browned kidneys; when sauce is hot, add ½ teaspoon each paprika and salt; simmer no longer than 3 minutes before serving. Vary by adding 1 cup cucumbers sliced paper thin.

Kidneys with onion: While kidneys are browning, cook with them 1 or 2 grated or shredded onions, ¼ crushed bay leaf; serve with or without sour cream.

Kidneys with tomato sauce: Omit sour cream and mushrooms; when kidneys have browned, add 1 cup tomato purée, ⅛ teaspoon basil, 5 drops Tabasco, salt, peppercorns. Vary by adding any tomato sauce (pp. 140–141).

FLAMING KIDNEYS IN BRANDY

Mix well in saucepan:

2 tablespoons vegetable oil, partially hardened margarine, or butter	3 tablespoons whole-wheat flour 1 teaspoon salt

When well blended, add:

¼ cup diced bell pepper ¼ cup chopped onion, preferably green with tops	1 cup mushrooms (optional) 1 cup water with 2 teaspoons instant chicken bouillon

While sauce simmers, remove white tissue and dice into ¾-inch cubes:

3 or 4 veal kidneys or	6 lamb kidneys

Five minutes before serving, stir kidneys into hot sauce. Center in a bed of rice on platter. Immediately before taking to table, pour ¼ cup cooking brandy over kidneys and light. Carry to table while flaming.

VARIATIONS:

Omit brandy; add 2 tablespoons sherry or white wine with kidneys 5 minutes before serving.

Add 1 clove garlic, crushed bay leaf, pinch each of basil and orégano.

Use beef bouillon or beef bouillon cubes with water instead of chicken bouillon.

Liver, the Nutritive King of Meats

Although most of the following recipes are for liver prepared in more unusual ways, I suspect the old stand-by for most of us is simply to sauté it with or without onions or bacon (p. 41). The important point is not to overcook it. Wheat germ browns quickly and adds a pleasant flavor when used for dredging. If care is taken that the oil does not become overheated, there are no grounds for the widespread belief that broiling liver is superior to sautéing it. Broiling usually dries out the meat more than sautéing does and seems more of a nuisance.

See roast liver (p. 46); braised (p. 55); broiled (p. 34).

LIVER AND ONIONS

Sauté 5 minutes in 1 tablespoon vegetable oil:

4 large chopped onions

Cut into ¾-inch cubes and add:

1 pound lamb, calf, or baby beef liver	2 tablespoons sherry or port wine
	1 teaspoon salt

Stir while cooking 2 to 4 minutes. Serve immediately.

VARIATIONS:

Instead of sautéing onions, pan-broil bacon, remove, drain off drippings, and sauté liver cubes dredged with wheat germ. Season with salt, freshly ground peppercorns, and pinch of basil or thyme. Crumble bacon over liver, stir, and serve.

Sauté with liver ½ cup each finely chopped bell pepper and celery; use or omit onions; season with ¼ teaspoon orégano or cumin seeds.

LIVER BAKED WITH WINE

Dredge 1 pound sliced liver in wheat germ and quickly brown on each side. Layer in oiled baking dish or casserole with:

3 or 4 thinly sliced onions	1 teaspoon salt
1 crumbled bay leaf	freshly ground peppercorns
½ teaspoon thyme	¼ cup dry red wine

Sprinkle generously with paprika, and bake at 350° F. for 15 to 20 minutes.

VARIATIONS:

Sauté gently without browning 3 or 4 strips bacon; remove, drain drippings, and brown liver; before baking, lay bacon over onions.

Omit thyme, bay leaf, and wine; add ½ cup juice from black cherries or ½ cup tomato purée and ½ teaspoon basil.

Add ¼ cup finely chopped celery and bell pepper or fresh chili pepper.

LIVER CASSEROLE WITH RICE

Cut ¾ pound baby beef, lamb, or veal liver into 1-inch cubes and shake in paper bag with:

3 tablespoons whole-wheat-pastry flour	1 tablespoon powdered milk

Brown in heat-resistant casserole in:

2 tablespoons vegetable oil

Sauté as liver is browning:

6 to 8 green onions with tops or	1 or 2 chopped onions or leeks

Beat or shake until smooth and pour over liver:

¼ cup powdered milk	1 cup fresh milk

Add and mix together:

1½ to 2 cups cooked brown or
converted rice
1 teaspoon salt

¼ to ½ teaspoon crushed black
peppercorns
pinch of savory, orégano, thyme

Simmer 10 to 12 minutes.

VARIATIONS:

Omit herbs and add ½ teaspoon or more curry powder.

Omit fresh and powdered milk; add 1 cup tomato purée or any tomato sauce (p. 140).

Use diced kidneys or brain instead of liver; brown kidneys no longer than 5 minutes.

Sauté with onions and liver 1 chopped stalk celery, red bell pepper, fresh pimento, or paprika, or green chili pepper.

Instead of rice use leftover spaghetti, macaroni, or noodles.

BAKED LIVER WITH SOUR CREAM

Cut 6 or 8 small pockets in sides of:

1 or 2 pounds unsliced baby beef, lamb, or veal liver

Place in each slit:

1-inch piece of bacon

bits of 1 minced clove garlic

Place in flat baking dish and put over top:

¼ cup French dressing or
1 cup sour cream

generous sprinkling of paprika

Insert meat thermometer in center of thickest portion; bake in moderate oven at 350° F. for 30 minutes, or until internal temperature is 150 to 160° F.

Serve hot.

LIVER WITH APPLES

Mix together well:

3 chopped unpeeled cooking apples   ¾ teaspoon salt
1 chopped large onion   freshly ground black peppercorns

Place in oiled baking dish:

1 pound sliced baby beef, pork, or veal liver

Cover liver slices with apple-onion mixture; top with:

4 slices bacon cut in half   generous sprinkling paprika

Add:

¼ cup hot water

Cook in moderate oven at 350° F. for 20 minutes.

VARIATIONS:

Instead of apples use 1½ cups shredded carrots; add ¼ crushed bay leaf, pinch of thyme, 3 tablespoons chopped parsley.

Liver with tomatoes: Omit apples; slice onions thin; season liver with salt and peppercorns, and cover with slices of beefsteak tomatoes; top with onion slices and bacon.

LIVER STEW

Cut 1 pound unsliced baby beef, lamb, or pork liver into 1-inch cubes; dredge by shaking in paper bag with whole-wheat-pastry flour; brown in hot vegetable oil and set aside on paper towel; sauté lightly in same utensil:

1 chopped onion   3 diced stalks celery
1 minced clove garlic   2 teaspoons salt
2 diced turnips and carrots   ¼ teaspoon crushed black pepper-
1 quartered unpeeled potato   corns

When vegetables start to become tender, add:

1 cup soup stock	2 tablespoons whole-wheat-pastry
pinch each of savory, rosemary,	flour shaken with
orégano	½ cup soup stock

Simmer 10 minutes, or until vegetables are tender; add and reheat liver.

Serve surrounded by brown or converted rice.

VARIATIONS:

Instead of soup stock, add tomato juice or purée; if sour, sweeten with 1 to 3 teaspoons dark molasses.

Add other vegetables, such as peas, corn, zucchini, or string beans.

When liver is to be ground, it should first be dredged in whole-wheat flour and sautéed to solidify the proteins; otherwise valuable juices may be lost when it is being passed through the meat grinder.

LIVER LOAF

Dredge 1 pound sliced lamb or baby beef liver in whole-wheat-pastry flour and sauté quickly on both sides in vegetable oil; put liver aside on paper towel.

Pass through meat grinder into utensil used for sautéing liver:

1 or 2 onions	1 clove garlic
1 stalk celery with leaves	1 chilled bell pepper or pimento

Cover utensil and sauté vegetables slowly for 8 minutes.

Meanwhile grind liver and add to vegetables with:

pinch each of marjoram or basil	¼ teaspoon crushed black pepper-
¼ cup each wheat germ and pow-	corns
dered milk	1 egg
1½ teaspoons salt	¼ cup tomato catsup

Mix thoroughly; put into a loaf pan brushed with vegetable oil; bake in a moderate oven at 350° F. for about 40 minutes; insert meat thermometer when nearly done; cook to internal temperature of 185° F.

VARIATIONS:

Use ground liver instead of beef or with beef in any meat loaf (pp. 108–110).

Omit part of liver and use brain, pork sausage, ground heart, leftover meats, or hamburger.

Liver paste: See page 228.

Stuffed peppers: Use half the basic recipe for stuffing bell peppers which have been steamed 10 minutes; bake at 350° F. for 15 to 20 minutes; pour 1 or 2 cups tomato sauce (p. 140) over peppers when nearly done. Vary by using canned chili peppers; stuff, flatten, dip in beaten egg, and sauté until light brown.

Heart

Since heart is a muscle meat, its flavor is similar to that of meats used for steaks and roasts. Persons usually enjoy it the first time they eat it. Uncooked heart can be used instead of beef in any recipe in which the meat is sliced, diced, or ground.

CHICKEN-FRIED HEART

Use 1 to 1½ pounds young beef, pork, or veal heart; wash under running water, drain, and cut across the fibers into ¾-inch slices; dredge with wheat germ or whole-wheat flour, pound well with tenderer, and dredge again; form into compact serving sizes and hold together with toothpicks or skewers.

Brown well on both sides in vegetable oil; reduce heat and sauté slowly about 5 minutes. *Do not cover.*

Put heart on serving platter; make country gravy seasoned with pinch each of savory and marjoram.

VARIATIONS:

If gravy is not desired, mix ¼ teaspoon each savory and marjoram with the flour used for dredging.

If lamb or veal heart is used, cut into ½-inch slices and dredge without pounding; season gravy with minced clove garlic, ½ teaspoon dill seeds.

Broiled heart: Pound slices of pork or beef heart; sprinkle with **minced garlic and lemon juice;** wrap in wax paper and refrigerate overnight; place on baking sheet, brush with **vegetable oil,** and broil slowly 10 minutes on each side. If lamb or veal heart is used, broil without pounding.

HEART MEAT LOAF

Use **2 pounds beef, pork, veal, or lamb heart;** wash quickly, drain, and snip off tough membranes.

Put through the meat grinder:

1 onion, 2 leeks, or 6 green onions and tops	1 clove garlic several sprigs parsley

Heat vegetables 5 minutes in **2 tablespoons vegetable oil** and any juices extracted by grinding.

Meanwhile pass heart through meat grinder; add to vegetables:

ground heart	2 teaspoons salt
¼ to ½ teaspoon crushed black peppercorns	1 egg
	⅓ cup wheat germ
pinch each of marjoram and savory	⅓ cup powdered milk
	½ cup tomato purée

Mix ingredients thoroughly, preferably with fingertips; place in flat baking dish brushed with oil, form into a loaf, and bake in a moderate oven at 350° F. for 30 minutes; cover top with any **tomato sauce or condensed canned tomato soup;** insert meat thermometer and bake 10 minutes longer, or until internal temperature is 185° F. This is a delicious meat loaf.

VARIATIONS:

Spread one-third of meat-loaf ingredients ¾ inch thick on baking dish; cover with mound of crumb dressing (p. 129) or leftover mashed potatoes; spread remainder of meat mixture over top.

Use 1½ pounds ground heart, ½ pound pork sausage, ground left-over ham, or ground sautéed liver.

Use ground heart instead of beef in any meat loaf (pp. 108–110) or patties (pp. 111–112).

Heart with chili: Substitute ground heart for beef in making chili (p. 179) or use half heart, half kidney.

Heartburgers: Grind with heart ¼ pound beef suet, 1 onion, 1 clove garlic; make into patties and sauté or broil. If lamb hearts are used, mix 1 teaspoon dill seeds with meat.

Heart cutlets: Prepare half the basic recipe, using 1 egg; mold into cakes; roll in sifted whole-wheat-bread crumbs and sauté until golden brown.

Stuffed peppers: Use ground heart instead of beef in recipe on page 215.

HEART IN CASSEROLE

Purchase 1 veal or 4 lamb hearts; slice across the fibers; dredge with whole-wheat-pastry flour; brown in vegetable oil in heat-resistant casserole; when slices are well browned, add:

1½ cups soup stock or tomato juice	2½ teaspoons salt
2 tablespoons vinegar	½ teaspoon crushed black peppercorns
2 teaspoons dark molasses	

Cover casserole and simmer until heart is almost tender, or about 1¼ hours; add:

1 chopped onion	pinch each of basil and savory
1 minced clove garlic	3 tablespoons whole-wheat-pastry
1 chilled diced bell pepper	flour shaken with
¼ crushed bay leaf	½ cup soup stock or tomato juice

Stir well; cover casserole and simmer 15 minutes.

VARIATIONS:

If oven is in use, combine all ingredients, cover casserole, and steam heart until tender, or about 2½ hours at 350° F.

Add any diced fresh vegetables in time to become tender when heart is done or add leftover vegetables in time to reheat.

Heart pot roast: See page 65.

Heart stew: See page 71.

Heart with fruit: Prepare heart as directed, using soup stock or vegetable-cooking water; omit herbs; add in time to become tender ¼ **pound dried apricots or prunes or thick rings of unpeeled apple.**

One of the easiest ways to include heart in your menus is to cook it in soup or soup stock each time you make either. Although some of the flavor of the meat is lost, the soup gains in flavor. Unless part of the heart is to be eaten in the soup, it should be cooked until it is barely tender and the cooking completed as it is reheated. The following recipes are designed to suggest ways of serving heart cooked in soup stock.

SAUTÉED HEART

Cut cooked heart across the fibers into ½-inch slices; form into compact serving sizes and hold together with toothpicks; dip in **egg stirred with ½ teaspoon salt, 2 tablespoons milk,** then in **wheat germ or sifted whole-wheat-bread crumbs.**

Meanwhile sauté lightly in **vegetable oil:**

2 **chopped onions**
1 **minced clove garlic**
pinch each of thyme and basil

dash of freshly ground peppercorns

Push onions to one side; brown heart well on both sides. Serve immediately.

VARIATIONS:

Cut heart into fingers ½-inch thick; moisten with milk, shake with flour, and brown; add salt, paprika, ½ to 1 cup sour cream.

Use or omit egg and crumbs; heat 1 or 2 cups any tomato sauce (p. 140) or cream sauce (pp. 135–138); slice or dice heart and reheat in sauce or serve with sauce over meat. Add mushrooms if desired.

Broiled heart: Cut cooked heart into ½-inch slices; hold in serving sizes with toothpicks; brush with **vegetable oil,** sprinkle generously with **paprika;** broil on oiled baking sheet until heated through. Vary by marinating overnight with **minced garlic and mixed herbs** or by sprinkling with **chopped chives** before serving.

Creamed heart: Prepare 2 cups any **cream sauce or brown sauce** (pp. 135–136), or reheat **leftover gravy;** dice cooked heart or cut into fingers and add to sauce in time to reheat before serving.

Heart pie: Follow directions for kidney pie (p. 71), substituting cooked heart for beef or kidneys.

Heart with apples and prunes: Sauté in vegetable oil 2 finely diced unpeeled apples; add 12 chopped cooked prunes, ½ teaspoon grated lemon rind. Slice cooked heart ¼ inch thick and reheat over fruit. Serve with fruit sandwiched between heart slices. Pork heart is especially delicious prepared in this way.

Heart with raisin sauce: Stir 1½ tablespoons whole-wheat-pastry flour into 1 tablespoon melted, partially hardened margarine or butter; add 1 cup steamed raisins and juice, 1 or 2 tablespoons dark molasses, 3 tablespoons lemon juice; reheat heart in sauce; serve sauce between and over heart slices.

Stuffed heart: See page 54.

Sweetbreads

Most cookbooks direct one to parboil sweetbreads, a procedure which invariably leaves them dry and which seems to me similar to boiling a steak before broiling it. If one wishes to add sweetbreads to salads or appetizers, they may be gently steamed on a rack for 15 minutes, but they should not be touched with water. The tiny amounts of connective tissue they contain when raw disappear almost completely by the time they are cooked.

Although sweetbreads are usually thought of as an expensive delicacy, they are one of the cheapest meats sold. They contain almost no fat and no bone or waste, and are excellent both when the budget is limited and for persons on low-fat diets. Since their flavor is so mild, they are particularly delicious when cooked with bacon or ham. When rolled in wheat germ, flour, or crumbs and sautéed, they are like chicken breasts without the bones.

BAKED SWEETBREADS

Pull 1 pound uncooked sweetbreads into bite sizes or dice into 1-inch cubes. Combine in heat-resistant casserole with:

2 tablespoons vegetable oil	1 crumbled bay leaf
½ cup each chopped onion and finely diced carrot	½ teaspoon each thyme and salt
1 minced clove garlic	1 cup soup stock or water and 2 chicken bouillon cubes

Cover casserole and bake at 350° F. for 30 minutes. Garnish with parsley.

VARIATIONS:

Add ¼ cup each chopped celery and bell pepper. Or omit onion and add 1 or 2 cups fresh mushrooms and/or ¼ cup diced pimento.

Bake with sweetbreads ½ to 1 cup diced leftover ham, veal, lamb, chicken, or turkey.

Heat ½ to 1½ cups leftover gravy. Add sweetbreads and seasonings. Add 2 tablespoons sherry or dry white wine.

Sweetbreads in bacon rings: Sauté **6 slices bacon** slowly without browning until most of the fat is rendered out; form bacon into rings, fasten with hardwood toothpicks, and set on baking sheet; fill centers with uncooked sweetbreads; brush surface of sweetbreads with **vegetable oil,** sprinkle with **paprika;** bake at 350° F. for 20 minutes or until bacon is crisp. **Salt.**

BROILED SWEETBREADS

Cut **1 pound raw sweetbreads** into 1-inch cubes or pull into small chunks; roll in:

1 egg beaten with   **wheat germ**
2 tablespoons milk or white wine

Alternate on skewers with:

1½-inch pieces raw or partially   **large mushroom caps**
sautéed bacon   **1-inch squares bell pepper**

Brush with **vegetable oil,** sprinkle generously with **paprika,** set on rack, and broil slowly 10 minutes; turn and broil 6 minutes longer. **Salt** and serve.

VARIATIONS:

Leave sweetbreads uncut; brush with oil, sprinkle with paprika, and broil to an internal temperature of 160° F. Serve with caraway, caper, dill, or Mornay sauce.

CREAMED SWEETBREADS

Melt in a saucepan:

> 2 tablespoons partially hardened margarine or butter

Add and stir well:

> 3 tablespoons whole-wheat-pastry flour

When well blended, add:

1 cup fresh or reconstituted milk   1 teaspoon salt
generous sprinkling paprika   1 or 2 teaspoons Worcestershire

Stir and heat to boiling. Meanwhile pull or cut sweetbreads into 1-
to 2-inch pieces, removing bits of fat and thicker membrane. Add to
sauce:

1 pound sweetbreads   1 or 2 cups fresh whole mush-
        rooms (optional)

Simmer 20 minutes. Serve on whole-wheat toast.

VARIATIONS:

Add ½ to 1 cup fresh or frozen peas, fresh baby lima beans, or finely
diced celery, bell pepper, or carrot; or 2 tablespoons diced canned pimento or grated onion.

Season with ¼ teaspoon tarragon, basil, thyme, sage, or rosemary.

Instead of sauce and mushrooms, simmer sweetbreads in 1 can
condensed mushroom soup; add Worcestershire, pinch of thyme, 1 or 2
tablespoons each diced pimento and finely chopped parsley. Taste for
salt.

Add 1 or 2 chicken or beef bouillon cubes or 1 or 2 teaspoons instant chicken or beef broth.

See Sweetbreads Newburg, page 167.

SAUTÉED SWEETBREADS

Cut 1 **pound sweetbreads** into serving sizes; hold small pieces together with hardwood toothpicks. Roll in:

wheat germ

Sauté in:

2 or 3 tablespoons vegetable oil, partially hardened margarine, or butter

Keep heat moderate. Turn sweetbreads until golden on all sides, cooking 15 to 20 minutes; sprinkle with:

freshly ground peppercorns　　　**paprika**
¾ teaspoon salt

Serve alone or on toasted whole-wheat bread over a thin slice of ham. If desired, cover with Mornay sauce (p. 137) and garnish with parsley.

VARIATIONS:

Remove browned sweetbreads and keep hot; prepare country gravy seasoned with ¼ teaspoon sage; add 2 teaspoons instant chicken broth or 2 chicken bouillon cubes. Serve gravy over sweetbreads.

Instead of wheat germ, roll in whole-wheat flour or beaten egg and sifted whole-wheat-bread crumbs, or dip in batter (p. 158) before sautéing.

If time permits, pack sweetbreads into a deep square refrigerator dish; freeze; turn out, cut into ½-inch slices, and sauté as in basic recipe.

Sauté with sweetbreads ½ to 1 cup fresh mushrooms, chopped onions, bell pepper, or celery.

Braised sweetbreads: Brown in heat-resistant casserole; add **1 cup leftover chicken gravy** or make sauce of **1 cup water, 1 or 2 teaspoons instant chicken broth, 3 tablespoons whole-wheat flour** mixed with **¼ cup water;** season with ¼ teaspoon each tarragon and basil; simmer 10 to 15 minutes or bake at 350° F. for 20 minutes.

Sweetbreads sautéed with ham: Cut sweetbreads into 1-inch cubes; sauté quickly; add **1 bell pepper** cut into thin strips, **½ to 1 cup diced leftover ham, 1 cup fresh or reconstituted milk, ½ teaspoon salt.** Simmer 10 minutes; add **2 tablespoons dry sherry** (optional). Serve over toast. Vary by simmering 1 teaspoon mashed caraway or dill seeds with sweetbreads.

Marinated Meats

Almost an endless variety of flavors can be obtained by marinating meats, or by soaking them 2 hours or longer in white or red wine, French dressing, or some highly seasoned liquid. For the seasoning actually to penetrate, the meat should be no more than ½ an inch thick, and preferably pounded with a cleat hammer or put through a butcher's tenderizer.

The meat may be merely scored (p. 62), however, and a seasoned ¼ inch of all outer surfaces can give a delightful flavor to the whole. For these reasons, almost any meat which cooks in a short time can be marinated. French dressing and any marinade containing salt or soy sauce draws the juices from the meat, leaving it dry. The marinade can be heated and served with the meat as a sauce.

Use each of the following marinades, if you wish to, then originate your own, using your favorite seasonings with whatever juices or wines you have on hand.

SEASONED MARINADE

Combine in a deep glass or pottery bowl:

1 cup tomato juice, sauce, or purée or	1 large shredded onion
½ cup each tomato juice and red wine	2 tablespoons Worcestershire
	¼ teaspoon freshly ground black peppercorns
1 minced clove garlic	generous dash of cayenne
½ teaspoon each marjoram and thyme	2 tablespoons chopped parsley

Cut meat into serving sizes, put into marinade, and soak 2 or 3 hours or refrigerate overnight.

SWEET MARINADE

Combine in a deep pottery or glass bowl:

1 cup juice from canned pineapple, peaches, black cherries, or other fruit; or frozen, diluted orange juice or ½ cup each fruit juice and sherry	1 tablespoon vinegar or lemon juice 2 tablespoons Worcestershire ½ teaspoon rosemary or basil 1 minced clove garlic

Cut meat into serving sizes, put into marinade, and soak 2 or 3 hours or refrigerate overnight.

VARIATIONS:

Add to seasoned or sweet marinade 1 chopped stalk celery, ½ bell pepper, green onions with tops, or several sprigs parsley.

Vary marinades by using ½ teaspoon savory, orégano, tarragon, or other herbs; powdered ginger or turmeric; or crushed dill, caraway, or coriander seeds.

MARINATED FLANK STEAK

Pound with a cleat hammer, or ask butcher to run through tenderizer, cutting *across* the meat fibers:

1 to 2 pounds flank steak

Cut into serving sizes, and marinate 2 to 3 hours at room temperature or refrigerate overnight. Drain, brush with **vegetable oil,** sprinkle generously with **paprika,** and broil under low heat 10 minutes on both sides. **Salt.**

Heat marinade and serve with meat as a sauce.

VARIATIONS:

Instead of broiling, sauté with a small amount of vegetable oil.

Instead of flank steak, use pounded, tenderized, or scored round steak, ham, liver, veal, or lamb steaks, broiling chicken, or any meat which will cook in 30 minutes or less.

If marinade is not served as a sauce, freeze and re-use; or use to season Swiss steak, pot roast, beef or chicken stew, or any meat gravy.

Marinated ham with orange rind: Use **ham steak ¾ inch thick;** score and marinate in **1 cup pineapple juice** to which is added **shredded rind of 1 orange.** Bake in sauce at 300° F. for 20 minutes, or to an internal temperature of 160° F. Immediately before serving, sprinkle lightly with **dry mustard.** Or use broiling chicken cut in serving sizes.

Skewer cooking, which breaks the monotony of more prosaic cooking, can be both novel and fun. It is especially nice for guest dinners. Since the meat is cut into small pieces, the seasonings in the marinade penetrate well.

Almost any fruits or vegetables can be combined with meat in skewer cooking, provided the cooking time is roughly the same. At first such cooking seems complicated, but after it is done once or twice, it is as easy as stringing beads. The inexpensive bamboo slivers (100 for 25 cents) work as well as the metal or miniature-saber skewers. When vegetables or fruits fall off during cooking, they are either cut into too small pieces or the meat is being overcooked.

If you wish to startle your friends, bring the skewers of broiled food to the table flaming. This trick is accomplished by preparing balls of cotton ¾ inch in diameter and dipping them into alcohol or lemon extract immediately before slipping them onto the ends of the skewers and lighting them.

SKEWERED BEEF

Pound with a cleat hammer or have butcher pass through tenderizer, cutting across the meat fibers:

1 pound flank steak

Cut meat into 1¼- by 2½-inch pieces. Marinate 2 hours or longer (pp. 100–101).

Fold or roll pieces of meat and alternate on skewers with:

small cherry tomatoes   **1½-inch squares bell pepper**
whole mushroom caps

Brush with **vegetable oil** and sprinkle generously with **paprika** on all sides. Broil under moderate heat for 10 minutes, turning once. Salt and serve immediately.

VARIATIONS:

Cut ½-inch wedges of sweet onion or unpeeled eggplant and use instead of mushrooms or with mushrooms, or use wedges of solid beefsteak tomatoes.

Dip mushroom caps and pieces of pepper into oil before broiling.

Sauté without covering in small amount of oil or cook on an outdoor barbecue; or bake in hot oven at 425° F. for 8 minutes.

Instead of beef, roll shrimp in wheat germ or wrap oysters in partially sautéed bacon and alternate with tomatoes and mushrooms; or use marinated veal or lamb, cubes of top sirloin, or other tender meat.

Shish kebab: Marinate **lamb shoulder or leg** cut into 1½-inch cubes; alternate on skewers with **eggplant, onion, and tomato wedges.**

Skewered meat with fruit: Alternate marinated **flank steak, veal, or lamb** with 1½-inch pieces firm banana, ⅓ slices canned pineapple, wedges of raw apple, or canned cling peaches cut in half.

Ways of Making Inexpensive Meats Interesting

For value purchased, the least expensive meats are the glandular ones. Meats discussed in the following group are inexpensive because little or no waste need be purchased. Dried meat is economical by virtue of its protein concentration. Luncheon meats and wieners, which contain far too many preservatives to be recommended wholeheartedly, usually do contain soy flour as a binder, which offers two to three times more protein than does meat itself. I include recipes for these meats only because I feel they will be used regardless of the possible detrimental effect of the chemicals they contain. Contrary to popular belief, however, they are not made from poor quality meat but from meat which is as carefully inspected as are the prime cuts of highest quality.

Since sealed dried beef keeps indefinitely, it may be kept on the emergency shelf and used when dinners must be quickly prepared. Chipped beef sold in bulk or plastic packages contains so much preservative that it cannot be recommended. If you wish to serve chipped beef, buy the kind that comes in jars.

CREAMED CHIPPED BEEF

Heat:

> 1 cup fresh milk or reconstituted milk

Add:

1 jar (7 ounces) chipped beef	freshly ground black peppercorns
1 teaspoon Worcestershire	generous sprinkling paprika

Soak beef 10 minutes if particularly dry.
Add thickening of:

2 tablespoons whole-wheat-pastry flour mixed with	¼ cup top milk

Stir thoroughly; simmer 10 to 12 minutes and serve on buttered toast; garnish with parsley.

VARIATIONS:

Season beef with ½ teaspoon crushed dill or caraway seeds or add ¼ cup diced American cheese a few minutes before serving.

Cook with beef 1 cup fresh or frozen peas or finely diced carrots or ½ cup mushrooms or chopped celery; or add 1 tablespoon grated onion, diced pimento, or chopped parsley.

DRIED-BEEF CURRY

Heat to simmering:

> 2 cups leftover country gravy or any brown sauce (p. 136)

Use 1 jar (7 oz.) beef; cut or tear into bite-size pieces. Add to sauce and stir well:

dried beef	2 teaspoons coriander seeds
½ to 2 teaspoons curry powder	⅓ cup crushed pineapple

When heated thoroughly, serve on whole-wheat toast or with converted rice.

VARIATIONS:

Omit gravy or sauce and seasonings and add dried beef to any tomato sauce (pp. 140–141).

Use lamb, chicken, veal, or any leftover meat instead of dried beef or with dried beef.

Omit curry and seasonings; heat dried beef in dill, caraway, celery, horseradish, or other seasoned cream sauce (pp. 136–138).

Sautéed dried beef: Sauté beef in vegetable oil 2 or 3 minutes; serve with eggs as substitute for bacon.

Of all the luncheon meats available, liver sausage offers the greatest nutritive value. It is excellent to keep on hand for box lunches and spur-of-the-moment dinners.

LIVER-SAUSAGE CRISPS

Cut liver sausage into ½-inch slices; dip in:

egg stirred with 2 tablespoons fresh milk	wheat germ or whole-wheat-bread or cracker crumbs

Sauté quickly in **vegetable oil** until brown on both sides.

Put slice of **raw leek or sweet onion and 1 ring of red bell pepper** on each slice of sausage; sprinkle lightly with **salt.**

VARIATIONS:

Sprinkle sliced liver sausage generously with paprika and broil on an oiled baking sheet; use low heat. Serve with pickle relish or barbecue sauce (p. 140).

Instead of liver sausage, use bologna, luncheon loaf, or other luncheon meat.

Wieners are cooked before being sold and need no further cooking; yet they are almost invariably cooked too long and at too high a temperature. They should be reheated only at low temperature and usually not longer than 5 minutes. Unless they are dipped in batter, attempts to brown them cause them to curl, shrivel, toughen, and lose flavor. When they are to be served alone, heat them by steaming over water or in the oven on aluminum foil.

SPANISH WIENERS

Prepare **2 cups Spanish sauce** (p. 141); let simmer 10 minutes.

Meanwhile hold **1 pound wieners** together and slice all at one time into ½-inch pieces; drop wieners into hot sauce, stir well, cover utensil, and let heat 5 minutes.

Serve at once.

VARIATIONS:

Instead of Spanish sauce use any tomato sauce (pp. 140–141).

French-fried wieners: Prepare **batter** (p. 158); dip whole or sliced skinless wieners in batter and fry in deep **vegetable oil** at 360° F. for 1 to 3 minutes, or until golden brown.

Paprika wieners: Prepare **2 cups medium cream sauce** (p. 135); add **1 pound wieners** cut into ½-inch pieces, **2 tablespoons chopped parsley, onions, or chives, ½ to 1 teaspoon paprika;** stir well, cover utensil, and let stand 5 minutes. Vary by adding wieners to any cream sauce or brown sauce (pp. 135–138) or to leftover gravy.

Stuffed wieners: Split wieners lengthwise and put on baking dish over aluminum foil; fill with **preheated moist bread stuffing** (p. 129); wrap each wiener with **bacon** and fasten with toothpicks; bake until bacon is well browned.

Wieners with barbecue sauce: Use long slender wieners, 2 for each person; cut a slit lengthwise in each wiener, open slightly, and arrange in low rectangular baking dish; pour **1 cup barbecue sauce** (p. 140) into slits; heat in moderate oven 10 minutes. Vary by serving with any **tomato sauce** (p. 140).

Wieners in blankets: Follow recipe for beef in blankets (p. 107); serve with sauce made of **2 teaspoons dry mustard** mixed with **2 tablespoons each yogurt and freshly ground horseradish.**

Wieners with cheese: Split wieners lengthwise, set on pan over aluminum foil; fill with **strip of Cheddar cheese;** bake in slow oven until cheese melts.

Wieners with eggs: Allow 2 wieners for each serving; pan-broil on grill 1 minute on each side, using high heat to make wieners curl into semicircles. Lower heat, arrange 2 wieners to form a circle, and drop **1 or 2 eggs** into each; add **1 tablespoon water;** cover utensil and steam slowly 12 minutes; sprinkle with **freshly ground black peppercorns, salt and chives.**

Wieners with cabbage: Follow any recipe for cooking **green or purple**

cabbage (pp. 367–369); heat wieners over cabbage 5 minutes before serving.

Wieners with omelet or scrambled eggs: Slice ½ pound of wieners into ½-inch pieces; add to omelet (pp. 244–246) or **scrambled eggs (p. 237).**

Wieners with sauerkraut: Mix 2 to 4 teaspoons caraway seeds with 1 quart sauerkraut; cook without added moisture; 5 minutes before serving, put wieners on top and heat through.

Wieners with sour cream: Heat 1½ cups sour cream over direct heat in serving casserole; add 1 tablespoon ground horseradish, ¼ teaspoon salt, 1 pound wieners cut into ½-inch pieces. Serve as soon as wieners are heated through. Vary by adding seasonings suggested for sour-cream sauces (pp. 143–144).

Ground meats spoil readily, because of the large amount of surface exposed to bacteria. They should not be kept longer than a day unless at a temperature of 40° F. or lower.

Ground meat in blankets is an adaptation of *piroshki,* or Russian meat pies. They take only a few minutes to make and are sufficiently like our pigs in blankets to be enjoyed readily by Americans. If a high-protein dough is used, these meat pies are nutritionally excellent, especially for children whose calorie needs are high.

GROUND BEEF IN BLANKETS

Grate and sauté in **1 tablespoon vegetable oil:**

1 or 2 onions   1 clove garlic

Cook slowly until onions are transparent; add:

½ pound (1 cup tightly packed)   ⅛ teaspoon thyme
    ground lean beef   generous sprinkling ground black
1 tablespoon catsup   peppercorns
1 teaspoon salt

Allow meat merely to heat through. Meanwhile roll **wheat-germ pie dough** (p. 509), **biscuit dough** (p. 424), or **any yeast dough** (p. 408) ⅙ inch thick; cut into 4-inch squares; put 2 tablespoons ground meat in center of each piece of dough.

Moisten edges of dough with back of wet spoon and pinch together like an apple turnover. If yeast dough is used, let rise a few minutes.

Brush utensil used for heating onions lightly with **vegetable oil**; sauté meat pies slowly; turn and brown the other side, cooking about 10 minutes on each side; serve piping hot; eat with fingers or cover with gravy or meat sauce.

V A R I A T I O N S :

Season ground meat with a pinch of basil, savory, marjoram, or orégano or with other herbs or crushed seeds.

Instead of ground beef use any leftover meat, supplemented with chopped hard-cooked eggs if needed.

Made dough from nutritious mix (p. 428).

Instead of beef use ground lamb or veal; season veal with basil and lamb with 2 tablespoons capers or 1 teaspoon dill seeds.

Set meat in blankets on greased baking sheet; bake 10 minutes or until brown.

Chicken in blankets: Instead of beef, use **leftover chicken** which has been finely chopped or creamed; serve with chicken gravy.

The secret of having a meat loaf hold together and slice well is to cook it to the internal temperature at which egg, the binder, becomes tough. Insert the meat thermometer into the center of the thickest portion when the loaf is nearly done.

M E A T   L O A F

Crumble:

2 slices whole-wheat bread into	½ cup fresh milk

When moist, add and mix well:

1 egg	½ pound pork sausage
1 or 2 shredded onions	1½ teaspoons salt
1 minced clove garlic	2 tablespoons chopped parsley
¼ cup wheat germ	¼ teaspoon each basil and freshly
1½ pounds lean ground beef	ground peppercorns

Mix thoroughly, preferably with fingertips; mold into a loaf in a shallow baking dish or pack into a greased loaf pan; sprinkle generously with paprika; bake in a moderate oven at 350° F. about 1 hour, or until temperature in center is 185° F.; insert thermometer when loaf is nearly done.

VARIATIONS:

Bake in greased ring mold dusted with wheat germ or sifted crumbs; turn onto platter and fill center with creamed peas, carrots, or onions.

Add ¼ to ½ cup powdered milk or instant tiger's milk (p. 447) and 3 tablespoons tomato catsup.

Instead of milk, use ¾ cup concentrated mushroom or tomato soup; decrease salt to ¾ teaspoon.

Add 2 slices or more of quickly sautéed ground liver; ground left-over chicken, ham, beef, turkey, or other meat; or use half beef and half ground lamb, veal, or beef heart.

Season with savory, sage, tarragon, marjoram, rosemary, or green onions and tops.

Omit pork and use 2 pounds ground beef. Just before putting in oven, place 4 strips of bacon over top.

Add one or more of the following: ½ cup finely chopped celery, bell pepper, shredded raw carrot, fresh or frozen peas; 2 tablespoons catsup or chili sauce; 1 tablespoon Worcestershire or dry mustard; ¼ cup soy flour, rice polish, or soy grits; add 2 tablespoons brewers' yeast if catsup or chili sauce is used.

Add not more than 1 cup leftover peas, string beans, diced carrots, or other leftover vegetables.

Pour over meat loaf 15 minutes before removing from oven 1 or 2 cups tomato sauce (p. 140), leftover gravy, or can of condensed tomato soup.

Double recipe and serve part of the loaf chilled with caper, dill, or other sauce with sour-cream or yogurt base (p. 143).

Instead of fresh milk add ½ cup tomato sauce, drained canned tomatoes, leftover gravy, sour cream, catsup, or chili sauce.

Fish loaf: See page 168.

Ham loaf: Use equal parts of beef and ground ham or cured shoulder, either leftover of fresh; decrease salt to ½ teaspoon; season with savory or 2 teaspoons caraway seeds; when almost baked, pour ½ cup spiced peach juice or sweet pickle juice over top.

Italian meat loaf: Add ¼ cup chopped or ground celery and leaves, ⅛ teaspoon celery salt, dash of nutmeg, ½ cup Parmesan cheese.

Lamb loaf: Use **ground lamb breast** instead of beef; season as in basic recipe and add one of the following: 3 tablespoons chopped pimentos; 1 teaspoon dill seeds or 1 tablespoon dill sauce; 2 to 4 tablespoons capers.

Meat loaf of big game: Instead of beef use **ground venison, bear, moose,** or **buffalo meat;** if meat is gamy, use **catsup, chili sauce, tomatoes,** or **sour cream** instead of milk; proceed as in basic recipe.

Meat loaf of heart: Use **ground beef, veal, pork,** or **lamb heart;** prepare and season as in basic recipe.

Mutton loaf: Choose **lean mutton** and grind with a small amount of suet, bacon, or salt pork; add ¼ teaspoon each marjoram and savory.

Pork loaf: Substitute **ground lean pork** for beef; omit the garlic and onions; sauté and add ½ cup each diced apples and celery, pinch of thyme, dash of nutmeg; proceed as in basic recipe.

Stuffed meat loaf: Place one-third of meat-loaf ingredients in baking dish; pat ¾ inch thick; cover with mound of **2 cups of any crumb, cereal, vegetable,** or **fruit stuffing** (pp. 129–133) or leftover macaroni, noodles, rice, or mashed potatoes; cover with remaining meat-loaf ingredients.

When the budget is limited, the question arises as to which is more economical, the seemingly inexpensive ground chuck containing much fat or ground stew meat or flank steak, which is low in fat but higher priced per pound. Hamburger meat invariably contains a third fat and is often half fat. If it is fed to the family, one runs the risk of producing coronary disease and other high-cholesterol illnesses. If it is browned, the high temperature may cause cancer-producing substances to be formed from overheated fat. If it is slowly cooked and the melted fat drained, probably a third of the purchase price is wasted and delicious juices containing vitamins and minerals are discarded.

Although each housewife must decide this issue for herself, it seems to me it is more economical, especially if one considers medical expense, to purchase lean ground meat and to rely more heavily on such inexpensive proteins as wheat germ, powdered milk, and soy flour to supplement the family nutrition.

GROUND-BEEF PATTIES

Pinch to bits:

Soak in:

2 slices whole-wheat bread

½ cup milk

Grate into milk and crumbs:

1 onion

Add and stir well:

1 pound (2 cups tightly packed) ground lean beef	freshly ground black peppercorns
1 teaspoon salt	pinch of sage, basil, savory
	⅓ cup wheat germ

Make into patties 1 inch thick, roll in **wheat germ or sifted whole-wheat-bread crumbs,** and brown both sides in **vegetable oil;** do not cover utensil at any time. Serve at internal temperature of 155 to 170° F.

VARIATIONS:

Instead of milk and bread crumbs use ½ cup each **cooked rice and tomato juice or purée;** add pinch of basil.

Instead of ground beef use **ground lamb or veal;** lean mutton ground with a little beef suet or bacon, seasoned with marjoram, savory, rosemary; or use any **ground wild game** seasoned with mixed herbs.

Sauté onion until transparent before adding to meat; vary by sautéing with onion 2 tablespoons chopped **bell pepper** and/or **celery.**

Ground beef broiled on toast: Prepare basic recipe or omit bread, milk, salt; spread ground meat ½ inch thick on hot toasted **whole-wheat or rye bread;** sprinkle generously with **wheat germ and paprika;** broil with slow heat until well browned, or about 10 minutes. Salt and serve topped with a thin slice of mild-flavored **onion.** Excellent for quick lunches.

Ground beef in pepper rings: Cut **bell peppers, fresh pimentos, chilis, or paprikas** into rings ¾ inch thick; dip in **vegetable oil** and place on baking sheet; pack meat patties firmly into pepper rings, sprinkle with **wheat germ and paprika;** broil under moderate heat 6 minutes on each side. Vary by using **onion rings** instead of peppers; pepper or onion should be crisp when served.

Ground-ham patties: Use **ground leftover ham** instead of beef; prepare as in basic recipe or substitute **rice and tomato purée** for bread and milk; serve with mustard and horseradish.

Ground-lamb or -veal patties: Substitute **lamb or veal** for beef in basic recipe; add **1 teaspoon dill seeds**; serve tomato gravy (p. 127) or tomato sauce (p. 140) over meat.

Heart patties: Use **ground beef, veal, pork, or lamb heart**; prepare as in basic recipe.

Meat balls: Make into round balls instead of patties; brown well, cover utensil, and let steam 8 to 12 minutes. Serve with macaroni, noodles, or spaghetti and Italian sauce (p. 140).

Select firm and thick-meated peppers for stuffing. Since fresh peppers are among the richest known sources of vitamin C, which can easily dissolve in cooking water, they should not be parboiled. But if they are baked to tenderness without first being steamed, the meat in the filling is invariably overcooked and flavor is lost. When prepared in the following manner, they are so delicious that I frequently serve them for guest dinners. The delectability can be further improved if they are stuffed in the morning and allowed to sit in the refrigerator several hours while the seasonings permeate the filling. Since the vitamin C content doubles with ripening, use red bell peppers whenever they are available.

STUFFED PEPPERS

Select **4 large red bell peppers** with firm flesh. Wash quickly, cut in half lengthwise, and remove seeds. Put on rack above boiling water and steam only until tender, or 10 to 15 minutes.

Meanwhile, mix thoroughly:

1 pound raw lean ground beef	freshly ground peppercorns
1 cup cooked rice	⅛ teaspoon each savory, basil, and
1 teaspoon salt	marjoram

Stuff peppers and set in baking pan. If time permits, put in refrigerator several hours to allow seasonings to penetrate filling. Sprinkle generously with **wheat germ and paprika**. Bake in oven at 350° F. for 20 minutes, or until internal temperature, taken by inserting meat thermometer momentarily, is 140 to 150° F. Be extremely careful not to overcook.

VARIATIONS:

Use whole green bell peppers when red ones are not available; pour 2 tablespoons undiluted canned tomato soup over each.

Home gardeners lucky enough to raise their own fresh pimento or paprika peppers may use either without cutting in half.

Instead of bell peppers use whole green chili peppers. Be careful to remove all seeds if mild flavor is desired. If hot chili taste is preferred, mix part or all of the seeds into filling.

Use raw ground flank, round steak, or heel of round mixed with diced leftover beef, pork, or chicken.

Add ½ teaspoon mashed caraway or dill seeds or other herbs rather than the ones suggested.

Instead of fresh beef use ground or finely diced leftover beef, turkey, chicken, ham, or lamb. Add 1 teaspoon dill seeds with lamb; use caraway seeds with ham; sage or thyme with chicken or turkey. Mix any leftover gravy with filling.

Fill steamed peppers with any hot creamed dish such as leftover macaroni and cheese, or creamed shrimp, oysters, chicken, or ham. Sprinkle with wheat germ, grated cheese, and paprika. If peppers are still warm, brown under broiler; otherwise heat in oven at 350° F. for 10 minutes.

When making meat loaf, prepare enough to stuff peppers; freeze until needed.

With little effort, pork sausage can be changed from a prosaic to an ever-varied and interesting dish. After making or buying sausage, add one or two seasonings; fry a small amount and taste it. Try different combinations, using any fresh or dried herbs, any member of the onion family, any sauces such as Tabasco or Worcestershire, or cumin, caraway, mustard, or celery seeds. Use seasoned pork sausage for lunches or dinners. Keep heat moderate and do not overcook.

SEASONED PORK SAUSAGE

Mix together thoroughly:

1½ pounds pork sausage	1 tablespoon chopped pimento or
1 or 2 teaspoons caraway seeds	green pepper
2 tablespoons chopped parsley	1 grated onion

Mold into cakes ½ inch thick; pan-broil slowly over low heat, draining fat as it is rendered out; insert meat thermometer momentarily in center of each cake; take up when internal temperature of 165° F. is reached.

VARIATIONS:

Omit onions and add garlic or 2 tablespoons chives; or use dill, cumin, or mustard seeds instead of caraway seeds; or season with basil and serve with tomato gravy (p. 127).

Pigs in blankets: Pierce casings of link sausages and pan-broil for 6 to 8 minutes; or season sausage as in basic recipe or any variation and make cakes the size and shape of large wieners; brown over slow heat for 10 minutes; prepare like beef in blankets (p. 107); sauté or bake.

Sausage with apples and sauerkraut: Brown seasoned sausage in heat-resistant casserole; remove and drain on paper; pour off all but 1 tablespoon fat; brown apple rings cut ½ inch thick; place 2 to 4 cups sauerkraut over apples; put sausage on top of sauerkraut; sprinkle generously with paprika; cover and steam sauerkraut 15 to 30 minutes. Vary by preparing sausage with apples and finely shredded cabbage; cook 8 minutes; or use slices of yam instead of apples with shredded green cabbage.

Tongue can be cooked most easily in soup stock as it is being prepared. During the winter months, however, when soup is frequently on the menu, cold tongue may be unappetizing. Following are recipes for reheating tongue cooked in soup stock.

If no stock is being made, tongue should be steamed on a rack above water until it is tender. Remove skin while meat is still warm and trim base. Slice diagonally, and serve hot or cold with horseradish or dry mustard mixed to a paste with a little water.

SWEET-SOUR LAMB TONGUES

Steam above water or simmer in broth about 1½ hours, or until tender:

8 or 10 lamb tongues

Remove tongues; add to 1 cup of stock or broth left from steaming:

1 minced clove garlic
1 chopped onion
1 crushed bay leaf
½ cup seedless raisins
2 tablespoons brown sugar
1 teaspoon salt

2 tablespoons whole-wheat flour mixed with ¼ cup water
freshly ground black peppercorns
1 or 2 tablespoons vinegar or lemon juice

Simmer 10 to 15 minutes. Meanwhile skin and slice or dice tongues. Add tongues to sauce, reheat, and serve over rice mixed with chopped parsley.

VARIATIONS:

Omit raisins, sugar, and vinegar; add ½ cup each chopped celery and bell pepper; or season with ⅛ teaspoon orégano, basil, rosemary, or other herbs.

Instead of lamb tongues use sliced or diced beef or veal tongue.

BROWNED BEEF TONGUE

Cut beef tongue diagonally into ½-inch slices; dip in:

1 egg, slightly beaten, mixed with 2 tablespoons fresh milk

Dredge with:

sifted whole-wheat-bread crumbs

Sauté until brown on each side; sprinkle with salt.

VARIATIONS:

Use pork or veal tongue; serve with any meat sauce (pp. 136–138).
Creamed lamb or mutton tongues: See page 55.

Pork tongue with apple rings: Cut tart red apples into rings ⅓ inch thick and brown in vegetable oil; put slices of pork tongue over apples, cover utensil, and cook until apples are tender; serve tongue topped with apple slices. Vary by spreading **thick applesauce sprinkled with nutmeg** between thin slices or over thick slices of pork tongue; reheat in oven.

Rolled pork or beef tongue with bacon: Slice tongue diagonally ⅛ inch thick; roll tightly, wrap a strip of **bacon** around each slice, and hold with toothpicks; bake until bacon is crisp. Vary by filling with **leftover vegetables or well-seasoned mashed potatoes.**

Tripe is usually the cheapest meat available. It contains little adequate protein and should be served with eggs, cheese, or other proteins on the menu with it. In cooking tripe, include a small amount of bone for flavor and calcium.

CREAMED TRIPE

Use **1 or 2 pounds veal, beef, lamb, or pork tripe and 2 small pieces bone.** Put tripe and bones in utensil with:

1 cup vegetable-cooking water   2 tablespoons vinegar

Simmer 2 hours for pickled or precooked tripe, 3½ hours for un-cooked tripe, or until tender and cut edge has a clear appearance; add a small amount more liquid if needed; remove from utensil and cool.

Prepare in same utensil, using moisture left from steaming:

2 cups cream sauce (p. 135)

After sauce has simmered 10 minutes, cut tripe into small strips or squares with scissors, dropping it directly into sauce; salt to taste; serve as soon as tripe has reheated. Tripe is especially good with **dill, caraway, cheese, celery, pimento, or onion sauce.**

VARIATIONS:

Instead of cream sauce use any brown sauce (p. 136), any tomato sauce (p. 140), leftover gravy, or any heated sour-cream sauce (p. 143); if sour-cream sauce is used, heat only to simmering; do not boil.

Broiled tripe: Steam tripe as directed; cut into serving sizes, place on oiled baking sheet, sprinkle with **paprika**, and cover with bacon slices cut into thirds; broil slowly until bacon is crisp.

Pepper-pot stew: Simmer tripe in 2 quarts water and 1 cup canned or diced tomatoes, 2 teaspoons salt, 1 tablespoon dark molasses; when tripe is tender, discard bone, remove tripe, cool, cut with scissors into tiny strips, and add to broth with ½ teaspoon crushed black peppercorns, 1 each diced onion, unpeeled potato, carrot, turnip, pinch each of thyme and savory; thicken with 4 tablepoons whole-wheat-pastry flour mixed with ½ cup water; cook until vegetables are just tender.

Sautéed tripe: Cut steamed tripe into serving sizes, dip in salted **egg diluted with milk,** then in wheat germ or sifted whole-wheat-bread crumbs; sauté until golden.

Stuffed tripe: Simmer whole tripe until almost tender; cool slightly and cut into two matching sections, dicing scraps; fill with onion stuffing (p. 131) to which scraps are added; brush surface with **vegetable oil** and bake in moderate oven at 350° F. for 30 minutes.

Tripe creole: Prepare as in basic recipe, using 2 **cups creole sauce** (p. 140) instead of cream sauce.

Make the Bony Meats Rich Sources of Calcium

Because such meats as spareribs, backbones, and pigs' feet contain much fat, they are satisfying, yet they supply only about a fifth as much protein as do lean meats such as liver, steaks, or roasts. Unless the meat is removed from the bones after cooking, as it is in head cheese, additional protein foods should be served at the same meal with bony meats.

If soaked and cooked in vinegar or other acid, these meat dishes can become outstanding sources of calcium, sometimes supplying as much in a single serving as can be obtained from 3 quarts or more of milk. When they are cooked without acid, almost no calcium dissolves out. The amount of calcium dissolved in the gravy or sauce is in proportion to the amount of acid used, the length of time the meat is soaked and cooked with acid, and the amount of bone exposed. Use as much acid in preparing these meats as you can without making them unpalatable. Whenever time permits, soak the bones before cooking. Larger amounts of calcium dissolve out when these meats are stewed than when they are steamed, although stewing causes loss of flavor. Make sure every drop of liquid used for soaking and cooking is eaten with the meat.

PICKLED PIGS' FEET

Select **8 pigs' feet;** clean thoroughly, put into cooking utensil, and add:

3 cups water   **1 cup vinegar**

Simmer about 3 hours, or until tender; do not allow meat to fall from bones; put pigs' feet in a glass baking dish; skim all fat from broth, and add:

¼ to 1 teaspoon pickling spices   **2 teaspoons salt**
½ cup vinegar, or enough to make   **¼ teaspoon crushed black pepper-**
quite tart   **corns**

Add more liquid if needed to bring total to about 3 cups; pour broth over pigs' feet; cover lightly and keep in refrigerator 3 to 5 days before serving. Under no circumstances seal pickled pigs' feet; the protein and calcium can neutralize the acid in the vinegar, and botulinus can thrive in the absence of air and acid.

Serve pigs' feet chilled.

VARIATIONS:

Instead of pigs' feet use 2 pounds or more of spareribs, backbones, or smaller bony sections of oxtail; simmer spareribs and oxtail about 2 hours, backbones 2½ hours. If only 2 pounds of meat are pickled, use half the amounts of other ingredients.

BRAISED PIGS' FEET

Select **4 pigs' feet;** ask butcher to cut in half lengthwise; pack into refrigerator dish and add:

1 to 2 cups tomato juice or canned   **½ cup white vinegar**
tomatoes

After soaking 24 to 48 hours, drain well, roll in whole-wheat-pastry flour, and brown surfaces; add liquid used for soaking and simmer 3 hours, or until tender; add:

¼ teaspoon crushed peppercorns	1 to 2 tablespoons dark molasses
1 minced clove garlic	2 teaspoons salt
1 chopped or grated onion	4 tablespoons whole-wheat-pastry
1 diced stalk celery	flour shaken with
2 diced pimentos or bell peppers	½ cup tomato juice

Stir well and simmer 10 minutes.

VARIATIONS:

Add a pinch each of basil and orégano, 1 or 2 teaspoons cumin seeds; or omit other seasonings and cook ginger root with pigs' feet or add 3 or 4 tablespoons chopped preserved ginger just before serving.

Use spareribs instead of pigs' feet. Simmer 1½ to 2 hours.

Stewed pigs' feet: Prepare like backbones (p. 120). Simmer 3 to 4 hours.

BARBECUED SPARERIBS

Select 2 pounds or more meaty, uncut spareribs or farmer's style containing part of the loin; put in flat baking dish and pour over meat:

2 tablespoons vinegar	2 cups tomato purée or
2 or 3 tablespoons dark molasses	chopped canned tomatoes

Let soak overnight or longer; pour off liquid, put spareribs on meat rack over baking pan, insert meat thermometer between bones, and set in preheated oven at 300° F.

Meanwhile add to liquid used for soaking:

dash each of Tabasco, allspice,	1 teaspoon salt
and nutmeg	1 minced clove garlic

After spareribs have baked 1½ hours, drain drippings; remove rack and set meat in pan, pouring sauce over it. Return to oven. Baste meat with sauce once or twice. Bake to an internal temperature of 170° F., or about 2 hours.

VARIATIONS:

If size of broiler compartment permits, barbecue slowly with direct heat. Set ribs bony side up during first half of cooking. Proceed as in basic recipe.

Select matching sections of spareribs; bake as in basic recipe; when well browned and nearly done, spread one section with sauerkraut, put other section on top, cover with sauce.

Braised spareribs: Prepare as braised pigs' feet (p. 118) or stewed backbones.

Spareribs with apples: Omit tomatoes or purée; brush spareribs well with vinegar; 30 minutes before serving cover with ½-inch rings of tart, cored but unpeeled apples; brush apples with vegetable oil and dark molasses; cook until well browned.

Stuffed spareribs: See page 47.

STEWED BACKBONES

Select **2 to 4 pounds pork backbones** cut at each joint. If meat is not to be cooked immediately, pack solidly into a refrigerator dish; pour over meat:

¼ to ½ cup white vinegar   ½ to 1 cup vegetable-cooking
1 or 2 tablespoons dark molasses   water, or enough to cover

After soaking for 24 to 48 hours, simmer in the same liquid 2½ hours, or until meat is tender; put backbones on serving platter, skim fat from broth, and add:

1 minced clove garlic   2 teaspoons salt
¼ teaspoon crushed black pepper-   ½ cup vegetable-cooking water
   corns   shaken with
1 whole cayenne or chili tepine   3 tablespoons whole-wheat-pastry
¼ crushed bay leaf   flour

Add more water if needed; stir well, cover utensil, and simmer 15 minutes.

VARIATIONS:

Soak backbones in vinegar and tomato juice or canned tomatoes instead of water; or omit vinegar and add with water ¼ to ½ cup dry white or red wine.

Shake ⅓ cup powdered milk with thickening.

Instead of backbones use pigs' feet or spareribs; simmer pigs' feet 3 to 4 hours, spareribs, 1½ to 2 hours.

I would probably never have prepared head cheese or scrapple had it not been necessary to test the following recipes. To my surprise, I found them unusually delicious. Head cheese is quite similar to pressed chicken in taste, and scrapple is a flavorful variation of old-fashioned fried mush. I was even more surprised at the tremendous amount of food one could obtain at little cost. Surely few other cuts of meat can offer so much satiety value for money spent as can hog's head. The heads are carefully cleaned at the slaughterhouses; hence the work of preparing these dishes is slight.

HEAD CHEESE

Select **hog's head,** wash thoroughly, put into large utensil, and add:

½ cup white vinegar	4 cups vegetable-cooking water

Simmer about 4 hours, or until meat starts to fall from bones; set head in colander, let head and broth chill overnight; it is much easier to work with and far less greasy if chilled.

Remove meat from bones; dice fine or pass through meat grinder, using large knife, tongue, brain, skin, all lean meat. Skim all fat from broth, heat to boiling, and add:

3 teaspoons salt	⅛ teaspoon each savory, sage,
½ teaspoon crushed black pepper-	marjoram, basil
corns	½ crushed bay leaf

Mix together:

half of the diced or ground meat	1½ cups hot broth, or enough to
½ cup powdered milk	moisten

Pack into oiled mold or loaf bread pans; chill until firm; slice and serve cold. Use remainder of broth and meat in making scrapple.

Serve with horseradish.

VARIATIONS:

Grind or dice fine and add to head cheese one or more of the following: sweet onion or leek; green pepper, pimento, or green chili pepper; celery; or add 1 or 2 teaspoons caraway seeds.

Dice fat meat taken from hog's head into ½-inch cubes; pan-broil until crisp and well browned; use for seasoning baked or string beans or green leafy vegetables; or add to scrambled eggs or to any food customarily seasoned with crisp bacon.

Scrapple: Add enough water to remaining broth to make 1 quart; bring to a rolling boil and stir in slowly 1¼ **cups yellow stone-ground corn meal** sifted with ½ **cup powdered milk;** stir constantly until mixture thickens, or about 5 minutes; add ½ **cup wheat germ** and remaining diced or ground meat; salt to taste; cool, pour into loaf pans, and chill. Slice and serve cold or dredge in whole-wheat flour or crumbs and sauté. Vary by using entire hog's head, cooking it in 2 quarts water and stirring 2½ **cups corn meal** into broth.

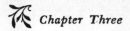

Chapter Three

Make Delicious Gravies or None at All

Tender, juicy, and delightfully cooked meat can be almost ruined by having gray, lumpy gravy served over it. Although there are two ways of making gravies, the causes of failure are the same in both varieties.

All kinds of gravy should have an appetizing color. Brown gravies may be achieved in three ways: by heating fat until it darkens; by browning bits of lean meat until some of the protein breaks down; or by heating flour until some of the starch changes to dextrin, a semisugar, which is partly caramelized. Since over-heated fat is dangerous to health, the first two procedures cannot be recommended; therefore the browning of flour should be relied upon to produce the color desired. The taste of undercooked flour can be avoided if all gravies are simmered at least 10 minutes after the flour is added.

One trick of mixing thickenings in a second is to put the liquid into a small jar, add the flour, fasten the lid securely, and then shake vigorously. The liquid must be put in first; otherwise the flour sticks to the bottom. This same procedure is excellent for mixing powdered milk or brewers' yeast with liquids. The time-honored method of mixing water or milk and flour together in a cup, however, is still adequate.

Lumps can be avoided by a moment's consideration of why lumps lump. If flour and liquid are not shaken or stirred to a smooth batter, the lumps in the thickening are cooked into small dumplings; this type of lump can be prevented by more thorough shaking or stirring. Lumps of a pudding texture are made by pouring smooth thickening drop by drop into boiling liquid; each drop is immediately cooked and preserved. Such lumps may be prevented if you keep the liquid to be thickened below the boiling point until the thickening is added and the mixture is thoroughly stirred.

Gravies made by adding flour to fat cannot lump if stirred sufficiently to coat each particle of flour with fat. As little as 1 tablespoon of fat can prevent the particles in 3 tablespoons of flour from sticking together if the two are well mixed. The liquid should be added slowly and the heat kept low until liquid, fat, and flour are blended.

In my opinion the most delicious gravy has a proportion of 1 tablespoon of fat to 2 tablespoons of flour. If you use more than 2 tablespoons of fat for each tablespoon of flour, you can expect the fat to separate; hence excess fat should be removed before the flour is added. An easy way to ruin gravy is to allow it to be greasy.

The problem of making gravy too thick or too thin can be met by memorizing once and for all the proportions of flour to liquid: 1 level tablespoon of flour is used to each $\frac{1}{2}$ cup of liquid, including the liquid used in mixing the thickening. If the flour is to be highly browned, allow an extra tablespoon.

When a liquid other than milk is to be added to gravies, tomato and other vegetables juices, vegetable-cooking water, or soup stock should be used instead of water. Because of the great nutritive value of milk, however, country gravy should be served more often than other varieties. Since the milk in gravy is to be heated, reconstituted rather than fresh milk may be used if the budget is limited.

Gravies can be made creamier in texture, superior in flavor, and richer in protein, vitamin B_2, and calcium if extra powdered milk is added. Since meat juices contain much nutritive value, no more gravy should be prepared than is likely to be eaten. Any leftover gravy may be used as cream or brown sauce, added to fresh gravy, meat loaf, or dressing, or reheated with fresh seasonings.

The earmark of good gravy lies in the seasoning. When a person becomes accustomed to well-seasoned gravy, chicken gravy without a pinch of sage or thyme, tomato gravy without orégano or basil, and beef gravy without savory, marjoram, or rosemary seem as flat as if the salt were omitted. The use of crushed peppercorns instead of stale ground pepper makes a striking improvement. Endless variations and delightful flavors can be achieved by adding seasonings. Chopped onions, celery, any variety of fresh peppers, and garlic may be slightly cooked in the fat before making the gravy. All gravy should be tasted for salt before being served.

GRAVY MADE WITH FLOUR ADDED TO FAT

Heat slightly:

> 2 to 4 tablespoons fat

Add and stir thoroughly:

> 4 level tablespoons whole-wheat-pastry flour

Brown to the color desired over moderate heat; reduce heat and add slowly while stirring:

2 cups fresh or reconstituted milk	1 teaspoon salt
¼ teaspoon crushed black peppercorns	¼ teaspoon minced fresh herbs or pinch of dried herbs

Simmer for at least 10 minutes; taste for salt; garnish with paprika.

VARIATIONS:

Instead of milk use tomato or other vegetable juice, vegetable-cooking water, or soup stock.

Add sage or thyme to chicken or turkey gravy; orégano, basil, or cumin seeds to gravy containing tomato; and savory, basil, rosemary, or marjoram to veal, lamb, or beef gravy.

GRAVY MADE WITH THICKENING
ADDED TO LIQUID

Heat to boiling:

1½ cups meat broth

Meanwhile shake to a smooth paste in a small sealed jar or stir together, adding liquid first:

½ cup cold milk, broth, or water   4 tablespoons whole-wheat-pastry
flour

Remove broth momentarily from heat; add thickening slowly, stirring constantly; when gravy is well blended, add:

1 teaspoon salt   ½ teaspoon minced fresh or a
¼ teaspoon crushed white or   pinch of dried herbs
black peppercorns

Simmer at least 10 minutes. If gravy is too thin, boil to evaporate excess moisture; if too thick, dilute with more liquid. Taste for salt. Garnish with paprika.

VARIATIONS:

If insufficient broth is available, add fresh or reconstituted milk, tomato purée or juice, vegetable-cooking water, soup stock, or water to which 1 bouillon cube per ½ cup has been added. If bouillon cubes are used, omit salt.

Shake ¼ to ½ cup powdered milk with 1 cup cold broth or other liquid to be used for gravy; add 5 minutes before serving.

For highly seasoned gravies, see brown sauces (p. 136).

Omit flour and salt; use canned tomato or mushroom soup diluted to desired consistency with milk or broth; season the tomato soup with a pinch of orégano or basil.

Beef gravy: Vary the seasonings by adding one or two of the following: marjoram, rosemary, savory, basil, or orégano; or chopped chives, green onions, leeks, parsley, or garlic; or crushed mustard, celery, caraway, or cardamon seeds; chili tepine, chili sauce, Worcestershire, or catsup; chopped celery, fresh pepper, or pimento.

Chicken gravy: Season with sage or combine with sage one or more of the following: **savory, basil, thyme, marjoram, chives, leeks, or a generous amount of ground paprika; chopped canned or fresh pimento or mushrooms.**

Duck, goose, or small-game gravy: Season like chicken gravy.

Gravy with big game: Season like beef gravy, combining 2 or more seasonings if the meat is gamy.

Lamb gravy: Season like chicken gravy or combine **chervil, rosemary, savory, and marjoram;** or omit herbs and add 1 teaspoon **dill seeds** or fresh dill, or 1 or more tablespoons **capers.**

Mutton gravy: Season like lamb or beef gravy, or combine several herbs or herbs and seeds; add a small amount of **Worcestershire and Tabasco.**

Pork or ham gravy: Season with any one of the following: **sage, savory, basil, thyme, chives, parsley, minced leeks;** or **celery or mustard seeds.** Season ham gravy with **mustard or caraway seeds.**

Tomato gravy: Use **tomato juice or canned tomatoes** instead of milk or other liquid; add **basil, orégano, chili powder, or Worcestershire.** If the tomatoes are sour, sweeten with 1 or 2 teaspoons dark molasses.

Turkey gravy: Season with **basil, sage, and thyme;** on rare occasions add a mere sprinkle of grated lemon peel and nutmeg or mace.

Veal gravy: Season like beef or chicken gravy.

Chapter Four

Dress Up Your Meats with Dressings

Dressings are easy to make, add interest and variety to a meal, and are excellent nutritionally provided your family can utilize the calories they supply. Yet aside from stuffing an occasional turkey and chicken, few housewives use them. Fish, rabbit, and any number of cuts of meat can be made more festive by delicious stuffing.

If you wish to stuff chops or steaks—delicious with onion, celery, or fruit dressing—have them cut double thickness; cut a pocket by inserting a knife in one side and rotating it without cutting the edge of the meat. Make a pocket between the bones and meat in such cuts as brisket, plate, shoulder, and breast of lamb or veal, or a standing rump roast. You can select matching sections of spareribs, round steaks, ham slices, flank, or plate, put the dressing between them, and tie them or hold them together with poultry skewers. Any roast having a bone in the center, such as a ham, a leg of lamb, roast cut from the chuck, or a fresh pork shoulder can be boned and the resulting space filled with dressing. And do not overlook stuffed meat loaves (p. 110).

Underestimate the amount of dressing which a pocket will hold. Since stuffing swells as steam is formed, pack it lightly into the available space. This point I'm afraid I shall never learn. I invariably think of how delicious the dressing will be, pack it in tightly, and then feel distressed when it bursts forth from its pocket and ruins the appearance of the meat.

One of the cutest culinary tricks I know is lacing up a roast (it isn't original). Close the pocket by slipping large trussing pins or hardwood toothpicks through either side of the opening about

1 inch apart. I have even used thin nails, for lack of something better. Then lace around both ends of the pins or toothpicks or nails with a string, as hiking boots are laced. After the roast is put on a serving platter, the toothpicks or pins or nails can be removed and the string falls away. If the meat or skin is thin, the "spikes" should be set farther back from the opening.

Achieve variety in your menus by stuffing many kinds and cuts of meat and by using many different types of dressings. Since only low heat reaches the stuffing, vegetables to be used should first be heated to destroy enzymes and thus retard the destruction of vitamin C during cooking.

One person may enjoy dressing made largely of crumbs with few vegetables, whereas another wants vegetables with little bread, and still another hates sage while someone else loves it; therefore the recipes for dressings do not give exact measurements. I personally like a large proportion of onions, celery, pimentos, and the like. A five-year-old guest at one of our Thanksgiving dinners reported later to his mother, "There were plants in my dressing."

Juggle the ingredients around to suit yourself. Do not waste time in measuring ingredients except by eye. The throw-it-together method, tasting it as you make it, usually produces the best stuffing.

CRUMB DRESSING

Dice, chop, or run through the meat grinder and sauté gently in 1 or 2 tablespoons vegetable oil:

1 or 2 onions	1 handful parsley
1 minced clove garlic (optional)	1 chilled bell pepper or pimento
1 to 4 stalks celery with leaves	(optional)

Cover utensil and steam 5 minutes; remove from heat and add:

2 or 3 cups diced or crumbled dry whole-wheat bread	1 teaspoon salt
¼ to ½ cup wheat germ mixed with ¼ cup powdered milk	pinch to ½ teaspoon sage, thyme, marjoram, or savory
1 to 2 cups broth	¼ teaspoon crushed black peppercorns

If for turkey, chicken, or other fowl, cook neck and giblets and add broth and chopped or ground gizzard, liver, heart, and meat from neck. Mix thoroughly; taste for seasonings; stuff lightly into the meat.

This recipe, or approximately 4 cups of dressing, is enough for stuffing 1 chicken, 1 rabbit, 1 large beef roast, or 2 matching flank steaks.

VARIATIONS:

If broth is not available, use milk, leftover gravy, or water with 1 to 3 chicken or beef bouillon cubes. If bouillon cubes are used, omit salt.

Add leftover vegetables, such as peas, diced carrots, or celery root; or substitute leftover potatoes or rice for part of the crumbs.

If more dressing is prepared than can be stuffed into the available space, bake in a separate utensil 20 to 30 minutes; serve in mounds around meat.

Dice ¼ pound bacon and pan-broil until crisp; drain on paper; mix the crisp bacon with the other ingredients. Use for poultry or fish.

Chestnut dressing: Boil unshelled chestnuts 15 minutes; drain, shell, and cut off brown skin while hot; substitute for 1 cup or more of crumbs. Use for poultry, veal, or pork.

Cornbread dressing: Use crumbled stale cornbread instead of crumbs; if cornbread is prepared for dressing, omit sugar. Use for pork, veal, or poultry.

Dressing for beef, pork, lamb, or mutton: Prepare 1 cup dressing for small chops; make half the recipe (2 cups) for other cuts; increase amounts of the vegetables and decrease the crumbs as desired. Vary by seasoning dressings for beef with basil, rosemary, or a pinch each of several herbs; dressings for lamb or mutton with 2 to 4 tablespoons capers or 1 to 2 teaspoons dill seeds; dressings for pork with 1 to 3 teaspoons caraway seeds.

Dressings for poultry: If the fowl weighs less than 10 pounds, prepare 1 cup dressing for each pound of dressed weight, or 4 cups for a 4-pound duck or chicken; if weight is more than 10 pounds, use 1 cup less than the pounds of dressed weight, or 15 cups for a 16-pound turkey.

Chicken or turkey dressing: Omit garlic; use **pimento**; vary by adding grated rind of 1 lemon, dash of nutmeg.

Duck dressing: Increase proportion of celery and onions, decreasing the crumbs. Vary by adding 1 cup diced tart apples, ¼ cup seedless raisins, or 3 teaspoons caraway seeds. Or stuff with steamed wild rice.

Eggplant dressing: Dice and sauté 1 unpeeled eggplant with other vegetables; add only enough crumbs to absorb moisture; prepare and season as in basic recipe. Use for stuffing pork, beef, or fish. Eggplant dressing is especially good with beef heart or liver.

Mushroom dressing: Omit garlic; decrease onion to 1 tablespoon; sauté 1 cup or more mushrooms with other vegetables; if canned mushrooms are used, add the liquid to crumbs. Use for poultry, pork, veal, or lamb.

Oyster dressing: Omit the garlic; decrease or omit onion; add to crumbs without heating 1 or 2 cups chopped or whole oysters and liquid. Use for poultry or fish.

Onion or celery dressing: Increase the amount of onion and celery to 2 or 3 cups; use only enough crumbs to absorb moisture; add other ingredients of basic recipe. Use for stuffing duck, pork, veal, or ham. For sweet mild dressing use leeks instead of onions.

Potato stuffing: Use mashed, riced, or leftover potatoes instead of crumbs; prepare as in basic recipe. For particularly delicious potato dressing, shred raw chilled potatoes directly into the fat, brown well before adding other vegetables; use a generous amount of **pimentos or celery salt** with the other ingredients. Vary by adding 1 to 3 tablespoons caraway seeds. Use for stuffing duck or pork.

Rice stuffing: Use cooked rice instead of crumbs; add the other ingredients of basic recipe. If for beef or mutton, add 2 tablespoons catsup. Use for any meat.

Stuffing for fish: Use half the amount of bread but the same amount of vegetables. Omit herbs and add 3 tablespoons butter or partially hardened margarine, ½ to 1 can tomato sauce, grated rind of 1 lemon or 1 to 2 teaspoons dill seeds; or use onion, celery, eggplant, or potato dressing.

Whole grains make delightful stuffings for almost any type of meat. When I stuff turkey, for example, I usually put crumb dressing on the inside and buckwheat stuffing above the breast. Persons who have not eaten buckwheat usually assume that buckwheat stuffing is made of wild rice. If you enjoy the taste of buckwheat pancakes, buckwheat stuffing is probably destined to be your favorite as it is mine.

BUCKWHEAT STUFFING

Bring to boiling:

2 cups water, broth, or consommé

Add so slowly that boiling does not stop:

1 cup buckwheat groats   1 teaspoon salt

Cover utensil and simmer 15 minutes. Add and stir well:

2 or 3 tablespoons butter or par-   1 cup fresh or canned mushrooms
tially hardened margarine   2 tablespoons chopped parsley
1 diced stalk celery and leaves   1 or 2 diced pimentos

Use for stuffing chicken, duck, wild fowl, pork, beef, or meat loaf.

VARIATIONS:

Use 1 cup millet or hulled barley instead of buckwheat; simmer for
30 minutes, or until tender. Season with ¼ cup each chopped onions,
bell pepper, and celery, ½ teaspoon sage, thyme, or other herbs.

Add to cooking water 2 or 3 chicken or beef bouillon cubes or 2 or
3 teaspoons instant chicken or beef broth; salt to taste.

Instead of pimentos and mushrooms, add 1 chopped onion and 1 or
2 stalks celery. If for fowl, use broth from stewing giblets for cooking
buckwheat; add diced or ground giblets if desired.

Rice stuffing: Prepare as in basic recipe, using **brown or converted
rice** instead of buckwheat; simmer brown rice 45 minutes.

Unground-wheat stuffing: Prepare as in basic recipe, using **cooked
unground wheat.** Use for stuffing meat loaf (p. 110) or beef, lamb, or
pork roast.

Wild-rice stuffing: Cook rice in broth, canned consommé, or in
water to which 2 chicken bouillon cubes are added. If bouillon cubes
are used, omit salt. Use for stuffing wild duck or other wild or tame
fowl.

Fruit stuffings can be delightful additions to meat. Unfortunately, they are little used. Thick broiled pork chops stuffed
with diced apple, crushed pineapple, or spiced crabapple can

be delicious. My favorite is flank steak stuffed with nuts and prunes. You may, of course, add crumbs to fruit dressings if you wish.

APPLE DRESSING

Estimate the amount of dressing needed. Select **tart apples,** such as Jonathans, which will not cook to a mush; chill thoroughly, core, and dice without peeling.

Brown the apples in **vegetable oil or fat from meat** to be stuffed. Add:

pinch of salt	**¼ to ½ cup walnuts, pecans,**
dash of nutmeg or cinnamon	**or almonds**

Stir well; use for stuffing ham, pork, or duck.

VARIATIONS:

Add ¼ cup seedless raisins for each cup of apples; steam with the apples until soft and plump; or use half apples and half diced and well-drained cling peaches, crushed pineapple, cooked dried apricots, or cooked prunes.

Apricot stuffing: Steam **dried apricots** in a small amount of water until soft and all water is absorbed; dice and prepare as in basic recipe. Use 1 or 2 cups for stuffing lamb, beef, pork, or small wild game.

Peach stuffing: Use **canned cling peaches;** drain well and prepare as in basic recipe. Use 2 cups for stuffing beef heart or flank steak; 1 cup for veal, pork, or lamb chops.

Pineapple stuffing: Drain **crushed pineapple** well in a strainer; sear until slightly brown; omit spices and nuts. Vary by adding **bits of crisp bacon.** Use 2 cups for stuffing boned ham or shoulder or fresh pork roasts; 1 cup for pork chops or matching ham steaks.

Prune stuffing: Pit **cooked prunes;** dice or leave whole; prepare as in basic recipe, keeping heat high until moisture has evaporated; add **grated rind of ¼ lemon or orange.** Use 2 cups for stuffing flank steak, beef heart, or breast of veal; 1 cup for pork chops.

Spiced-fruit stuffing: Dice any spiced or sweet-pickled fruit, such as **figs, crab apples, cling peaches, or prunes;** do not heat; use or omit nuts. Use 1 cup for stuffing small cuts such as pork chops, matching ham steaks, or flank steak to be broiled.

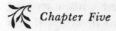 *Chapter Five*

Sauces to Be Served with Meats, Fish, or Vegetables

One of the easiest ways to make food interesting is to serve it in or with a sauce. Sauces make further seasoning unnecessary; they banish monotony; and few take as long as 10 minutes to prepare.

Sauces have not gained the popularity in America which they deserve. The reason, perhaps, is their names: sauce Bercy, which is essentially clear chicken gravy; poulette sauce, or chicken stock thickened with egg yolks; sauce Allemande, Béarnaise sauce, and so on. One of the cookbooks in my possession offers a little masterpiece of a recipe for making soubise sauce: you are to add 2 cups of velouté sauce. It took considerable searching to discover that velouté sauce was thickened chicken or veal gravy, and that soubise, which means smothered, refers to smothered onions added to the sauce. Surely a rose by any other name would smell as sweet. You may recognize recipes for foreign sauces in the following pages, but their foreign names are largely missing.

Almost anyone who cooks at all finds gravy easy to make. Actually most sauces are identical to gravies except that one starts with butter or margarine instead of meat drippings. In fact, a sauce could be said to be the variety of "gravy" made when no drippings are available. Instant and powdered chicken and beef broth and bouillon cubes make it possible to prepare delicious French sauces with almost no effort.

Cream sauces may be easily cooked over direct heat. Making them in a double boiler usually leaves a raw-flour taste and wastes time and fuel. Compared with the usual variety of cream sauces, which taste strikingly like wallpaper paste, sauces made with whole-wheat flour have a delightful flavor. The richness contributed by extra powdered milk makes the addition of cream superfluous. Use cream sauces frequently as a means of working milk into your menus.

MEDIUM CREAM SAUCE

Melt in a saucepan:

> **2 to 4 tablespoons partially hardened margarine,**
> **or 1 or 2 tablespoons each butter and vegetable oil**

Add and mix thoroughly without browning:

> **¼ cup whole-wheat-pastry flour**

Add gradually, stirring rapidly:

> **2 cups fresh or reconstituted milk**

When milk and flour are well blended, add:

> **¼ to ½ teaspoon crushed white or**   **¼ teaspoon paprika**
> **black peppercorns**   **1 teaspoon Worcestershire (op-**
> **1 teaspoon salt**   **tional)**

Simmer at least 10 minutes to destroy all raw-flour taste.

Add vegetables, meats, cheese, or seasonings mentioned in variations.

VARIATIONS:

For thin cream sauce, use 2 tablespoons each flour and fat, keeping other ingredients the same; for thick cream sauce, use ½ cup flour and ¼ cup fat.

If fresh milk is used, stir into it ⅓ cup instant powdered milk; or use ¾ cup instant milk mixed with 2 cups water.

Brown sauce: Put ⅓ cup flour into pan and brown before adding fat; use soup stock, meat broth, canned consommé, or 4 beef or chicken bouillon cubes with 2 cups water; salt to taste. Since brown sauce is essentially brown gravy, use leftover gravy when available.

Mushroom sauce: Add 1 or 2 cups sliced fresh mushrooms to cream sauce 5 minutes before serving; or add 1 or 2 cans button mushrooms, using liquid instead of part of the milk in the sauce. Or heat 1 can condensed cream of mushroom soup (1⅛ cups) and add ⅓ cup instant powdered milk blended with ½ cup fresh milk; salt to taste; omit the other ingredients of basic recipe. This is an excellent sauce to prepare when time is limited.

Unless otherwise stated, as a base for any of the following sauces use:

2 cups medium cream sauce or   *2 cups medium brown sauce or*
2 cups mushroom sauce or   *leftover brown gravy*

Merely add the following ingredients to one of the three basic sauces. When seeds are to be used, simmer them in the sauce and, if time permits, let it stand ½ hour or longer. Reheat and serve the food in the sauce, serve the sauce over the food, or serve the sauce separately. When meat, fish, fowl, or vegetables are served in the sauce, salt to taste.

Caper sauce: 4 to 6 tablespoons capers, 2 tablespoons chopped parsley. Serve with fish, lamb, brains, or sweetbreads.

Caraway sauce: Simmer in basic sauce 1 or 2 tablespoons crushed caraway seeds; let stand and reheat. Serve over steamed cabbage or sauerkraut, with fresh or leftover pork or ham.

Celery sauce: Simmer 5 minutes in basic sauce 1½ cups finely chopped celery or 1 teaspoon celery seeds. Serve with baked or broiled fish, hard-cooked eggs, baked or steamed unsliced liver or heart.

Cheese sauce: Remove basic sauce from heat and add 1½ cups diced nippy cheese 3 minutes before serving. Serve over broccoli, cauliflower, spinach, or other vegetables; or add ½ to 1 teaspoon crushed anise or dill seeds and serve over steamed or broiled fish.

Cheese-pimento sauce: Use pimento cheese or add 4 tablespoons diced pimentos, generous dash of cayenne, 1 to 2 teaspoons crushed coriander seeds.

Curry sauce: 1 minced clove garlic, 3 tablespoons grated onion, ½ to 4 teaspoons curry powder, generous sprinkling cayenne. Serve with shrimp, fish, chicken, lamb, rice, or potatoes.

Dill sauce: 2 tablespoons or more minced fresh dill or 1 to 3 teaspoons crushed dill seeds. Serve with fish, lamb, veal, eggs, or potatoes.

Egg sauce: Just before serving add 1½ teaspoons Worcestershire, ¼ cup lemon juice or tarragon vinegar, 2 to 4 diced or sliced hard-cooked eggs. Serve over steamed spinach, broccoli, or any green leafy vegetable; decorate baked fish with sliced eggs and pour sauce over it.

Horseradish sauce: Just before serving add ¼ cup freshly grated horseradish and 1 or 2 teaspoons dry or prepared mustard. Serve with fresh or leftover ham, pork, beef, heart, tongue, liver, or kidney.

Hot tartar sauce: Heat ⅔ cup medium cream sauce; add ⅓ cup mayonnaise, 2 tablespoons tarragon vinegar, ½ cup chopped pickles, 1 grated onion, 1 teaspoon dry mustard. Serve with fish.

Mock Hollandaise sauce: Heat 1 cup medium cream sauce; just before serving beat in 2 egg yolks, 2 tablespoons partially hardened margarine or butter, ¼ cup lemon juice. Serve with asparagus, broccoli, artichokes, steamed spinach or other greens, fish, or hard-cooked or poached eggs.

Mornay sauce: To one cup thin cream sauce, add 3 minutes before serving 2 egg yolks beaten with 2 tablespoons sherry, dash of nutmeg.

Mustard sauce: Just before serving add 2 to 4 tablespoons dry mustard. Serve with tongue, heart, baked liver, corned beef, ham, or pork.

Olive sauce: ½ cup chopped ripe or sliced stuffed olives; salt to taste after olives are added. Serve with fish, eggs, broccoli, asparagus, spinach, or other green vegetables, broiled tomatoes or eggplant; leftover veal, lamb, or ham.

Onion sauce: 2 cups chopped onions, a generous dash of cayenne; cook the onions in sauce only 5 minutes. Serve over steamed sliced heart or tongue, unsliced baked liver, hard-cooked eggs, leftover lamb, veal, or pork.

Pimento sauce: ½ cup chopped canned or sautéed fresh pimentos; 2 tablespoons chopped parsley. Serve with fish, eggs, lamb, liver, or leftover pork.

Piquant sauce: Sauté 3 chopped onions, 1 minced clove garlic, 2 finely diced carrots; make basic sauce, using same utensil; add pinch of thyme, a dash of nutmeg; just before serving add 4 tablespoons chopped parsley, ¼ cup lemon juice or tarragon vinegar. This is a delicious sauce. Serve with fish, lamb, heart, liver, tongue, veal, rice, spinach, or any greens.

Sauce delicious: 1 grated onion; just before serving, beat in 2 egg yolks, 2 tablespoons lemon juice or sherry, 4 tablespoons Parmesan cheese. Serve with tongue, heart, sliced beef, fish, broccoli, spinach, or other steamed green vegetable.

One of the biggest misconceptions is that Hollandaise sauce is difficult to make. Egg protein starts to thicken at 130° F. In the presence of an acid, such as lemon juice or vinegar, it thickens, or curdles, very quickly. If you heat Hollandaise sauce above 135° F. you can expect it to curdle. Even if you do not use a thermometer, you can make beautiful Hollandaise in about 5 minutes if you keep the heat low and take the sauce from the heat as soon as it thickens.

EASY HOLLANDAISE SAUCE

Combine in a saucepan:

2 egg yolks
2 tablespoons lemon juice or vinegar

¼ teaspoon freshly ground white
peppercorns
½ teaspoon salt

Fasten the cooking thermometer to edge of saucepan so that bulb of the mercury reaches top of sauce; put saucepan over low direct heat and beat constantly with a wire whisk or 6-pronged fork. Add in 4 portions:

¼ pound (½ cup) partially hardened margarine or butter

As soon as 1 portion of margarine or butter is beaten in, or melted, add another portion. Remove from heat as soon as it is thick. Do not allow sauce to heat beyond 135° F. at any time.

Serve at once with broccoli, asparagus, artichoke hearts, or baked or broiled fish, veal, or broiled chicken.

VARIATIONS:

If heat cannot be controlled, cook in top of double boiler, over but not touching boiling water.

Use 1 tablespoon lemon juice and 1 tablespoon sherry or dry white wine; or make with tarragon or wine vinegar.

Add any of the following: 1 teaspoon or more grated onion; dash of nutmeg; ½ teaspoon dry mustard; 1 tablespoon chopped parsley or minced tarragon leaves.

If to be served with fish, add ½ teaspoon or more grated lemon rind or dill or anise seeds.

LEMON OR VINEGAR SAUCE

Combine and heat over simmer burner:

¾ cup soup stock
1 tablespoon grated onion
1 teaspoon salt

⅛ teaspoon freshly ground peppercorns

When hot, beat in:

3 tablespoons partially hardened margarine or butter

2 egg yolks

Simmer 2 or 3 minutes, or until thick; *do not boil*. Remove from heat and add:

2 tablespoons tarragon or wine vinegar or
3 tablespoons lemon juice and ½ teaspoon grated rind

Serve at once over baked or broiled fish, steaks, broccoli, steamed spinach, or other cooked greens. This is a delicious sauce.

VARIATIONS:

Add any of the following: 2 teaspoons horseradish or dry or prepared mustard; 2 drops Tabasco and 1 finely diced cucumber; 2 tablespoons chopped fresh dill or 1 teaspoon dill seeds; 3 tablespoons chopped chives or ground parsley.

T O M A T O   S A U C E

Sauté lightly in vegetable oil:

1 or 2 chopped onions
1 minced clove garlic
1 chopped stalk celery with leaves

1 green pepper
1 finely diced carrot

Stir well and add:

2 cups tomato purée or chopped
  fresh or canned tomatoes
1 teaspoon salt
pinch of basil and/or orégano

1 teaspoon dark molasses or sugar
  (optional)
¼ to ½ teaspoon crushed black
  peppercorns

Cook slowly 10 minutes, stirring occasionally. Before serving add 2 tablespoons chopped parsley. Serve with macaroni, spaghetti, noodles, rice, lamb, pork, fish, beef, broiled eggplant, or Spanish omelet.

V A R I A T I O N S :

Season with one or more of the following: ¼ crushed bay leaf; 3 or 4 whole cloves; 1 teaspoon Worcestershire or dry mustard; bits of crisp bacon; a pinch of thyme, marjoram, rosemary, or savory; ¼ teaspoon crushed mustard or celery seeds or 1 teaspoon cumin seeds.

Without telling your family, stir in ¼ cup instant tiger's milk (p. 447).

Barbecue sauce: Add to basic recipe a dash each of Tabasco, allspice, and nutmeg; 2 tablespoons each vinegar and dark molasses.

Chili sauce: Use 2 each large onions and green chili peppers or bell peppers; add ¼ teaspoon crushed mustard seeds, 1 tablespoon each dark molasses and vinegar, a generous dash of nutmeg. If bell peppers are used, add 1 to 3 teaspoons chili powder.

Creole sauce: Omit carrots and celery; sauté ½ cup fresh mushrooms with onions and peppers; use 1 cup each tomato purée and brown sauce or leftover brown gravy; add 8 or 10 sliced stuffed olives.

Italian sauce: Add a pinch each of rosemary, basil, and orégano; use 1 can Italian paste diluted with 1 cup water instead of tomato purée.

Mexican sauce: Use 2 fresh chili peppers or add 1 to 3 teaspoons chili powder; add 1 teaspoon cumin seeds.

Spanish sauce: Before salting add 1 teaspoon beef extract or 1 bouillon cube; or use 1 cup brown sauce instead of 1 cup tomatoes; season with ¼ crushed bay leaf, and a pinch of basil.

Uncooked sauces are usually served with chilled foods. If they are served with hot foods, their charm lies in having the sauce thoroughly chilled and the food piping hot. The following creole sauce is a delicious one.

UNCOOKED CREOLE SAUCE

Pare 2 raw tomatoes and squeeze out as much juice as possible; use the pulp for the sauce, or use chilled tomato purée. Combine:

1 chopped onion	½ teaspoon salt
1 diced bell pepper or pimento	⅛ teaspoon freshly ground peppercorns
2 finely diced raw tomatoes without juice or	pinch each of orégano and basil
¾ cup chilled tomato purée	

Let stand in refrigerator 20 minutes or longer. Serve over kidneys, chops, steaks, jellied fish, cold sliced tongue or heart, broiled or sautéed liver or cold baked liver.

VARIATIONS:

Add any of the following: finely diced celery; chopped chili pepper; minced clove garlic; 2 tablespoons or more French dressing; or omit herbs and add minced fresh dill or 1 teaspoon mashed dill seeds.

Fresh herbs and other seasonings may be added to butter, partially hardened margarine, or a little vegetable oil, which may then be used for seasoning meats, fish, and vegetables. Herb butter makes a delicious sandwich spread. Since the freshness of the herbs is retained, such fats may be kept for weeks in a tightly sealed jar in the refrigerator.

HERB BUTTER

Pulverize dried herbs by rolling between palms of hands or mince fresh herbs before using. Combine:

¼ pound (½ cup) soft butter, partially hardened margarine, or vegetable oil
1 tablespoon chopped parsley
1 tablespoon minced chives

½ teaspoon each fresh or pinch of dried savory, marjoram, basil, or tarragon
1 minced clove garlic
¼ teaspoon paprika

Blend well, pack into a small jar, and cover; keep in refrigerator. Serve on fish, steak, chops, baked or steamed potatoes, or other vegetables; add to fat-free bouillon; use for sandwiches.

VARIATIONS:

Add any of the following: 1 tablespoon minced canned pimento, anchovy paste, or grated onion; any single minced fresh herb or any two or more herbs, omitting herbs in basic recipe.

Garlic butter: Melt butter or partially hardened margarine with 1 or 2 mashed garlic cloves; let stand 20 minutes or longer; discard the garlic. Use on toasted rye bread, steaks, or serve melted with mussels.

Lemon butter: Melt fat; omit other ingredients; add 3 tablespoons lemon juice, grated rind of ½ lemon. Serve with fish or green vegetables.

Spiced sauce: Heat 2 tablespoons fat prepared as in basic recipe; add 1 tablespoon each catsup, Worcestershire, wine vinegar or lemon juice, ½ teaspoon dry mustard. This sauce is delicious over broiled or sautéed kidneys, brains, liver, steamed heart, or any barbecued meat.

An almost endless variety of delicious sauces can be made by adding seasonings to sour cream or to thick yogurt. The sauces made with yogurt are considerably lower in calories than those prepared with cream. Serve these sauces with meat and fish aspics, cold sliced meat, chilled fish fillets, or chilled steamed vegetables. They can add much to hot-weather dinners and buffets.

SOUR-CREAM OR YOGURT SAUCE

Combine and stir well:

1 cup sour cream or thick yogurt
2 tablespoons lemon juice or vinegar
½ teaspoon grated lemon rind
(optional)
1 teaspoon salt
1 teaspoon Worcestershire

½ teaspoon dry mustard
2 to 4 tablespoons grated onion
(optional)
2 tablespoons finely chopped parsley
dash of cayenne

Serve with cold meats, fish, aspics, or chilled vegetables.

VARIATIONS:

Instead of sour cream or yogurt, whip ½ cup sweet cream no earlier than ½ hour before serving; add the seasonings of basic recipe; or whip ⅓ cup chilled evaporated milk, add seasonings and 3 tablespoons mayonnaise. For reducing diets use evaporated-milk sauce.

Add any one or more of the following: 1 minced clove garlic; 1 tablespoon minced fresh or pinch of any dry herb; ¼ cup or more chili sauce, catsup, Parmesan or other nippy grated cheese; ground mixed pickles, or sliced stuffed or diced ripe olives; 1 chopped green chili pepper; 2 to 4 tablespoons chives, capers, or minced fresh dill; 1 diced cucumber or 2 diced hard-cooked eggs with 3 tablespoons chili sauce; 1 or 2 teaspoons dry mustard, or dill or anise seeds. If anise is used, serve with fish; add 2 teaspoons caraway seeds if to be served with cold pork. The sauce is customarily given the name of the principal seasoning.

Almond sauce: Omit seasonings except salt and lemon juice; add ¼ cup slivered almonds, ½ cup finely diced unpeeled red apple, dash of nutmeg. Serve with cold fowl or lamb.

Citron-cherry sauce: Omit seasonings; add ¼ cup each finely diced citron and maraschino cherries. Serve with beef, lamb, or pork.

Lemon sauce: Use lemon juice; add grated rind of 1 lemon. Use or omit other seasonings. Serve with fish.

Mint sauce: Omit seasonings; add 4 tablespoons minced leaves of fresh mint; let stand 30 minutes. Serve with lamb, mutton, or fruit aspic.

Mustard-horseradish sauce: Use 2 teaspoons dry mustard; add 2 tablespoons freshly ground horseradish. Serve with tongue, heart, liver, kidney, cold meats, ham, or pork.

Onion sauce: Add 2 finely diced onions or leeks. Serve with fish, mutton, pork, or cold baked liver.

Pineapple-curry sauce: Omit seasonings; add ½ cup well-drained crushed pineapple, 1 to 3 teaspoons curry powder, 2 tablespoons shredded coconut. Serve with cold lamb, chilled rice, or leftover chicken.

Tartar sauce: Add to ½ cup mayonnaise or to basic recipe ½ cup ground mixed pickles, dash of Tabasco, pinch of chervil, basil, ½ teaspoon dill or anise seeds; if mayonnaise is used, dilute with 2 tablespoons tarragon vinegar. Serve with fried shrimp or other sea food.

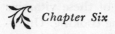

Chapter Six

Get Acquainted with Fish

The consumption of fish in America has increased rapidly. Since fish are not given hormones and tranquilizers nor fed on commercially fertilized soils covered with poison sprays, as are our meat animals, their flesh is far more wholesome as food than most of our meats. It is to be hoped that our nation will eventually become a fish-eating people. In years past, about a third of the fish caught were discarded as trash fish, though fishermen considered many of them delicious. One such fish, the monkfish, when served recently to a group of dietitians was judged to be ham. It behooves each housewife to become acquainted with many kinds of fish and to learn how to prepare them so that they will be consistently delicious.

Fish contains approximately the same amount of protein as does meat and has a comparable content of essential amino acids, or health-building qualities. All fish are rich sources of phosphorus, and ocean fish and sea foods are excellent sources of iodine; fresh-water fish often have goiters because of lack of iodine. Since fish are active and the B vitamins are necessary for energy production, their flesh is a rich source of these vitamins provided the juices are not lost before or during cooking. Unfortunately, vitamins A and D are stored almost entirely in fish liver, which is rarely eaten.

Serve fish and sea foods not only in the place of meat but in addition to it, especially when your protein requirements are high or when you serve meats or meat substitutes low in protein. Steamed fish or other sea food may be prepared in advance, kept frozen until needed, and served in salad or an appetizer on the same menu with meat.

Since the muscles of fish are tender and delicate, juices are easily lost after fish is cut or the skin removed. Much flavor is lost even during a short period of soaking. Shrimps, scallops, oysters, and other shellfish contain a sweet substance known as glycogen, which is lost readily if these foods are washed slowly, soaked, or cooked in water. Fish should be washed thoroughly but rapidly, and dried immediately. During cooking it should not be touched unnecessarily with any liquid which is not to be eaten. Salted fish which must be soaked to be edible cannot be recommended for its nutrition.

Fish cookery differs markedly from that of meat. Fish, except for roe, contains little fat, but this small amount consists almost entirely of valuable unsaturated fatty acids. Whereas well-marbled beef averages 33 per cent fat and ham 50 per cent, many fish contain only 1 per cent or less. The so-called fat fish, such as shad, mackerel, herring, and lake trout, average 7 to 10 per cent fat, and salmon alone sometimes reaches 14 per cent. Since fat is a poor conductor of heat, the lack of fat allows heat to penetrate fish more rapidly than it does meat. Furthermore, fish is usually flat in shape, with a large amount of surface through which heat can pass quickly. The cooking time of fish, therefore, is based not on pounds of weight, as it is in meat, but upon thickness.

With the exception of abalone, the connective tissue between the muscle fibers of fish is in extremely thin sheets. When submitted to heat, these thin sheets break down almost as soon as they are warm. The problem of cooking fish, therefore, is exactly opposite to that of cooking meat: the trick is to cook the proteins of the muscle fiber without allowing the connective tissue to break down. If the connective tissue of fish does break down in cooking, juices carrying vitamins, minerals, sweet glycogen, and delicious flavors are quickly lost. The fish is left dry and unappetizing.

Older recipe books mention moist fish, meaning fish which contain some fat, and dry fish, meaning lean fish. It should be clearly understood that such a thing as a dry fish does not exist. The flesh of all fresh fish contains from 65 to 80 per cent moisture. If the fish is properly cooked, these juices are held in, and the flavor and deliciousness are retained.

The juices of ocean fish and sea food contain the same amount of salt as does ocean water. Steamed shrimps, for example, which have not been overcooked or soaked before cooking, taste not only quite sweet but well salted. Fresh-water fish likewise must have salt to live. Since added salt draws out juices, flavor, and nutritive value, most fish should be salted only when it is served. When fish is rolled in flour or crumbs or dipped in batter, any of which catches juices as they are drawn out, it may be salted before being cooked. Because the cooking time is short, seasonings other than salt should be added at the beginning of cooking so that the aromatic oils may be extracted.

You can cook fish that is consistently juicy if you know the temperature at which fish proteins are cooked and the connective tissue is broken down. Fish loses its raw flavor as soon as the fiber proteins become firm, or at an internal temperature of 140° F. The proteins become progressively more firm as the heat increases.

Since the sheets of connective tissue in fish are extremely thin, they start breaking down around 150° F. If the fish is cooked beyond this internal temperature, the connective tissue breaks down rapidly. As in meat, the contracting proteins act as a hand squeezing water from a sponge, and the juices, flavor, and much nutritive value are squeezed through the broken connective tissue. The fish or sea food is robbed of flavor and left dry. To cook fish perfectly so that no juices are lost and yet all proteins are well cooked, the internal temperature should be checked with a meat thermometer whenever possible; the fish should be taken up as soon as the internal temperature reaches 145 to 150° F. Fish is most enjoyed at this degree of doneness.

There are many so-called tests for doneness: The fish is supposedly done when it curls, flakes, or comes to the surface during French frying. These are actually tests for overcooked fish after connective tissue has already broken down and juices have been lost. Since fish cooks when little more than warm, it continues to cook after it has been put on the serving platter. For this reason you should be most careful not to cook it beyond 150° F. Do not precook fish which is to be creamed, French fried, or added to casseroles.

To boil fish is nothing less than criminal treatment of good food. Not only do flavor and nutritive value quickly soak out, but the temperature is 62° F. above that at which juices are lost. For example, shrimps when boiled shrink to half their original size. Stewing likewise soaks out flavor, and it is not recommended unless the fish is stewed in sauce with which it is to be served. Even in this case, the fish is usually far more delicious if steamed above the sauce. Moist heat penetrates about twice as quickly as does the dry heat of broiling and roasting, and therefore it is extremely difficult to steam or stew fish without overcooking it.

No attempt should be made to brown fish without the aid of paprika, flour, crumbs, or batter. When fats which burn easily, such as margarine and butter, are used to coat fish before roasting or broiling, a delicate suggestion of a golden color may be attained without overcooking. Further browning causes marked deterioration of flavor. Beauty should be achieved instead through garnishes. A rich brown can be most easily obtained by sprinkling the fish generously with paprika before cooking it.

Frozen fish should be thawed slowly at room temperature and then cooked immediately. If heated while still frozen, fish becomes overcooked on the outside while the center is still chilled; the expansion of steam is so great that the fish usually falls to pieces. Since juices are invariably lost when frozen fish is thawed, use fresh fish rather than frozen whenever possible.

If the thousands of recipes for preparing fish were stripped of their seasonings, they would be reduced to four basic recipes:

broiled, baked, fried, and steamed. The seasonings are no more than sauces cooked with the fish. Time and effort can be saved by learning the basic ways of cooking fish, using the method which appeals to you, and serving the sauce you happen to enjoy. Since most fish are lean, fish sauces are usually rich in fat.

The principles and methods of cooking fish remain identical regardless of the type of fish; the same is true of shellfish. Bass and mackerel are baked the same way; trout and squid are fried alike. A fish having approximately the same size or cut in the same manner as another can be substituted in any recipe. To feel that you must have a separate recipe for each variety of fish limits your horizon. Many excellent fish for which no recipes exist have recently appeared on the market. But new recipes are not needed. If you are buying fillets, buy one from a kind of fish which is new to you. If you are making salad or creamed fish, add a small, unfamiliar fish to the familiar ones you plan to use. The ones you have not yet discovered may be far more delicious than your favorites. By such an approach, by careful cooking, and by the use of a wide variety of sauces and seasonings, monotony can be avoided indefinitely.

When you plan to serve fish, decide first whether you wish to bake, fry, broil, or cream it. Then glance through the sauces, and decide how you would like it seasoned. Prepare the sauce and cook the fish in it; or pour the sauce over the cooked fish; or serve each separately. By following such a procedure you will need no recipes except basic ones. In general, large fish are usually baked, small ones are fried, and fillets and steaks are broiled or sautéed.

In buying fish, allow ⅓ pound per person if it contains no bones and ½ pound if it is not trimmed.

Since the kinds of fish available in different parts of the country vary widely, with a few exceptions I have purposely not suggested specific types of fish with each recipe but rather the size and type of cut. Each of the following fish can be delicious when well cooked and interestingly seasoned:

FISH

anchovies	flounder	shad
barracuda	haddock	shad roe
bass, black	hake	shark
striped	halibut	skate
bloater	mackerel	smelt
bluefish	monkfish	squid
bonito	mullet	sturgeon
bream	muskellunge	sturgeon roe,
bullhead	perch	or caviar
butterhead	pickerel	sucker
carp	pike	swordfish
catfish	pompano	terrapin
cod, black	red snapper	trout, fresh-water
ling cod	salmon	sea trout
rock cod	salmon roe	tuna
yellow cod	sand dabs or sole	turbot
eel	sardine	whitefish

SHELLFISH

clams	lobster	prawns, or giant shrimp
crabs	mussels	scallops
crawfish	oysters	shrimp

How to Clean Fish

Clean fish on several layers of newspapers. If it is slimy, rinse
quickly with hot water. Use the blunt edge of a knife or a fish
scaler and remove the scales by forcing under them from tail
toward head. If the fish is to be cooked whole, leave head and
fins on and do not cut skin unnecessarily.

A fillet is a slice from which the bones have been removed. To
prepare fillets, skin the fish before cutting it open. Cut off head,
tail, and fins with kitchen shears. Use small scissors and slit skin
down the backbone and lengthwise along center of abdomen.
Start at gills and gently remove skin from head toward tail, cutting with scissors when necessary. Cut through abdominal wall

and remove organs. Wash inside of fish quickly and dry immediately. Remove bones by cutting along both sides of the backbone from the inside of the fish; loosen flesh from bones by pushing it back with dull edge of a knife. If fish is large, cut in half along backbone before removing ribs.

The ribs from any small fish to be cooked whole may be taken out by cutting them from inside the body cavity along either side of the backbone. A knife can be slipped under the ribs, cutting them free. The backbone should be left to retain the shape of the fish.

To prepare fish steaks, clean the fish, remove organs, and slice across the grain without skinning or removing bones.

To clean shrimp to be used in any way except for salad and appetizers, wash quickly and remove shells before cooking. Cut along sand vein to depth of $\frac{1}{16}$ inch. Wash out sand vein. Dry shrimp immediately.

Clean lobster and crab by washing thoroughly. Unless they are to be steamed whole and eaten chilled, cut open lengthwise and crack shells with hammer or nutcracker. Remove meat from crab claws and body; from the claws, tail, and body of the lobster. Discard intestinal vein; remove stomach and liver by holding under running water.

To remove odor of fish from hands, wash with soda or vinegar.

Fish Can Be Cooked without Odor

How many hundreds of times have you heard housewives remark, "I don't cook fish because I don't like the odor in the house"? The fact is that when fish is properly cooked, there is no odor. The substances which cause the unpleasant odor volatilize, or evaporate, at temperatures above 150° F.; fish should not be allowed to exceed this temperature. Whenever you smell fish cooking, you may be sure it is being overcooked.

On one occasion, two assistants and I prepared dozens of fish recipes in a small apartment, cooking practically every variety of fish and sea food sold on the market. During the course of the day, nine friends dropped in, and each was greeted at the door with the question, "Do you know what we are cooking?" To our delight each friend answered with a puzzled expression, "No. Why?"

If for no other reason than to prevent the escape of unpleasant odors, a meat thermometer should be used in cooking fish.

For ways of serving fish other than those listed here, see the following recipes:

Fish appetizers (p. 258)	**Fish omelet** (p. 245)
Fish salads (p. 232)	**Fish soufflé** (p. 195)
Fish chowders and bisques (p. 312)	**Fish to be served cold** (p. 222)

To bake fish means to cook it on a rack with dry heat surrounding all surfaces. If it is put on a pan or aluminum foil instead of a rack, moisture quickly collects, steams the lower part of the fish, and invariably overcooks it. To facilitate handling and lifting the fish out intact in case it overcooks, it may be laid on a thin cloth. A piece of aluminum foil may be placed under the rack to catch drippings.

When baking fish, achieve variety by using different kinds of stuffing (pp. 130, 131) and by serving it with different sauces (pp. 135–144). Since the skin prevents evaporation, small whole fish may be stuffed and baked as well as large ones. If you wish to "bake" fish in a sauce, prepare any sauce and pour it over the fish before it is put in the oven.

BAKED, STUFFED FISH

Select **any whole fish weighing 2 to 3 pounds**, such as salmon, trout, shad, mackerel, fresh tuna, or herring; or use several small fish.

Clean the whole fish without removing tail, fins, and head. Let the fish reach room temperature. Stuff with **rice, mushroom, eggplant, celery, or onion dressing** (p. 131), preferably still hot.

To facilitate lifting cooked fish onto platter, place on a cloth and put on a wire rack over foil-covered baking dish; set fish with its back up. Insert a meat thermometer into thick flesh behind gills; brush with **vegetable oil.** *Do not salt.*

Set in preheated, slow oven at 300° F. Allow approximately 20 minutes for heat to penetrate fish 1 inch thick, 30 minutes for fish 2 inches thick, 35 minutes for fish 3 inches thick; take fish from oven when the internal thermometer reading is 145 to 150° F.

Lift fish to serving platter by rolling from cloth; garnish with **sprigs of parsley and lemon sections.**

Serve with caper sauce p. (136), dill sauce (p. 137), **or herb** butter (p. 142).

VARIATIONS:

If the stuffing is cold when fish is put into the oven, insert a meat thermometer in the stuffing and cook to 140° F.

Tie a string from head to tail of fish to hold it in a semicircle, or fasten with skewers in the shape of an **S.**

Baked fillets of fish: Select fillets from **halibut, red snapper, trout, or other fish.** Insert a thermometer into one fillet. Brush or spread with **herb-seasoned butter or vegetable oil;** lay on a wire rack, not on a pan; sprinkle generously with **paprika.** Bake as in basic recipe. Serve with olive sauce.

Browned fillets: Dip fillets in **milk and wheat germ or sifted whole-wheat-bread crumbs;** insert thermometer, lay fish on rack, brush with **vegetable oil,** and sprinkle with **crushed dill seeds and paprika;** bake as in basic recipe. Serve with Hollandaise sauce (p. 138).

Fillets baked with barbecue sauce: Dip the fillets in any **tomato sauce,** such as barbecue, Spanish, or Italian sauce, or in **catsup;** roll in **wheat germ or sifted crumbs** and lay on rack; insert the meat thermometer, dot with **butter or partially hardened margarine;** sprinkle generously with **paprika** and bake as in basic recipe. Serve with barbecue, Spanish, or Italian sauce.

Stuffed fillets: For guest dinners, select 2 matching fillets weighing about 1½ pounds each; spread one with **onion or celery dressing** (p. 131) **or crumb stuffing** (p. 129), lay the other fillet on top. Lace sides together with string and poultry skewers, insert thermometer into fillet; brush with **vegetable oil,** sprinkle generously with **paprika,** and bake. Serve with hot cheese sauce (p. 136). To serve only four persons, select thick fillet, such as halibut; cut pocket in side for dressing; or stuff matching sand dabs.

FISH "BAKED" IN SAUCE

Clean **2 or 3 pounds fish,** using 1 large fish, several small ones, or fish fillets or steaks; stuff whole fish if desired.

Prepare in a heat-resistant baking dish **2 cups medium cream sauce** seasoned with **capers, cheese, dill, mushrooms,** or **other seasoning** (p. 135). Set fish in sauce.

Insert meat thermometer in the center of a steak or fillet or into thick muscles behind gills of whole fish, placing thermometer near the edge of utensil; dip sauce over fish.

Sprinkle over the top of fish:

¼ cup wheat germ or toasted   **generous amount of paprika**
whole-wheat-bread crumbs

Put into a preheated slow oven at 300° F. Allow approximately 10 minutes for heat to penetrate fish or fillets 1 inch thick, 15 minutes for fish 2 inches thick, 20 minutes for fish 3 inches thick. Check thermometer reading frequently. Remove from oven as soon as internal temperature reaches 145 to 150° F.

Garnish with **sprigs of parsley and lemon wedges.**

VARIATIONS:

Instead of cream sauce use any sauce with a sour-cream base (p. 143).

If sauce is cold when fish is put into the oven, double the baking time.

Instead of cream sauce use any tomato sauce, such as barbecue, chili, Spanish, or Italian sauce (p. 140).

Baked fillets with pickles and onions: Brush a shallow baking dish with **vegetable oil** and put in a layer of thinly sliced **onions or leeks,** a layer of sliced **dill pickles,** then the fish fillets; omit sauce; put slices of **lemon** on top, sprinkle with **paprika;** bake as in basic recipe, allowing 20 minutes for fillets 1 inch thick. Vary by sprinkling fish with **dill or anise seeds.**

Baked fish with mushrooms: Sauté in utensil to be used for baking **1 cup chopped mushrooms** and **2 tablespoons onions;** add the fish and **½ cup sauterne or sherry.** Bake as in basic recipe.

Baked fish with oysters: Put a layer of **uncooked fish fillets** in bottom of a baking dish brushed with **vegetable oil;** add layer of **fresh oysters,** grated **onion,** chopped **parsley, salt,** and **paprika;** repeat until dish is filled; dot the top with **partially hardened margarine** and sprinkle with **wheat germ and** paprika; insert a meat thermometer in the center of dish; bake in moderate oven at 350° F. for about 40 minutes, or until internal temperature is 145 to 150° F.

Baked roe: Select shad or other roe; wash and dry, being careful not to break membrane. Dip in **milk,** roll in wheat germ, place on a flat baking dish, insert a meat thermometer, and bake to 150° F., or about 30 minutes. Cover with a sauce a few minutes before taking from oven; sprinkle with **parsley.**

Fish with fried rice: Prepare **fried rice** (p. 191) in a heat-resistant baking dish; when rice is almost tender, cover the top with **fillets** about 1 inch thick; insert a meat thermometer; dot the fish with **partially hardened margarine,** sprinkle with **paprika,** and bake as in basic recipe. Serve with tossed salad (p. 266).

Broiling is one of the easiest and most successful methods of cooking fish. As a rule, the fish should not be more than 1½ inches thick; as long as this qualification is met, any fish can be broiled. Small fish, such as fresh-water trout, may be stuffed and broiled whole. Larger fish should be cut in half along the backbone or sliced into steaks or fillets of serving sizes.

Fish to be broiled successfully should be set on a wire rack. If it is put on a baking sheet or pan, the utensil becomes hot; juices collect and change to steam which penetrates quickly; overcooking can scarcely be prevented. If you wish to cook the fish in a low baking dish, broil only the top surface; do not turn it.

BROILED FISH

Select steaks or fillets not more than 1½ inches thick; unless the steaks are to be rolled in crumbs, do not remove skin. Leave small fish whole.

Carefully punch a hole for the meat thermometer in thickest part of the flesh. If whole fish are being broiled, insert thermometer into flesh behind gills. Move thermometer about to make sure it does not touch bone. Set fish on broiler rack.

Brush fish with **vegetable oil;** *do not salt;* sprinkle generously with paprika.

If using gas heat, set broiler pan on top ledge so that fish is about 1 inch from heat; keep the flames very small. If using electricity, set about 5 inches from heating unit. *Leave the broiler door open.*

Use pancake turner and turn fish after 8 to 10 minutes, or when half the thickness has become opaque. Read the thermometer frequently and take up the fish as soon as 145 to 150° F. is reached. Allow 15 minutes for cooking fish 1 inch thick, 18 minutes if 1½ inches thick.

Garnish with **chopped parsley.** Serve with herb butter seasoned with fresh dill, tarragon, and chives (p. 142), or with lemon butter (p. 142), or sauce of sour cream (p. 143).

VARIATIONS:

If a browned crust is desired, dip in milk or 1 egg stirred with 2 tablespoons fresh milk and then in sifted whole-wheat-bread crumbs, wheat germ, whole-wheat flour, or yellow cornmeal; sprinkle with paprika.

If egg or milk is used, season with freshly ground peppercorns and a pinch of sage, tarragon, fennel, thyme, or basil; or add 1 teaspoon dry mustard, paprika, minced fresh herbs, or crushed anise.

Broiled lobster: Drop the whole lobster into rapidly boiling water; boil 2 minutes, allow to simmer 10 minutes longer. Remove from water, split, clean (p. 151); crack claws. Dot with **partially hardened margarine or butter,** sprinkle with **browned crumbs and paprika.** Broil under low heat 8 to 10 minutes. Vary by filling cavity before broiling with **creamed lobster** (p. 164) prepared from the claws; or after broiling place a lettuce leaf in cavity and top with sliced lemon.

Broiled roe: Choose **shad, bass, barracuda, or other roe** with membrane unbroken; roll in **vegetable oil and wheat germ.** Broil on a baking sheet about 20 minutes on one side, or to an internal temperature of 150° F. *Do not turn.* Serve with melted butter or partially hardened margarine to which lemon juice, chives, and ground parsley are added.

Broiled scallops: Place 4 to 7 scallops on each of 4 skewers; brush with **vegetable oil or partially hardened margarine,** sprinkle with paprika; broil 3 to 4 minutes on each side. Serve with dill sauce (p. 137). Alternate scallops with mushroom caps if desired.

Broiled shrimps: Shell whole shrimps, leaving tails on. Dust with **whole-wheat flour and paprika;** set on oiled baking sheet and broil under low heat 4 or 5 minutes without turning. Serve with melted margarine or butter to which is added 1 minced clove garlic and finely chopped parsley. If large prawns are used, pierce one with a meat thermometer and serve as soon as temperature reaches 140° F.

Fish with herbs: If fish steaks or fillets are to be held several hours before cooking, sprinkle surfaces with **minced fresh dill or tarragon or crushed anise or dill seeds;** pile steaks or fillets on top of each other so that seasonings can penetrate from both surfaces. Broil as in basic recipe.

Seasoned broiled fish steaks or fillets: Spread surfaces of uncooked fish with **mayonnaise.** Broil with or without rolling in **wheat germ, crumbs, or flour.** Vary by sprinkling with **shredded nippy cheese or Parmesan cheese** 3 minutes before taking from broiler.

Nutritionally, little can be said for deep-fat frying as a method of cooking. Aside from supplying more calories than most people can use, fish cooked by this method is almost invariably dried out. The fat is often overheated to the point that cancer-producing substances may be formed. Furthermore, a high temperature causes any vitamin E in the fat to be destroyed, brings about changes in the unsaturated fatty acids similar to rancidity, and can harm the vitamins A, E, and several B vitamins in the food being cooked. The solid fats customarily used for deep frying may elevate the blood cholesterol.

Except for the excess of calories, the disadvantages can be largely overcome by watching both the temperature of the cooking fat, which should never be allowed to go above 360° F., and the internal temperature of the fish, which should be kept between 145° and 160° F.; and by using deep vegetable oil to which is added every time it is used the contents of a 100-unit capsule of vitamin E. If the vitamin E is not added each time, the vegetable oil oxidizes and an unpleasant rancid odor and flavor can be detected after it has been heated only once. Such oil is dangerous to use again, and should be discarded.

Until you have used a meat thermometer when French-frying fish, you can hardly believe how delicious the fish can be or how quickly it can cook. For example, jumbo shrimps require only 1 minute in fat at 360° F. to reach the internal temperature of 140° F., and continue to heat to 160° F. before they begin to cool. Shrimps fried 2 minutes at 360° F. are only half the size of those cooked 1 minute, and are not nearly as delicious. After fish or sea food is removed from the fat, the piping-hot crust causes cooking to continue until the crust has cooled. The cooking time of fried fish, therefore, must not be thought of as the time it is immersed in fat; instead, the fish cooks from the time it is put into the hot oil until it is actually cooled.

Cold fish put into heated fat lowers the temperature of the oil from 100° to 200° F. In order not to cool the fat so much that the fish overcooks before the crust can become delightfully brown, only a small amount of fish or sea food should be browned at one time.

The problem of crust flaking off during the cooking can be prevented by dipping the fish or sea food in wheat germ or crumbs and letting the crust dry before browning. Restaurants which specialize in sea foods often dip their fish several hours before time to fry them. The crust will also have less tendency to flake off if powdered milk is used in the batter.

BATTER FOR FRENCH-FRIED FOODS

Sift together:

⅓ cup whole-wheat-pastry flour   1 teaspoon salt
¼ cup powdered milk

Add and stir well:

¼ cup fresh milk   1 egg

Dip fish or sea food in batter; set on aluminum foil and let dry 10 minutes or longer. Place only enough for one serving in wire basket at a time. Fry in deep **vegetable oil** at 360° F. Repeat procedure.

VARIATIONS:

If especially light batter is desired, beat egg white until stiff and fold in.

Vary batter by adding any of the following seasonings: 1 teaspoon crushed dill, anise, or celery seeds or minced fresh basil or dill.

FRENCH-FRIED FISH

Use cod, flounder, lake haddock, barracuda, red snapper, halibut, or other fish.

Clean and trim fish, removing skin and bones; cut into sticks or serving sizes not more than 1 inch thick.

Dip in batter or shake in a paper bag containing:

½ cup wheat germ or	1 tablespoon powdered milk
¾ cup sifted whole-wheat-bread crumbs	1 teaspoon salt

Let dry 10 minutes or longer.

Heat 3 cups or more vegetable oil in pan used for French frying; fasten cooking thermometer to side of utensil. Drop contents of capsule containing 100 units of vitamin E into the fat to prevent oxidation or rancidity. Set basket in fat to heat and put meat thermometer into 1 piece of fish; when fat reaches 360° F., place 1 to 3 pieces of fish (one pierced by thermometer) in basket, lower into hot fat and brown; take up when internal temperature reaches 145 to 160° F. Drain fish on paper towels and keep in a warm place.

Reheat fat to 360° F. and continue frying until the remainder of fish is browned.

If 100 units of the vitamin have been added for each quart of oil, cool oil, pour into bottle, and refrigerate; use for general cooking or deep frying. If no vitamin E has been added, discard oil.

Garnish the platter with parsley and pickled beets. Serve fish with caper or horseradish sauce with sour-cream of yogurt base (p. 143) or with uncooked creole sauce (p. 141).

VARIATIONS:

Dip fish in 1 egg stirred with 2 tablespoons fresh milk, 1 tablespoon powdered milk, 1 teaspoon salt; roll in wheat germ, whole-wheat flour, or sifted bread crumbs.

Shrimp: If fresh shrimp are used, *do not precook before frying;* remove the shells and sand veins (p. 151); dry quickly, dip in batter seasoned with 1 teaspoon dill or anise seeds. Fry as in basic recipe; allow them to be in the hot oil only 1 minute. Serve with chili sauce; mix dry mustard with a little water and put 1 teaspoon in center of each serving of sauce.

Mock scallops: Use halibut fillets or fillets of other white-fleshed fish; cut into 1¼-inch cubes; dip in batter seasoned with dill, adding 1 teaspoon sugar. Fry 1 minute as in basic recipe.

Scallops: Dip in batter. Fry 1 minute as in basic recipe or in shallow fat.

Fish croquettes: Add 2 cups of any steamed and flaked or leftover fish to ½ cup thick cream sauce (p. 135) seasoned with 1 or 2 tablespoons capers or 1 teaspoon dill or anise seeds; add ½ teaspoon each salt, Worcestershire, and paprika, 1 tablespoon grated onion, 1 egg. Stir well, mold into croquettes, roll in wheat germ, and fry as in basic recipe 1 to 2 minutes. Vary by adding ½ cup shredded American cheese. Do not miss this recipe; these are delicious croquettes. Well-drained canned salmon or tuna can be used.

Potato-fish croquettes: Use ½ to 1 cup leftover mashed potatoes instead of cream sauce. Vary by adding 2 tablespoons chili sauce as well as the seasonings in fish croquettes.

Only small fish which are to be cooked whole, such as mackerel, smelt, squid, and fresh-water bass or trout, should be fried rather than sautéed. In order that all contours of the fish may be evenly browned, the fat used should be the depth of half the thickness of the fish. Although butter browns easily and gives a delicious flavor it usually causes fish to stick; partially hardened margarine has proved more satisfactory. As in deep-fat frying, cooking continues as long as the fish is warm. The fat should be hot before the fish is put into it, and the fish should be taken up the minute it is delicately golden.

FRIED FISH

Clean **2 pounds or more small whole fish.** Mix well and use for dredging fish:

¼ cup whole-wheat flour or yellow   1 teaspoon salt
corn meal

Heat:

½ cup or more vegetable oil or partially hardened margarine

Lay fish in hot fat; turn as soon as golden, or in 2 to 5 minutes; brown the other side; *do not cover utensil;* take up immediately after both sides are browned.

Serve with caper or dill sauce (pp. 136, 137).

VARIATIONS:

Dredge in ½ cup wheat germ or sifted whole-wheat-bread crumbs.

Fried skate and roe: Fry fish as in basic recipe; fry roe more slowly, cooking 10 to 12 minutes, or to 160° F. Serve with vinegar sauce (p. 139) or lemon butter (p. 142) poured over fish.

Stuffed squid: Choose small squid 5 to 6 inches long; remove tentacles and bone, or shell, from inside of back; stuff with **crumb dressing** (p. 129) and fry as in basic recipe.

Fish which has a flat surface, such as fish steaks and fillets, should be sautéed, or cooked by easily controlled direct heat, rather than fried. When the slices are sufficiently thick, use a thermometer and take up the fish when the internal temperature is 145 to 160°F.

SAUTÉED FISH

Select 4 **fish steaks or fillets,** such as bonito, cod, halibut, barracuda, shark; roll in **wheat germ,** dip in **batter** (p. 158), or shake in a paper bag containing:

¼ cup whole-wheat flour or yellow corn meal or ½ cup sifted whole-wheat-bread crumbs	1 tablespoon powdered milk freshly ground white peppercorns 1 teaspoon fresh basil, tarragon, or
1 teaspoon salt	dill

Insert the meat thermometer in the center of one serving parallel to surface.

Heat grill and brush with **vegetable oil;** set fish on grill; *do not cover at any time.*

Turn fish as soon as the undersurface is golden brown; take it up when the thermometer reading is 145 to 160° F. or when fish has cooked 8 to 10 minutes.

Sprinkle with lemon juice and garnish with parsley.

VARIATIONS:

As soon as fish is taken up, heat in same utensil 3 tablespoons each lemon juice or vinegar, water, and chives; pour over fish.

With almond sauce: Set fish on platter and heat in same utensil 2 **tablespoons each partially hardened margarine or butter, lemon juice, and soy sauce; add ½ cup slivered almonds.** Pour sauce over fish. This is an especially nice way to serve sand dabs.

Although there is much danger of overcooking when fish is steamed, the method is preferable to baking if time is limited. Steamed fish should be cooked with the utmost care and the time closely checked. To prevent loss of flavor and sweetness, the fish should be set on a rack so that water cannot soak out the juices. Since the penetration of moist heat is extremely rapid, the internal temperature should be checked with a meat thermometer.

If the oven is in use, fish may be steamed in an ordinary paper bag in the oven. The thermometer should be inserted and the bag closed with string or paper clips in such a way that thermometer readings may be taken. The dead-air space inside the bag acts as an insulator and causes the temperature to be from 50° to 75° F. below that of the oven; the fish is steamed slowly and stays delightfully moist and juicy.

STEAMED FISH

If the fish is more than 2 inches thick, cut in half along the backbone or into slices of uniform thickness.

Put into a utensil below rack:

½ cup water

Insert a meat thermometer in a piece of fish; as soon as water boils, put fish on rack, cover utensil, and note the time.

If fish is 1 inch thick, steam no longer than 3 to 4 minutes; if 2 inches thick, steam 6 to 8 minutes. Add 2 to 3 minutes if fish is chilled.

Check internal temperature near end of cooking time; remove from steam immediately when internal temperature reaches 145 to 160° F. Sprinkle with paprika and chopped parsley.

Serve with olive sauce (p. 137) or tartar sauce (p. 144).

VARIATIONS:

If fish is to be used for appetizers (p. 258) and salads (p. 232), remove skin and bones after steaming, and separate into flakes.

Use leftover steamed fish for making patties (p. 168), creamed dishes (p. 164), or casseroles (p. 165).

Fish steamed in a paper bag: Put fish fillets, steaks, or whole fish on 2 or more paper towels. Season fish with **fresh basil, fennel, dill, or thin slices of lemon, onion, or dill pickle.** *Do not salt.* Insert a meat thermometer; slip the fish into an ordinary paper bag, fold over the opening and fasten with string so that the thermometer extends and may be read easily. Put in a preheated oven. Remove when internal temperature reaches 145 to 160° F. Serve with any sauce or lemon butter (p. 142). Whole fish for salads and appetizers may be steamed in this manner.

Steamed fillets: Cut fillets into serving sizes and steam as in basic recipe. Serve with Hollandaise sauce, tartar sauce, or any sauce having a cream-sauce base. Any cream sauce can be prepared in same utensil to be used for steaming fish; set rack over the sauce, cover utensil, and steam the fish as in basic recipe. Serve cream sauce over the fish.

Steamed lobster, crabs, or crawfish: Wash thoroughly and steam as in basic recipe; cook crawfish 5 to 6 minutes, crabs 8 to 10 minutes, and lobster 10 to 12 minutes. Shellfish will continue cooking as they cool. Split in half, clean, and serve with lemon butter (p. 142) or tartar sauce (p. 144).

Steamed shrimp, clams, and mussels: Wash thoroughly, but do not remove shells; put on a rack over boiling water, cover utensil, and steam no longer than 2 minutes; remove from heat and take off lid of utensil to let steam escape; cover utensil again and let stand 3 to 4 minutes to cook from heat inside shells. Use steamed shrimp for salads or appetizers; serve clams and mussels hot with lemon butter or garlic butter (p. 142).

Although creamed dishes and casseroles may be prepared with leftover or canned fish or sea food, a far more delightful flavor can be gained by making these dishes with uncooked fish or sea food. When the uncooked fish or sea food is diced, it should be added to the hot cream sauce or casserole dish only 3 minutes before serving. Fish should not be heated above 160° F.; simmering liquid can quickly overcook it. Any cream sauces or brown sauces may be used in preparing creamed fish and fish casseroles.

A friend who attempted to prepare the following recipe felt sure that the uncooked diced fish would be raw if not heated longer than 3 minutes; therefore she allowed the cream sauce to boil a minute or two after the fish was added. The diced fish contracted into tiny tough lumps and the fish juices diluted the sauce into a thin soup. If you are skeptical about the cooking time, pierce a small cube of fillet with a meat thermometer, making sure the mercury is in the exact center. Serve the creamed fish when the temperature reaches 140° F. The temperature will continue to rise to 160° F. or more before it is served. It is hard to realize how quickly fish can overcook until you have checked the temperature with a thermometer.

CREAMED FISH WITH DILL

Prepare **2 cups dill sauce** (p. 137), using thick cream sauce as the base.

No more than 3 minutes before serving, add to the simmering sauce:

2½ cups diced uncooked fish fillets   **1 teaspoon salt**

Reheat sauce to simmering; *do not boil.*
Garnish lightly with chopped parsley.

VARIATIONS:

Pour hot creamed fish into scallop shells; sprinkle top with wheat germ, Parmesan cheese, and paprika. Set on baking sheet and brown under broiler.

Instead of fresh fish use flaked leftover or canned fish. Salt to taste.

Take from their shells uncooked shrimp or oysters, or use quickly steamed crab, lobster, clams, or mussels; add to dill sauce, dicing crab or lobster into 1-inch cubes. If canned shellfish is used, substitute the liquid for part of the milk in the sauce.

Omit dill from sauce and add 1 or 2 teaspoons anise seeds.

Omit cream sauce; add chilled steamed fish or seafood to 2 cups sour-cream or yogurt sauce; season with dill, anise, or capers, and paprika.

Add fish or shellfish to any cream sauce or brown sauce (p. 136) such as caper, celery, cheese, curry, mock Hollandaise, or hot tartar sauce.

Prepare the sauce in a heat-resistant casserole; add fish, wipe edges of casserole, and sprinkle the top with wheat germ, grated cheese, and paprika. Brown under broiler.

Casserole with potato chips: Prepare sauce in a heat-resistant casserole; add diced fillets or canned tuna and small package potato chips; sprinkle with wheat germ and paprika and brown surface under the broiler. Vary by combining 1 can condensed mushroom soup, potato chips, and diced fillets or flaked tuna; omit salt; heat in a moderate oven 30 minutes.

Curried shrimp: Prepare as chicken curry (p. 74), adding 2 to 3 pounds uncooked, shelled shrimps no earlier than 3 minutes before serving. If jumbo shrimps are used, pierce one with meat thermometer and serve shrimps when internal temperature is 140° F. This dish is food for the gods.

In making fish casseroles, vegetables may be quickly cooked, a sauce prepared in the same utensil, and the fish or sea food added. By varying the kinds of fish, sea foods, sauces, and vegetables, an unlimited number of casserole dishes can be prepared. Follow this procedure and create your own recipes.

FISH IN CASSEROLE

Use a heat-resistant casserole or baking dish and sauté lightly in 3 tablespoons partially hardened margarine or vegetable oil:

1 cup finely diced carrots   1 tablespoon chopped onion
1 chopped bell pepper

Add and mix well:

1½ teaspoons salt   ¼ teaspoon crushed white pepper-
3 tablespoons whole-wheat flour   corns

Stir in slowly:

1½ cups canned or diced fresh to- ½ cup chili sauce
matoes

Cook until slightly thick and lay across the top:

1½ pounds fresh fillets, fish steaks, or small whole fish

Insert meat thermometer in the center of steak or fillet or in the flesh behind gills of whole fish.

Sprinkle top with **wheat germ or whole-wheat-bread crumbs, paprika,** and dots of **partially hardened margarine.**

Put in the oven at 325° F. and bake about 12 minutes, or until the internal temperature of fish reaches 145 to 150° F.

VARIATIONS:

Add diced uncooked fish fillets or flaked steamed or leftover fish to boiling tomato sauce 5 minutes before serving; wipe edges of casserole, sprinkle top with Parmesan cheese and wheat germ. Brown under broiler. Vary by using fresh or canned shellfish.

Sauté with other vegetables ½ cup fresh or canned mushrooms or chopped celery.

Add a pinch of basil, tarragon, dill, or fennel, or 1 teaspoon dill or anise seeds.

Sauté vegetables and prepare 2 cups any cream sauce, brown sauce (p. 136), or tomato sauce (p. 140); add diced fish or shellfish or cover with fresh fish, and bake as in basic recipe. Vary by adding peas, string beans, cauliflower, potatoes, leeks, or other vegetables.

Add any diced leftover vegetables to casserole before adding fish.

Fish or sea food in rice casserole: Prepare **fried rice** (p. 191) in a heat-resistant casserole, using ½ cup uncooked rice; when rice is tender, stir in 1 teaspoon salt, 2 cups uncooked diced fish fillets or fresh or canned crabmeat, lobster, clams, oysters, or shrimp. Sprinkle with **wheat germ or whole-wheat-bread crumbs** and brown under broiler.

Fish or sea food with eggplant: Prepare **eggplant creole** (p. 340) in a heat-resistant casserole; 3 or 4 minutes before serving stir in 2 tablespoons chopped parsley, 1 teaspoon salt, 2 cups diced uncooked, steamed, or canned shrimp, clams, oysters, lobster, or crab, diced uncooked fillets, or flaked steamed or leftover fish. Cover with wheat germ or buttered crumbs; brown under broiler.

Fish or sea food in corn and tomato casserole: Prepare as in basic recipe, omitting carrots; when sauce is thick, add a **No. 2 can of corn,** 1 teaspoon salt, 2 or 3 cups diced uncooked or canned shrimp, crab, lobster, or other shellfish, diced fish fillets, or flaked leftover fish; heat to simmering, sprinkle top with **wheat germ or buttered crumbs.** Brown under broiler.

Fish or sea food with mixed-vegetable casserole: Combine and simmer 8 minutes in a casserole with 2 tablespoons partially hardened **margarine or butter, 1 cup each shredded unpeeled carrots and pota-**

toes, 1 grated onion, 1 finely chopped pimento, 2 tablespoons chopped parsley; 3 minutes before serving add 1 teaspoon salt and 2 cups diced uncooked or canned shrimp or other sea food, fish fillets, or flaked, canned, or leftover fish. Top with wheat germ, Parmesan cheese; brown under broiler.

SEA FOOD NEWBURG

Sauté 2 or 3 minutes in ¼ cup partially hardened margarine, butter, or oil:

   1 to 2 cups fresh mushrooms (optional)

Add and heat, stirring constantly:

¾ cup fresh or reconstituted milk   3 cups sea food or diced, uncooked
¾ teaspoon salt   fish fillets
dash cayenne and nutmeg

When sea food is hot, add and stir thoroughly:

3 beaten egg yolks   3 tablespoons sherry

As soon as eggs begin to thicken, serve in a nest of brown or converted rice into which has been mixed ¼ cup chopped parsley. Sprinkle with paprika and garnish with sprigs of parsley.

VARIATIONS:

Use whole raw, frozen, or drained canned oysters or shrimp; Eastern scallops; diced steamed whole lobster or fresh or frozen lobster tails; steamed or canned crab; uncooked fresh or frozen halibut or other white fish fillet; or leftover steamed fish.

If canned sea food is used, drain ¾ cup liquid and blend into it ⅓ cup instant powdered milk; use instead of fresh milk.

Brains Newburg: Steam brains until quite firm; chill, dice into 1-inch cubes, and proceed as in basic recipe.

Lobster Newburg: If steamed lobster tails are used, dice meat into 1-inch cubes. Garnish rice with ends of tails and sprigs of parsley.

Shrimp Newburg: Use fresh shrimps when available; shell and add without precooking. If canned shrimps are used, instead of milk add liquid from shrimps mixed with ⅓ cup instant powdered milk.

Sweetbreads Newburg: Dice uncooked sweetbreads into 1-inch cubes or pull into bite sizes; sauté gently for 10 minutes before adding mushrooms; or use diced steamed sweetbreads and proceed as in basic recipe.

FISH LOAF

Mix together:

2 cups diced uncooked fish or 1½ cups flaked steamed or canned fish
¼ cup powdered milk
2 tablespoons chopped parsley
1 grated onion

1 chopped pimento
1½ teaspoons salt
dash of cayenne
freshly ground white peppercorns
2 eggs
½ cup fresh milk

Pack in a shallow baking dish brushed with **vegetable oil** and sprinkle with **wheat germ or whole-wheat-bread crumbs.**

Bake in a moderate oven at 350° F. for 35 to 40 minutes; test the center with meat thermometer; serve when internal temperature reaches 150° F.

VARIATIONS:

Add ¼ to ½ cup wheat germ to other ingredients of loaf.

Add any leftover vegetables, such as peas or diced carrots, potatoes, string beans, or shredded uncooked carrots.

Omit onion and pimento and add 1 teaspoon dill or anise seeds or 2 tablespoons minced fresh dill or fennel.

With the exception of canned salmon, few varieties of fish are customarily used in making patties. Actually any steamed, canned, or flaked fish may be used. Patties of leftover fish may be prepared for sautéing, then wrapped, frozen, and kept for a hurry-up dinner.

FISH PATTIES

Mix thoroughly:

1 slightly beaten egg
½ teaspoon salt
1 teaspoon mashed dill seeds

¼ cup wheat germ
1 to 2 cups flaked canned, steamed, or leftover fish

Form into patties. Roll in **wheat germ** and sauté slowly about 8 minutes on each side. Serve with lemon wedges.

VARIATIONS:

Add ¼ cup powdered milk.

Omit dill seeds and season with 1 teaspoon anise seed or ⅛ teaspoon basil or crushed rosemary.

Add 1 grated onion, 1 diced pimento, 2 tablespoons finely chopped bell pepper or celery, or ½ to 1 cup shredded Cheddar cheese.

If canned tuna is made into patties, drain oil and use for sautéing.

It seems strange to me that a sea food so expensive as crab is the only one customarily served highly seasoned, or deviled. Many varieties of fresh, canned, or leftover flaked fish may be improved by such seasoning, whereas crab, although delicious when deviled, needs little or no improving.

If you wish to keep a few cans of crabmeat, tuna, or other sea food on hand, you can delight unexpected guests in a few minutes by preparing the following recipe.

DEVILED SEA FOOD

Combine, stir well, and heat to simmering:

½ cup milk or cream	¼ teaspoon thyme (optional)
1 grated onion	2 tablespoons sherry or white wine
1 teaspoon salt	(optional)
2 teaspoons Worcestershire	1½ cups sea food
generous dash cayenne	½ cup wheat germ

After removing from heat, stir in **1 teaspoon dry mustard**. Put into scallop shells or heated ramekins and set in flat baking pan over ¼ inch of hot water. Sprinkle with:

wheat germ	paprika
Parmesan cheese (optional)	

Brown under broiler and serve immediately.

VARIATIONS:

If more convenient, omit initial heating; prepare recipe in advance and bake at 350° F. for 10 to 15 minutes, or just long enough to heat through.

Sauté lightly before adding milk ¼ cup each finely chopped celery and bell pepper; or add 1 or 2 pimentos.

Use fresh, frozen, or canned crabmeat; shelled, uncooked and diced or drained canned shrimps; any flaked steamed or leftover white fish; or flaked canned tuna. Add finely chopped celery and bell pepper to leftover fish and canned tuna.

Just before putting into shells or ramekins, stir in ¼ cup instant tiger's milk (p. 447).

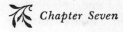 *Chapter Seven*

Meat Substitutes and Extenders for
Limited Budgets

Most of the so-called meat substitutes, such as dry beans, peas, rice, and macaroni, are actually not substitutes for meat. They supply only about 4 to 6 grams of protein per serving, compared with an average of 18 to 20 grams in a serving of meat or fish. The proteins they contain lack several essential amino acids and hence do not have the health-building value of meats, fish, eggs, or milk. Generous amounts of meat, cheese, or other adequate proteins should be added to these so-called "meat substitutes" whenever possible. It is difficult, however, to add sufficient protein to make them nutritionally equivalent to meat. When you serve these foods, plan your menus to include other sources of protein, such as fish or glandular-meat appetizers; meat, fish, cheese, or eggs added to the salad; high-protein bread; or perhaps a dessert made of milk and eggs.

The one exception among legumes which is a true meat substitute is soybeans. They cannot be made to taste identical with the usual variety of beans, but can be delicious when well prepared. Soybeans differ from other beans in that they contain about three times more protein, a small amount of sugar, and no starch. They supply essential amino acids, calcium, and B vitamins. Whether the budget is limited or not, they can be served frequently to nutritional advantage.

171

If soybeans are frozen after they have soaked and before they are cooked, the cooking time is decreased about 2 hours and they taste more like navy beans. Since soybeans are relatively new to Americans, seasonings should be heavily relied upon to make them palatable. There are now available dried green soybeans which many housewives have found to be more delicious than other varieties and which cook in a somewhat shorter time. One must not expect any soybeans, however, to taste like navy beans.

A satisfactory means of working soybeans into your menus is by using soy grits, in which each raw bean is broken into 8 or 10 pieces. They are inexpensive and bland in flavor, cook in a few minutes, and can be added to any number of foods without altering the taste. They can be substituted for cooked soybeans; thus the long cooking is avoided and the seasonings are more evenly distributed. Precooked soy grits are available, but those quickly cooked at home probably retain greater nutritive value.

COOKED SOYBEANS

If convenient, soak in an ice tray 2 hours or longer in 2 cups water:

1½ cups dry soybeans

Place in freezing compartment and freeze until solid, preferably overnight. Remove from refrigerator and drop into:

1 cup hot soup stock or vegetable-cooking water

Cover utensil and simmer 2½ to 4 hours; add more soup stock or water if needed. When nearly tender, add:

½ teaspoon crushed black peppercorns
2 teaspoons salt
2 tablespoons vegetable oil
1 or 2 minced cloves garlic
1 chopped onion

½ to 1 cup tomato purée or 2 to 4 tablespoons catsup or chili sauce
1 tablespoon Worcestershire
1 bay leaf

Continue cooking until tender; remove lid of utensil, allowing excess liquid to evaporate; add:

2 to 4 tablespoons chopped parsley

Serve either hot or cold.

VARIATIONS:

Soak beans overnight without freezing; simmer 4 to 5 hours in water used for soaking. Or omit soaking and cook until tender.

Pass cooked soybeans through meat grinder and substitute for meat in making meat loaf (p. 108) or patties (p. 111); add 2 teaspoons meat extract before salting; use tomato purée or catsup for liquid in loaf; omit liquid from patties. Soybean loaf and patties are surprisingly good.

Instead of soybeans use 1½ cups or less uncooked soy grits; add 1½ cups boiling stock or vegetable-cooking water and the seasonings of basic recipe or any variation; simmer 10 to 15 minutes.

Add any of the following groups of seasonings to cooked soybeans about 15 minutes before serving or to uncooked soy grits; prepare soy grits as directed above.

"Baked" soybeans: 2 to 4 tablespoons dark molasses; if needed, increase heat to evaporate moisture until consistency is that of baked beans. Stir in 1 tablespoon dry mustard and 2 chopped onions 5 minutes before serving.

Chinese soybeans: ¼ cup dark molasses, 2 chopped onions, 1 teaspoon powdered ginger or 3 tablespoons diced preserved or candied ginger, 1 diced apple, 2 tablespoons soy sauce; salt to taste after soy sauce is added; serve while apple and onion are still crisp.

Creamed soybeans: 2 diced pimentos, 2 finely diced carrots, 3 tablespoons chopped parsley, pinch of basil, 1 cup or more undiluted evaporated milk; evaporate moisture before adding milk; sprinkle generously with Parmesan cheese.

Savory soybeans: 2 finely diced carrots, 2 chopped onions, 1 diced stalk celery; pinch each of rosemary, savory, marjoram.

Spanish-style soybeans: 2 chopped fresh chili peppers or bell peppers with 1 or 2 teaspoons chili powder, ¼ cup tomato catsup, 1 or 2 chopped onions, ½ cup shredded American, Jack, or Parmesan cheese.

Soybean chili: Instead of kidney beans use cooked soybeans in preparing chili (p. 179). A friend adds red coloring to the soybeans to prevent them from being detected.

Soybeans with bacon: Add 2 chopped onions, a pinch of savory, a dash of smoke flavoring; crumble and add 2 or 3 pan-broiled strips of bacon just before serving.

Soybeans with beef: 3 or 4 drops Tabasco, 1 cup leftover diced beef or beef heart, tongue, or liver, 2 diced leeks or onions, pinch of marjoram.

Soybeans with chicken: Diced leftover chicken; a pinch of thyme, sage, or basil; season with chicken fat if available.

Soybeans with green onions: ½ to 1 cup each green onions with tops and chopped celery; a pinch each of savory, basil, marjoram; 2 tablespoons Worcestershire.

Soybeans with ham: 1 or 2 teaspoons caraway seeds, ½ to 1 cup each chopped onions and diced leftover ham or smoked tongue.

Soybeans with tomatoes: 2 to 4 tablespoons dark molasses, 1 cup canned or fresh tomatoes, or ½ cup tomato catsup, 1 each chopped onion, bell pepper, stalk celery; a pinch of basil; 5 minutes before serving add 1 tablespoon dry mustard.

Soybeans with wieners or sausage: ½ cup tomato catsup or chili sauce, 1 diced onion, 4 or 5 sliced wieners; or pan-broil, drain, and cut sausage links into 1-inch lengths and add.

Soybeans with vegetables: 1 cup canned tomatoes, 1 each diced carrot, onion, green pepper; ¼ teaspoon celery seeds, 1 tablespoon dark molasses.

You can use soy grits frequently as a meat extender by adding them to soups, cereals, or any moist food. When the moisture in a recipe is limited, however, the grits should be soaked or precooked unless it is desirable to have a nut-like texture, as in cookies.

SOFTENED SOY GRITS

Combine:

1 cup boiling vegetable-cooking water or soup stock	1 cup uncooked soy grits

Soak until all moisture is absorbed; if a softer texture is desired, simmer 5 minutes. Cool and store in a covered jar in the refrigerator.

Add ¼ cup of the cooked soy grits to omelet, scrambled eggs, or any soufflé (p. 194); ½ cup to meat loaf or meat patties, to any casserole, croquettes, cooked beans, corn pudding, chili, creamed meats, stuffing for peppers, or other meat substitutes.

Use either uncooked or softened soy grits in desserts, depending upon texture desired.

The cooking time of dry beans, peas, and lentils varies widely, depending on the age of the legumes and the locality in which they were grown. When these legumes are soaked before cooking, vitamins and minerals pass into the water; therefore they should be cooked in the water used for soaking. Under no circumstances should they be parboiled and the liquid drained.

Soaking legumes is unnecessary if the dry legume is quickly washed and dropped into boiling water so slowly that boiling does not stop. As in popping corn, the starch grains burst and break the outside covering of the legume. After the covering and starch grains have burst, water is absorbed rapidly and the cooking time is shortened. When all the beans, lentils, or split peas have been put into the water, the heat should be lowered immediately to prevent the protein from becoming tough. A simmering temperature should then be maintained until the beans are tender. Soda, which destroys a number of the B vitamins, should not be used in cooking legumes.

If salt, fat, or molasses is added at the beginning of cooking, the cooking time is prolonged. Fat coats the outside covering and prevents moisture from passing readily into the legume. The acid in molasses toughens the outside covering. Salt attracts water away from the legume rather than into it. Add these seasonings and others only after the legume is starting to become tender.

So-called baked beans are not actually baked but are cooked by the heat of simmering liquid. They can be "baked" over a simmer burner far more quickly and with less fuel cost than in an oven. The difference in taste between boiled and baked beans lies in the seasonings and the amount of liquid lost through evaporation. Any dried beans may be prepared in a heat-resistant casserole and have the appearance of baked beans.

DRIED BEANS

Bring to a rolling boil:

1 quart water

Wash quickly without soaking:

2 cups dry navy beans, lima beans, kidney beans, or other dry beans

Add beans so slowly to boiling water that boiling does not stop; reduce heat immediately after all beans are in the water. Do *not* add soda.

Simmer until beans are almost tender, or 2 to 2½ hours; add and stir well:

½ teaspoon crushed black pepper-corns	½ to 3 teaspoons salt seasonings suggested under varia-
3 or 4 tablespoons vegetable oil or 2 thin slices of salt pork	tions if desired

Add more water if needed; if more moisture is left than is desired, finish cooking without covering utensil. Allow 2½ to 3 hours as total cooking time for dry navy beans, 2 to 2½ hours for lima or kidney beans.

Taste for seasonings.

VARIATIONS:

Soak beans overnight and bring slowly to boiling in water used for soaking, or soak in ice tray for 2 hours, using 2 cups water; freeze 2 hours and cook 1½ to 2 hours; add 1 cup vegetable-cooking water or soup stock during cooking.

If recipe is doubled, use 4 cups beans to 6 cups water.

Prepare beans as in basic recipe; when they start to become tender, add salt, peppercorns, oil or pork, and the following seasonings:

Black-eyed beans: 1 minced clove garlic, 2 chopped onions, and small whole cayenne pepper; discard the pepper before serving.

With ham: 1 chopped pimento, a pinch of basil, diced leftover ham; or cook with a ham bone or ham stock; or add smoke flavoring to taste.

With onions: 2 sliced onions, 2 teaspoons Worcestershire; add 1 tablespoon dry mustard 2 minutes before serving. Or add onions just in time to heat through.

With sausage: ½ cup tomato purée, catsup, or chili sauce, ½ pound pork sausage made into small balls, 2 or 3 chopped stalks celery with leaves, 2 chopped onions, 1 minced clove garlic; omit fat of basic recipe; just before serving add 2 tablespoons sherry. Vary by including fat and using sliced wieners instead of sausage; add 5 minutes before serving.

Fried kidney beans, Mexican style: Omit fat; mash half the beans; heat ¼ cup vegetable oil and add beans, 2 minced cloves garlic, pinch of orégano and/or 1 teaspoon cumin seeds; simmer 10 minutes, turning frequently with a pancake turner; just before serving add 1 cup grated or shredded Jack, American, or Swiss cheese. These beans are delicious; don't miss them.

Kidney beans Creole: 1 each finely chopped onion and green pepper; 1 minced clove garlic; instead of 1 cup water use 1 cup tomatoes.

Kidney beans with chives: Add 5 minutes before serving 3 tablespoons finely chopped chives, 2 tablespoons each Worcestershire and chopped parsley.

Lima beans, "baked": 2 chopped onions, 1 to 3 tablespoons dark molasses, 1 tablespoon dry mustard, leftover ham scraps or smoke flavoring to taste; prepare in a heat-resistant casserole; remove lid and let excess moisture evaporate; brown slightly under broiler. Vary by placing 4 partially sautéed bacon strips on top before browning.

Lima beans, creamed: Evaporate excess moisture; use partially hardened margarine or butter; add a pinch of basil, 2 diced pimentos, 3 tablespoons chopped parsley, 1 cup top milk or evaporated milk shaken with ½ cup powdered milk.

Lima beans with lentils: Cook together 1 cup each lima beans and lentils, adding lentils after lima beans have cooked 1½ hours; add 1 diced carrot, 1 each chopped onion, green pepper, pimento, 1 minced clove garlic, ½ cup catsup or chili sauce.

Lima beans with vegetables: 2 finely diced carrots, 1 chopped onion or leek, 2 tablespoons parsley, 1 tablespoon Worcestershire.

Navy beans, "baked": 2 tablespoons dark molasses, ¼ cup brown sugar; use ¼ pound salt pork; cook in a heat-resistant casserole; evaporate excess moisture; stir in 1 teaspoon dry mustard immediately before serving.

Navy beans "baked" with tomatoes: 2 cups tomatoes, 3 tablespoons each dark molasses and brown sugar, 1 or 2 finely chopped onions, 1 minced clove garlic; cook in a heat-resistant casserole; evaporate excess moisture.

Navy beans with bacon: Pan-broil slowly 4 slices bacon without browning and use part of the drippings to season beans; finish cooking the beans until tender; put into a shallow baking dish, cover with thin slices of fresh tomatoes, sweet onion or leeks, strips of bacon; set under a slow broiler until tomatoes are cooked; serve when onions are hot but still crisp.

Navy beans with ham: Cook with a ham bone, with the skin from cured ham or bacon, or in ham stock; just before serving add scraps of leftover ham, 2 teaspoons each Worcestershire and dry mustard; if no ham is available, add smoke flavoring to taste.

Savory navy beans: A pinch each of basil, savory, and thyme; 1 each chopped onion, stalk celery with leaves; minced clove garlic; 1 pimento or ripe bell pepper or green chili pepper.

Split peas and lentils may be served often, particularly when the budget is limited. If cheese, meat, or other adequate protein is added to them, they become excellent meat substitutes. They are so easy to cook that either can be used for hurry-up dinners.

SEASONED LENTILS OR SPLIT PEAS WITH MEAT

Bring to boiling:

2½ cups soup stock or vegetable-cooking water

Add so slowly that boiling does not stop:

1 cup lentils or split peas	1 crumbled bay leaf
1 chopped onion	½ teaspoon thyme

Reduce heat and simmer 30 minutes. When lentils or peas are tender, add:

¼ teaspoon ground peppercorns	1 or 2 cups diced fresh fish or left-
2 tablespoons vegetable oil or par-	over beef, lamb, or veal
tially hardened margarine	1 teaspoon salt

Serve as soon as meat is heated through.

VARIATIONS:

Sauté 2 strips bacon until crisp. Instead of oil add 2 tablespoons drippings to lentils or peas and stir in crumbled bacon just before serving.

Dice 1 strip salt pork; cook with lentils or peas.

Season with ½ teaspoon basil, marjoram, rosemary, or savory; or simmer 2 teaspoons caraway seeds with either peas or lentils.

Instead of other meat, add ½ pound sliced wieners or 1 cup diced ham.

Creamed lentils or split peas: Add 1 cup top milk blended or shaken with ½ cup powdered milk; 2 diced pimentos, 2 tablespoons chopped parsley, ¼ teaspoon thyme; use partially hardened margarine or butter.

Lentils or split peas with chicken: Add 1 diced carrot, 2 chopped pimentos, a pinch each of sage and basil; chicken fat, partially hardened margarine, or butter; leftover diced chicken.

Lentils or split peas with cheese: Add 1 diced carrot, 1 chopped onion, 2 stalks celery with leaves, 1 green pepper, 2 tablespoons chopped parsley, ½ cup tomatoes or tomato sauce; just before serving add ¼ cup grated Parmesan or other cheese. Vary by adding 3 or 4 smoked pork sausages, 1 cup diced ham, or bits of crisp bacon.

CHILI WITH MEAT AND BEANS

Heat in large utensil:

¼ cup vegetable oil

Add and sauté lightly:

¾ cup chopped onions
½ cup chopped green pepper

2 minced cloves garlic

When onions are transparent, add:

2 cups cooked or canned kidney beans
1 pound ground meat
1 to 3 teaspoons chili powder
1 or 2 teaspoons cumin (optional)

1 cup soup stock, tomato purée, or liquid from beans
2 teaspoons salt
2 teaspoons minced fresh or ½ teaspoon dried orégano

Mash about half the beans to allow starch to thicken broth. If convenient, let beans stand without further cooking for one hour or longer. Reheat and serve.

VARIATIONS:

If available, use 3 diced fresh chili peppers or 1 dried chili instead of ground chili powder; discard the dried chili before serving.

Use cooked soybeans instead of kidney beans or add ½ cup or more soy grits to basic recipe.

Stir in ½ cup instant tiger's milk just before serving.

Macaroni, spaghetti, and noodles are available prepared from whole-wheat flour and from whole-wheat flour combined with soy flour. Gluten-flour products made especially for diabetics can also be purchased. Although delicious, these foods usually cost two or three times more than do their refined counterparts. All macaroni, spaghetti, and other pastas must be made of high-protein wheat, otherwise they would fall apart in the cooking. If the budget is too limited to buy the unrefined products, try to add enough wheat germ, cheese, and powdered milk to compensate for the nutritional losses.

In addition to unrefined brown rice, there is available a nutritionally rich white rice, known as converted rice. It is prepared by treating the unmilled grain with steam under pressure. As the steam penetrates the rice, the B vitamins dissolve in it and are carried into the starchy centers. The rice is then milled. It cooks quickly and does not differ in taste or appearance from devitalized white rice. Both of these products are far superior nutritionally to refined rice. If you sincerely wish your family to maintain excellent health, use them instead of rice from which the minerals and vitamins have been removed. Keep them covered in a dry, cool place.

It has been found that as much as 20 per cent of the B vitamins are lost when rice is washed by being dipped from one pan of water to another. Wash rice quickly under running water. Since most of the minerals and the B vitamins may pass into the cooking liquid, water in which rice, macaroni, or spaghetti is cooked should not be drained off. The liquid should be carefully measured and no more used than is actually needed.

The proportions in cooking rice, macaroni, cereal, or any starchy food which packs solidly should be memorized: use 2 cups boiling water or other liquid and 1 teaspoon salt to 1 cup of the starchy food to be cooked. In cooking spaghetti, merely estimate the volume of the spaghetti and use twice as much water.

To cook rice, macaroni, and other starchy food so that each grain or particle is separate, drop the food so slowly into hot liquid that boiling does not stop. The starch grains burst quickly, as they do when corn pops, and the cooking time is shortened. Furthermore, when the starch in the food is cooked immediately, it does not have time to soak out to thicken the cooking liquid or hold the particles together; hence washing the food after it is cooked is unnecessary. The reverse of this procedure can be used when thickening is needed. Instead of making cream sauce when preparing macaroni and cheese, for example, and thus adding starch to starch, put the macaroni into cold milk; some of the starch from the macaroni soaks into the milk and when heated thickens the sauce. To prevent rice or macaroni from boiling over, add a small amount of fat.

Rice, macaroni, noodles, and spaghetti can be cooked more quickly and economically over a simmer burner than in an oven. Since shorter cooking time allows greater retention of B vitamins, the longer oven cooking is not recommended.

When the main dish of the meal is macaroni, spaghetti, noodles, or rice, the protein intake for the day is usually far too low. Try to add as much meat, cheese, milk, or other proteins to these foods as you possibly can. Vary your recipes, using different leftover meats, fish, or sea foods with various seasonings and vegetables.

The following recipes for rice, noodles, and the various kinds of Italian pastas are actually interchangeable. I have divided them only to prevent confusion. Since Italian cheeses are expensive, I have suggested using generous amounts of American cheese for added protein with only enough Italian cheese to supply flavor.

SHELL MACARONI WITH CHEESE

Bring to boiling in heat-resistant casserole:

2 cups vegetable-cooking water

Add so slowly that boiling does not stop:

1 teaspoon salt   2 cups shell macaroni

Cover utensil; if water starts to foam or boil over add ½ teaspoon
margarine or butter; lower heat and simmer 10 minutes, or until almost
tender. Stir, evaporate off most of the remaining moisture, and remove
macaroni from heat; add:

1½ cups fresh or reconstituted   ⅔ cup instant powdered milk
  milk   1 cup cubed Cheddar-type cheese

Stir until well mixed. Sprinkle top generously with:

wheat germ   Parmesan cheese (optional)
paprika

Brown in moderate oven at 300° F. for 15 minutes.

VARIATIONS:

Instead of shell macaroni, use 2 cups elbow macaroni or 5 ounces
spaghetti, rigatoni, or noodles; or use 1 cup converted or brown rice;
cook converted rice 12 minutes and brown rice 30 minutes before adding milk and other ingredients.

Lasagne with cheese: Use a rectangular 10- by 7-inch baking tin,
and boil over direct heat 6 ounces (12 strips) lasagne in 2½ cups salted
water; use similar but larger pan or cookie sheet for lid. Cook lasagne
10 minutes and lift onto paper towels. In same baking tin mix fresh
and powdered milk as in basic recipe; put into milk alternating layers
of lasagne and shredded cheese sprinkled lightly with basil. Cover
with topping and bake as directed. Vary by sprinkling both lean ground
meat and cheese between layers of lasagne; season with basil.

Shell macaroni with beans: Omit milk and cheese; add 2 tablespoons
partially hardened margarine or butter, 1 can kidney beans; or use 2

cups cooked pinto, navy, garbanzo, or other varieties of beans. Season with freshly ground black peppercorns, 1 shredded onion, and crumbled sautéed bacon if desired; or add 1 quart soup stock and serve as soup.

Follow the basic recipe, using macaroni, rigatoni, spaghetti, noodles, or brown or converted rice; use or omit cheese; add the ingredients suggested below. When fresh vegetables are used, cook them with the rice, macaroni, spaghetti, or noodles, adding them only in time to become tender; stir sea food or leftover meat into the sauce just before adding topping.

With chicken: 2 diced pimentos, 2 tablespoons ground parsley, 1 cup diced leftover chicken, 2 tablespoons chicken fat or partially hardened margarine, pinch each of sage and basil. Vary by adding 1 cup peas.

With clams: 1 can minced clams with broth, 2 tablespoons each partially hardened margarine and chopped parsley, few sliced stuffed olives. This is a delicious and inexpensive dish.

With ham: 1 cup diced leftover ham, 1 tablespoon each dry mustard and ham drippings. Vary by adding 1 or 2 teaspoons caraway seeds instead of mustard.

With liver: 2 tablespoons each partially hardened margarine and chopped celery, 1 chopped onion, 1 chopped bell pepper, pinch each of savory and marjoram; 1 cup diced sautéed liver.

With mushrooms: ½ cup or more sliced fresh or canned mushrooms.

With oysters: 1 pint fresh or canned oysters, 2 tablespoons chopped parsley, 2 tablespoons chili sauce. Vary by omitting chili and adding 1 teaspoon dill or anise seeds; or use shrimp, lamb, or veal instead of oysters.

With peas: 1 cup fresh or frozen peas, 1 chopped leek or sweet onion, 1 diced pimento; stir 1 cup cheese into sauce.

With salmon or other fish: 1 each finely chopped onion and pimento or green pepper, 1 stalk chopped celery and leaves, 2 tablespoons each partially hardened margarine and chopped parsley, 2 cups canned salmon, diced fresh fillet, or flaked steamed fish.

With seeds: Add 2 to 4 teaspoons poppy seeds 15 minutes before serving; include cheese. Poppy seeds are particularly delicious with rice or noodles. Or add 1 to 3 teaspoons crushed dill seeds with any recipe in which cheese is used, and caraway seeds with ham or pork sausage.

With shrimp: 1 cup or more of uncooked fresh or canned shrimp and the broth, 2 diced hard-cooked eggs, 2 teaspoons minced onion, 2 tablespoons partially hardened margarine, dash each of cayenne, nutmeg, and celery salt.

With vegetables: ½ cup each diced carrots, finely chopped celery and onion, 2 or 3 strips crisp bacon broken to bits; add bacon just before sprinkling on topping.

Many recipes for spaghetti sauce state that it should be simmered for 5 hours; actually nothing is thus accomplished except that liquid is evaporated off (less could be added in the first place) and the aromatic oils are extracted from the seasonings. Nutritive value, of course, is lost.

Instead of cooking any highly seasoned sauce for 5 hours, let it stand in the refrigerator for that length of time. The standing brings about a vast improvement in flavor.

SPAGHETTI WITH BEEF

Use a large utensil and sauté 5 minutes in 2 tablespoons vegetable oil:

½ cup each chopped bell pepper and finely diced carrot

1 or 2 minced cloves garlic
1 to 3 chopped onions

Add:

4 cups peeled and diced raw tomatoes or
1 large can tomatoes with juice
½ cup tomato paste (optional)

2 teaspoons dark molasses or sugar
1½ teaspoons salt
¼ teaspoon each freshly ground peppercorns, basil, and orégano

If canned tomatoes are used, cut into small pieces and add 1 cup consommé, soup stock, or water.

Bring sauce to a boil and add so slowly that boiling does not stop:

8 ounces (half a large package) spaghetti

If you do not wish spaghetti to be broken, put ends into boiling liquid and curve remainder into pan as soon as ends soften. Cover utensil and cook slowly for 10 minutes. Crumble in and stir to break into small pieces:

1 pound lean ground beef

If time permits, set aside for 4 hours or longer; the meat is immediately cooked by the hot liquid. Reheat and turn onto serving platter; sprinkle with:

¼ cup chopped parsley   3 tablespoons Parmesan, Romano
                                     or mozzarella cheese

VARIATIONS:

Use ⅔ pound ground beef and ⅓ pound pork sausage; if high in fat, sauté pork and beef first; pour off drippings and proceed as in basic recipe.

Just before serving stir in ¼ to ½ cup instant tiger's milk.

To cook spaghetti separately, drop 8 ounces spaghetti into 3 cups boiling water; boil 10 minutes, or until it cuts easily with a spoon; transfer to hot platter. Evaporate off most of the water, and add remainder to sauce. Serve sauce over spaghetti.

Add any of the following: 1 cup fresh or 1 can mushrooms; ½ cup chopped celery; 1 teaspoon cumin seeds; 3 or 4 slices diced salami, other Italian sausage, or smoked wieners; ½ teaspoon mashed rosemary; ½ cup or more diced Cheddar, Swiss, Jack, or other varieties of cheese; or 1 can pizza sauce; omit herbs if pizza sauce is used.

Use 8 ounces whole-wheat, whole-wheat and soy, or gluten spaghetti or macaroni; the macaroni may be plain, elbow, or shell. Or use 6 ounces rigatoni or 1 cup brown or converted rice; cook converted rice 15 minutes with other ingredients; cook brown rice 40 minutes in 2 cups stock before adding other ingredients.

Use 1 small can tomato sauce or tomato paste with 1 cup soup stock instead of fresh or canned tomatoes.

Omit ground beef and 1 teaspoon salt; add only in time to heat 1 cup or more diced leftover chicken, beef, liver, tongue, veal, or lamb; add any leftover gravy or broth to sauce.

Lasagne with meat and mushrooms: Boil for 10 minutes over direct heat in a rectangular 10- by 7-inch baking tin about **6 ounces (9 to 12 strips) lasagne** in 2½ cups salted soup stock, tomato juice, or **vegetable-cooking water;** use similar but larger pan or cookie sheet for lid. Lift all but 3 strips of lasagne onto paper towels; layer over lasagne and remaining stock ⅓ **pound crumbled ground lean beef;** ⅓ **can tomato or pizza sauce, 3 or 4 sliced fresh mushrooms or shredded onion;** sprinkle with salt, freshly ground peppercorns, and basil; repeat, forming 2 more layers; add more stock if needed to cover lasagne. Sprinkle top generously with **wheat germ, paprika,** and **Parmesan cheese.** If time permits, refrigerate for 4 hours or longer. Slowly reheat to simmering over top burner and bake at 300° F. for 10 minutes or brown top under broiler.

Spaghetti with leftover roast beef: Remove meat and pass through grinder; simmer bones in **3 cups water,** strain, and cook spaghetti in stock; instead of canned tomatoes use **1 can tomato paste** with remaining stock; use seasonings of basic recipe; add ground meat only in time to reheat.

Spaghetti with meat balls: Omit ground meat and ½ teaspoon salt; make recipe for **meat loaf** (p. 108) or **meat patties** (p. 111) using only ¼ **cup milk;** add **2 tablespoons Parmesan cheese.** Form into 1½-inch balls, set on spaghetti after it has cooked 3 minutes; cover utensil and steam meat balls 8 minutes before stirring into sauce. If browning of meat is desired, roll meat in **wheat germ,** set on greased baking sheet, sprinkle with **paprika,** and brown under broiler before adding to spaghetti and sauce.

Stuffed rigatoni: When preparing meat balls use ⅓ of the seasoned meat to stuff 5 or 6 ounces uncooked rigatoni; stuff by jabbing each piece of rigatoni into the raw meat. Put into plastic bag and freeze. To 1 cup leftover brown gravy, add **1 can tomato paste, 1 cup water,** ½ **teaspoon salt,** and seasonings of basic recipe; cook rigatoni in sauce no longer than 10 minutes, being careful not to overcook.

The following recipe is an adaptation of a Jewish dish which can be made quickly and is usually enjoyed the first time it is eaten.

NOODLE PUDDING

Use heat-resistant casserole and bring to boiling:

2 cups vegetable-cooking water   **1 teaspoon salt**

Add so slowly that boiling does not stop:

5 or 6 ounces noodles

Cover utensil; if water starts to boil over, add ½ teaspoon partially hardened margarine or butter; lower heat and simmer 10 minutes. Evaporate off most of the remaining water and add:

1 to 1½ cups fresh or reconstituted milk	1 cup cottage cheese
⅔ cup instant powdered milk	1 tablespoon sugar
	¼ cup sour cream

Wipe edges of utensil. Sprinkle generously over noodles:

wheat germ	paprika

Bake in moderate oven at 350° F. for 10 minutes, or just until heated through. Be careful not to overbake.

VARIATIONS:

Season with 2 teaspoons poppy seeds.

Add 2 eggs with cold milk; stir thoroughly before adding other ingredients. Bake 12 to 15 minutes.

Instead of sour cream add ¼ cup yogurt and 1 or 2 tablespoons partially hardened margarine.

Add ½ cup each raisins and sugar, 1 or 2 eggs, 1 teaspoon cinnamon, dash of nutmeg; bake 15 minutes and serve for dessert.

Noodles with chicken: Omit cottage cheese, sugar, and sour cream; add with milk 2 or 3 chicken bouillon cubes, 1 tablespoon partially hardened margarine or chicken fat, 1 or 2 cups diced leftover chicken; salt to taste; or add powdered milk to leftover chicken broth. Add dash of nutmeg or serve sprinkled with slivered almonds.

Chicken noodle ring: Prepare as above, adding 2 beaten eggs and slightly more salt. Pour into a greased ring mold and bake 20 minutes at 300° F.

Noodles with ham: Instead of cottage cheese, sugar, and sour cream, add to milk ¾ cup or more diced or ground leftover ham, ½ cup each chopped green pepper and celery or onions and diced Cheddar cheese. Add topping and bake at 300° F. for 30 minutes.

With veal, lamb, or beef: Prepare as noodles with ham, adding 1 cup diced or ground leftover veal, lamb, or beef. Stir powdered milk into leftover gravy when available; add 1 tablespoon partially hardened margarine, butter, or meat drippings.

Noodles with tuna or shrimp: Omit cottage cheese, sugar, and sour cream. Stir in with fresh and powdered milk 1 can tuna; or add 2 tablespoons partially hardened margarine or butter and 1 or 2 cups

fresh or canned shrimps. If canned shrimps are used, drain liquid into cooking water and decrease fresh milk. Add ½ teaspoon **crushed dill seeds** if desired.

Home-made pizzas can be far more delicious and nutritious than the commercial varieties. Since the dough does not have to rise, they may be made quickly, especially if you use whole-wheat-bread mix and prepared pizza sauce. If you are dealing with teen-age appetites—and most housewives who make pizzas are—the pizzas disappear with lightning speed.

The following recipe makes two 13-inch pizzas or three 9-inch ones; any not eaten may be frozen and reheated.

PIZZA

Mix thoroughly without heating:

1½ pounds lean ground meat
2 cups tomato purée or 2 cans tomato sauce
1 shredded onion

½ teaspoon each basil, orégano,
  and freshly ground black peppercorns
1½ teaspoons salt

Set sauce aside. Combine and let stand 5 minutes:

1 cup warm water
1 tablespoon, package, or cake
  baker's yeast

1 teaspoon honey (optional)
1 tablespoon vegetable oil
1 teaspoon salt

Add without sifting:

2 cups high-protein stone-ground whole-wheat flour

Beat dough until smooth and elastic. Add ½ cup more flour, or enough to make a stiff dough; turn onto a floured canvas or bread board and knead until smooth.

If two large pizzas are to be made, cut dough in half; set one aside and make the other into a ball. Roll into a round sheet and transfer to a greased 13-inch pizza pan; pull and stretch dough gently to fit pan, turning up edges ⅛ inch. Sprinkle seasoned meat over dough, spreading it well to margins. Bake in a preheated oven at 450° F. for 15 minutes, being sure to put pizza to be served immediately on lower rack. The bottom of the crust must be crisp. Remove from oven, and sprinkle over top:

½ to 1 cup shredded Cheddar cheese   **1 to 2 tablespoons grated Parmesan or Romano cheese**

Return pizza to be served immediately to oven until cheese melts. Serve piping hot.

Slide pizza from pan and repeat procedures.

If smaller pizzas are to be made, divide dough into 3 equal parts, form each into a ball, roll and fit into greased 9-inch cake pans, allowing edges to turn up slightly. Spread with sauce and proceed as for larger pizzas.

If pizza is not to be eaten immediately, omit cheese; chill, wrap, and freeze. Before serving, thaw completely, set on lower rack of oven, and reheat at 350° F. for 10 minutes, or only until heated through. Add cheese as in basic recipe. If cheese is submitted to high heat, it becomes stringy and nutritive value is lost.

VARIATIONS:

For quick pizza dough, use 3 cups whole-wheat-bread mix (p. 406) with yeast and 1 cup of water; or for 1 large pizza or 2 small ones, make 1 biscuit recipe, using either flour (p. 424) or nutritious mix (p. 428); flatten dough and spread over pan with fingers.

Bake on cookie sheet instead of in pizza pan.

Crumble meat over uncooked pizza, cover with 1 can pizza sauce and spread with back of spoon; proceed as in basic recipe.

Add to meat one or more of the following: 1 or 2 minced cloves garlic; ½ cup finely chopped bell pepper or celery, or 4 or more sliced mushrooms; ⅓ cup chopped parsley; ½ teaspoon crumbled rosemary. Or put thin slices of bell pepper over cheese.

If ground meat contains much fat, sauté lightly and drain before adding other ingredients of sauce.

Omit ground meat; stir into sauce chopped salami, anchovies, Italian sausage, or smoked wieners; or mix 1 tablespoon oil with sauce and lay anchovies or sliced sausages over top. Or after baking, lay 1 cup uncooked or 1 can drained shrimps over pizza and sprinkle with mozzarella cheese; return to oven for 5 minutes after heat has been turned off.

Instead of Cheddar cheese, lay over pizza thin slices of Jack, mozzarella, Swiss, or other types of cheese; or use Cheddar with mozzarella, Romano, or any Italian cheese.

Instead of sauce cover pizza dough with chopped fresh or drained canned tomatoes; shred onions over tomatoes, and sprinkle with basil, orégano, and other seasonings.

If dough has risen before sauce is spread over it, pierce at 1-inch intervals with a fork.

Stir into sauce ½ to 1 cup instant tiger's milk (p. 447); the flavor is disguised by the tomato and seasonings.

SPANISH RICE WITH MEAT

Sauté lightly in 2 tablespoons vegetable oil:

> ½ cup each chopped onions, celery, and bell pepper or
> fresh chili pepper

Add:

1 cup soup stock or vegetable-cooking water	1 large can tomatoes and juice 1½ teaspoons salt

Bring to boiling and add so slowly that boiling does not stop:

> 1 cup converted rice

Lower heat and add:

½ teaspoon cumin seeds 1 teaspoon sugar (optional)	½ teaspoon each basil and orégano

Cover utensil and simmer 15 minutes; crumble in:

> ½ pound lean ground beef

Add freshly ground peppercorns and more soup stock or salt if needed. If time permits, let stand for 4 hours or longer. Simmer 10 minutes longer or reheat and serve.

VARIATIONS:

If meat high in fat is used, sauté slowly and pour off drippings before sautéing vegetables; proceed as in basic recipe.

Just before serving stir in ¼ to ½ cup instant tiger's milk.

Instead of fresh beef add 1 or 2 cups diced leftover chicken, beef, lamb, veal, or other meat; or sauté pork sausage and drain off fat before adding other ingredients.

Use 1 cup brown rice, cooking it in 2 cups stock for 25 minutes before adding vegetables; omit sautéing; cook 20 minutes longer. Or use 2 cups cooked brown rice.

Add any one or more of the following: ½ teaspoon rosemary; 1 or 2 teaspoons chili powder; ½ cup finely diced carrots; or crumbled sautéed bacon. Or omit meat and stir in ½ to 1 cup diced or shredded cheese just before serving.

Put any leftover rice in disposable baking pan; sprinkle top with wheat germ and shredded cheese; cool, wrap, and freeze. Thaw later and reheat as casserole dish.

Instead of rice use 6 ounces noodles. Simmer 20 minutes.

FRIED RICE

Wash quickly:

> **1½ cups brown rice**

Fry in:

> **3 tablespoons vegetable oil**

Keep heat high, stir frequently, and cook until rice is well browned; add slowly:

2 cups soup stock or vegetable-cooking water	**1½ teaspoons salt**

Simmer 30 minutes and add:

¼ to ½ teaspoon crushed black peppercorns	**1 minced clove garlic**
	pinch each of basil and orégano

Cook until tender; allow about 45 minutes for the total cooking time. Just before serving stir in:

> **1 cup diced American, Swiss, or Jack cheese**

VARIATIONS:

Before browning rice, pan-broil 3 or 4 strips bacon; remove when crisp, break into bits, and add just before serving.

When rice begins to be tender, stir in 2 beaten eggs and the cheese;

turn into oiled ring mold; bake at 325° F. for 15 minutes, or to the internal temperature of 185° F. Serve with creamed spinach, peas, or other vegetable, or creamed meat in center.

If converted rice is used, brown the rice, reduce heat, and sauté vegetables; add soup stock and cook 15 to 20 minutes.

Omit or decrease cheese and add 1 cup of any of the following just before serving: diced leftover beef, chicken, heart, tongue, lamb, or veal; fresh or canned shrimps, oysters, or other shellfish and juice; diced uncooked fish fillets or flaked steamed fish; omit orégano if sea food is used and add 1 teaspoon dill or anise seeds.

Instead of rice, use noodles; omit browning; add seasonings of basic recipe or any variation and ½ cup whole ripe olives.

Add 1 teaspoon cumin seeds and 1 cup canned or diced fresh tomatoes.

CHILI RELLENO,
OR STUFFED CHILI PEPPERS

Shred:

2 cups Jack or American cheese

Stuff firmly into:

6 or 8 canned chili peppers

Beat until fluffy:

2 whole eggs

Add and beat slightly:

½ teaspoon salt   **2 tablespoons powdered milk**
1 tablespoon whole-wheat flour

Flatten the peppers and dip in egg; fry 3 or 4 at a time in:

¼ cup vegetable oil

Be extremely careful to keep heat low; brown peppers lightly on both sides. Serve plain or set on hot serving platter and keep in a warm place; heat 2 cups Spanish sauce (p. 141) and pour over peppers. We consider these peppers a choice delicacy.

VARIATIONS:

Select fresh green chili peppers with thick meat; put peppers under broiler and sear with high heat on all sides; wrap quickly in a damp towel and steam until skin is loose; remove skin, but do not remove seeds unless mild flavor is enjoyed; make a slit on one side, fill, and prepare as in basic recipe.

Stuffed bell peppers or pimentos: Remove stem end and seeds from 4 large red or green bell peppers or fresh pimentos; steam over boiling water until tender; stuff and proceed as in basic recipe. Or set upright; stuff half full of **shredded cheese**; drop **1 egg** on top of each pepper; season with **salt and dash of cayenne**. If pimentos are small, use 8; stir **4 eggs** together, add ¼ **cup milk, 1 teaspoon salt,** and pour over cheese in pimentos. Bake in a moderate oven at 350° F. for 12 to 15 minutes.

Well-made soufflés are one of the most nutritious of all meat substitutes and are superior to muscle meats in that they supply larger amounts of the essential amino acids. The temperature inside a soufflé when ready to serve is usually not high enough to harm the proteins and B vitamins.

Few recipes offer such an opportunity to work eggs, cheese, milk, and other nutritious foods into the menu as do soufflés. Powdered milk, wheat germ, soy flour, and soy grits may be added to improve the nutritive value without harming the flavor. Since cheese blends well with other foods, it may be added to almost every variety of soufflé. Serve soufflés frequently, especially when cooking for one whose health is below par.

A soufflé should be baked in much the same way as an angel-food cake, or at 300° F. If the oven becomes too hot, the soufflé, being largely protein, toughens and shrivels. Since soft-cooked eggs loll about in a relaxed manner, an undercooked soufflé naturally falls. If the soufflé is allowed to cool before it is served, the steam inside it contracts and causes it to shink. The soufflé will be a success if you control the baking temperature, give it plenty of time to cook, and serve it immediately.

Since almost any leftover meat, fish, or vegetable can be added to a soufflé, it is a good entree to serve whenever leftovers accumulate. Create your own recipes according to the foods you have on hand.

CHEESE SOUFFLÉ

Heat to simmering:

1 cup whole milk

Meanwhile beat together or blend in liquefier and add to the hot milk:

½ cup cold milk
¼ to ½ cup powdered milk
3 tablespoons whole-wheat flour

1½ teaspoons salt
⅛ teaspoon freshly ground white peppercorns

Simmer 5 minutes, stirring constantly; remove from heat, cool slightly; add and stir well:

4 egg yolks
¼ teaspoon dried basil
1 to 2 cups diced American cheese

2 or 3 tablespoons finely chopped parsley
1 or 2 teaspoons Worcestershire

Beat stiffly and fold in:

4 egg whites

Pour into greased casserole and place in a slow preheated oven at 300° F.; set an upright oven thermometer on same level with soufflé and check temperature carefully; bake 45 to 50 minutes. If it cannot be served immediately, turn off heat, open oven door a moment to cool, then let casserole remain in closed oven.

VARIATIONS:

Instead of cheese add 1 to 2 cups finely diced cooked tongue, heart, leftover beef, pork, or veal, 1 grated onion, a pinch each of savory and marjoram.

Add one or more of the following: ½ cup fresh or canned mushrooms; ¼ cup diced fresh or canned pimentos, chopped ripe olives, or sliced stuffed olives; 1 each finely chopped onion, celery stalk, or bell pepper. If fresh vegetables are added, simmer 5 minutes in milk before adding the other ingredients.

Add any leftover vegetable, such as peas, diced carrots, artichoke heart, chopped kale, broccoli, spinach, asparagus, celery, or string beans.

Omit flour; instead of fresh milk use 1½ cups leftover gravy, medium cream sauce (p. 135), brown sauce (p. 136), or condensed tomato or mushroom soup. Reduce salt to ½ teaspoon if canned soup is used. Or use tomato juice or purée instead of fresh milk, adding flour and powdered milk.

Add ½ cup wheat germ or ¼ cup precooked soy grits or soy flour. If tomatoes are used instead of fresh milk, 1 to 3 teaspoons of a bland brewers' yeast may be mixed with powdered milk and flour.

Follow the basic recipe, merely adding the ingredients suggested below; decrease the amount of cheese as desired, but omit it only when 1½ cups or more of meat or fish are added. Simmer the fresh vegetables in the hot cream sauce until heated through.

Carrot soufflé: 2 cups raw shredded carrots, 1 each finely chopped onion and green pepper or pimento.

Chicken soufflé: 1½ cups diced steamed chicken, 1 cup uncooked fresh or frozen peas, 2 diced pimentos, a pinch of sage; use liquid left from steaming chicken instead of fresh milk. Make soufflés of leftover turkey or rabbit in the same manner.

Corn soufflé: 1 to 1½ cups fresh, frozen, or canned corn; heat in milk only if corn is fresh; reduce cheese to 1 cup.

Crab, lobster, or shrimp soufflé: 1½ to 2 cups diced or flaked crab, shrimp, or lobster, 1 teaspoon anise or dill seeds; use liquid from canned sea food instead of part of the milk. Omit cheese.

Fish soufflé: 1 to 2 cups diced uncooked fish fillets or flaked leftover fish, 1 tablespoon minced fresh dill or 1 teaspoon dill or anise seeds, 1 or 2 diced pimentos.

Ham soufflé: 1 cup or more diced leftover ham, 2 tablespoons green onion with tops or chives, a pinch each of basil and savory; vary by adding 1 or 2 teaspoons caraway seeds.

Liver soufflé: Use leftover liver or dredge ¾ pound lamb, beef, or veal liver in wheat germ or whole-wheat flour and sauté quickly; remove the liver and heat milk in same utensil; grind liver or dice fine; add with ½ cup chopped onions or leeks, a pinch each of savory, marjoram, and rosemary. Vary by adding 1 or 2 teaspoons dill or caraway seeds.

Mushroom soufflé: ½ to 1 cup sliced fresh or canned mushrooms; use the liquid from canned mushrooms instead of part of the milk; use mild-flavored cheese.

Pea soufflé: Use 2 cups chilled fresh peas or thawed frozen peas; add chopped pimentos if desired; use mild-flavored cheese or omit cheese. This is a wonderful soufflé.

Potato soufflé: 1 cup or more leftover mashed potatoes, 1 grated onion, 1 or 2 teaspoons dill or caraway seeds.

Spinach or broccoli soufflé: 2 to 3 cups finely chopped raw spinach or ground uncooked broccoli, 1 grated or chopped onion; use 1 cup cheese. This is the best soufflé yet; it has the freshness of a spring garden. Vary by using kale, chard, New Zealand spinach, or other greens.

Soufflé of sweetbreads or brains: 1 cup or more finely diced steamed brains or sweetbreads, 3 drops Tabasco, 2 tablespoons pimento or chopped celery.

Spanish soufflé: Use tomato purée, canned tomatoes, or diced fresh tomatoes instead of fresh milk; add 1 each chopped onion, green chili pepper or bell pepper; 1 teaspoon chili powder, 1 minced clove garlic, 1 to 3 teaspoons brewers' yeast (optional), a pinch each of orégano, basil, and cumin seeds. Vary by adding diced ham, beef heart, liver, brains, chicken, or fish instead of cheese.

Whole, unground wheat is excellent to use as a meat extender. If hard wheat is purchased, the protein content is similar to that of rice, macaroni, and other meat extenders. The cooked wheat may be served with any cream sauce (p. 135), mixed with fresh meat, fish, or cheese, and made into patties, croquettes, or casserole dishes. Its flavor soon comes to be enjoyed; it may be served frequently when the budget is limited. The cooking time varies with the age and kind of wheat used.

COOKED WHOLE WHEAT

Place in a wire strainer and wash quickly under running water:

1½ cups whole, unground wheat

Add slowly to:

3 cups boiling soup stock or vegetable-cooking water

Reduce heat and simmer about 3 to 4 hours or until tender; add:

2 tablespoons partially hardened   1 teaspoon salt
  margarine or butter

Serve as a substitute for potatoes or rice; or eat with milk as a cereal.

VARIATIONS:

Soak wheat overnight; cook in same liquid used for soaking.

Cook wheat in a pressure cooker 30 minutes, or until tender.

Add seasonings suggested in any recipe for soybeans, split peas, or lentils; or substitute an equal amount of cooked wheat for rice, macaroni, or noodles in any recipe; use instead of rice in any casserole dish (p. 205), croquettes (p. 206), meat patties (p. 111), or cheese loaf (p. 228); add to omelets or scrambled eggs.

Although the recipe for tamale pie seems complicated, it can be prepared in about 15 minutes. Unfortunately, several utensils must be used in making it, but if you happen to enjoy Mexican food, the dishwashing is justified.

TAMALE PIE

Sauté lightly in **vegetable oil:**

1 chopped green pepper, preferably fresh chili pepper	1 chopped onion

Add:

1 cup canned or diced fresh tomatoes	1 to 3 teaspoons chili powder
8 to 12 ripe olives (optional)	pinch of orégano and basil
1¼ teaspoons salt	½ to 1 teaspoon cumin seeds (optional)

Simmer 10 minutes, remove from heat, and stir in:

½ pound ground lean beef	1 cup fresh, frozen, or canned corn

Set filling aside. Prepare corn-meal mush by sifting together or mixing thoroughly:

1 cup yellow stone-ground corn meal	½ cup powdered milk
	1 teaspoon salt

Add and mix:

1 cup cold milk

Stir constantly while adding corn-meal mixture to:

2 cups simmering milk

Stir until mixture thickens, or about 5 minutes, being extremely careful to use low heat after thickening starts. Immediately pour half the mush into a flat greased baking dish, spreading evenly; add and spread the filling and cover with remaining mush; sprinkle generously with paprika. Bake in oven at 350° F. for 15 minutes, or until brown.

VARIATIONS:

Instead of preparing mush, blend together 2 slightly beaten eggs, $\frac{1}{2}$ cup milk, $\frac{1}{2}$ teaspoon salt, 1 cup yellow corn meal. Proceed as in basic recipe; bake for 30 minutes at 350° F.

Instead of ground fresh meat use 1 or 2 cups diced or ground leftover ham, chicken, veal, lamb, heart, tongue, or liver.

Add $\frac{1}{2}$ cup softened soy grits (p. 174) to corn-meal mush, to filling, or to both.

Corn-meal mush: Prepare as in basic recipe; serve as a cereal or pour into a square mold, chill, slice, dredge in whole-wheat flour, and sauté until golden brown on both sides. This is delicious mush which browns much more easily than the ordinary variety. The protein content can be still further increased by adding $\frac{1}{2}$ cup soy grits.

Rice or spaghetti pie: Instead of corn-meal mush use **fried rice** (p. 191) seasoned only with salt; prepare as in basic recipe; or use **leftover macaroni, spaghetti, or rice.**

Tamale loaf: Sauté vegetables and add tomatoes and seasonings; mix corn meal and powdered milk with $1\frac{1}{2}$ cups soup stock and add to heated moist ingredients; when thick, add corn and meat. If tomatoes are sour, sweeten with **1 to 3 teaspoons dark molasses.** Bake as in basic recipe.

ENCHILADAS

Sauté slowly in **1 tablespoon vegetable oil** for 10 minutes:

1 chopped onion	1 teaspoon cumin seeds
$1\frac{1}{2}$ pounds lean ground meat	$1\frac{1}{2}$ teaspoons salt

Add:

1 small can (1 cup) tomato purée   1 or 2 teaspoons chili powder

If time permits, let meat stand with seasonings for 1 hour or longer; reheat.

Use 12 prepared corn-meal tortillas; roll into each and set in baking dish:

3 tablespoons seasoned meat	1 to 2 tablespoons grated Cheddar
1 tablespoon chopped green onions	cheese

Sprinkle over top:

1 large can drained kidney beans	1 to 2 cups grated cheese
chopped green onions with tops	generous sprinkling paprika

Brown in oven at 350° F. for 15 minutes, or until cheese is melted.

VARIATIONS:

Instead of tomato purée add ½ can of concentrated tomato soup to meat and pour remaining soup over enchiladas before adding beans; decrease salt to 1 teaspoon.

Use any finely diced or ground leftover meat with fresh meat or instead of fresh meat.

The trouble with learning to make cheese blintzes is that your family and friends will probably never let you stop making them. Reheated blintzes, in my opinion, are unworthy of the name, yet to serve them fresh and piping hot you need as many hands as an octopus has arms. Despite these difficulties, for pure gastronomic delight, blintzes cannot be recommended too highly.

CHEESE BLINTZES

Beat, preferably with an electric mixer:

1 pound, or 2 cups, crumbled dry cottage cheese, or hoop cheese	1 teaspoon salt
1 egg	3 tablespoons each sugar and powdered milk

Set aside. Prepare thin pancakes (p. 418), being sure to fold in stiffly beaten egg whites last. Bake pancakes on grill until golden on one side, turn and put 2 tablespoons of filling into each. Fold over and transfer to a large frying pan containing 4 tablespoons or more partially hardened margarine or butter. Brown on all sides over low heat.

Simultaneously continue to bake and fill more thin pancakes.

Serve piping hot with chilled sour cream or yogurt. The traditional way of serving blintzes is to put both sour cream and strawberry jam over them at the table. The lily, however, need not be gilded.

VARIATIONS:

Although delicacy of texture is lost, pancakes may be prepared in advance and filled with cheese mixture. Brown just before serving.

Apple pancakes: Make filling of 2 cups thinly sliced firm apples which will not lose shape when cooked; steam to tenderness and add ½ to ¾ cup sugar, 1 tablespoon whole-wheat flour, generous sprinkling of nutmeg and cinnamon. Proceed as in basic recipe. Serve with sour cream as dessert.

Cheese-filled pancakes: Shred 2 cups American, Jack, or Swiss cheese; add 4 tablespoons each chopped ripe or stuffed olives and minced chives. Fold into pancakes, sprinkle with grated cheese, and heat in oven or under broiler until cheese melts.

Spinach-filled pancakes: Steam until tender 1 bunch spinach, using high heat to evaporate off moisture; shred and add 1 each chopped onion and clove garlic, 1 teaspoon salt, 1 egg, 1 cup diced leftover ham, chicken, veal, or lamb. Fill pancakes and brown on all sides. Put on baking sheet, sprinkle top with shredded Cheddar cheese, and set in moderate oven or under broiler until cheese melts.

The recipe for cheese cutlets is almost identical to that for the filling for cheese blintzes. Cheese cutlets, a Russian dish, are inexpensive, highly nutritious, and usually enjoyed the first time they are eaten.

CHEESE CUTLETS

Blend in an electric mixer:

1 egg	2 tablespoons sugar
1 pound (2 cups) crumbled hoop cheese, or dry, unsalted cottage cheese	1 tablespoon whole-wheat-pastry flour
	¾ teaspoon salt

Form cheese mixture into flat patties ½ inch thick. Roll in wheat germ or whole-wheat flour. Sauté in partially hardened margarine or butter until golden brown on each side.

Serve instead of meat.

VARIATIONS:

Serve hot cutlets topped with chilled sour cream. Or top with 1 tablespoon each sour cream and strawberry preserves.

CHOW MEIN

Sauté lightly in **vegetable oil:**

2 chopped onions   4 stalks chopped celery

Cook 8 minutes and add:

1 or 2 cups lean leftover pork roast, diced in ½-inch cubes   1 cup fresh or 1 can sliced mushrooms and juice

1 pound fresh or a No. 2 can bean sprouts and juice   2 tablespoons or more soy sauce

Stir well; **salt** to taste after soy sauce is added; simmer only until heated through.

Heat in moderate oven:

1 can Chinese noodles

Arrange noodles in form of nest on hot serving platter; put chow mein in center.

VARIATIONS:

Add 1 can sliced water chestnuts.

Instead of pork, use leftover beef or chicken cut in thin strips.

Chicken chow mein: Omit pork; sauté onions and celery in **partially hardened margarine, chicken fat, or butter;** add with bean sprouts and mushrooms 1 or more cups diced leftover chicken, ½ cup well-drained crushed canned pineapple. Serve with noodles or rice.

Pork chop suey: Omit noodles and mushrooms; use **1 pound fresh or leftover pork cut into strips 2 inches long, 1 cup each chopped onions and celery;** proceed as in basic recipe, adding bean sprouts and soy sauce. Serve with steamed rice.

EGG FOO YUNG, OR EGG AND VEGETABLE PATTIES

Chop or cut fine or pass through the meat grinder:

2 onions   4 strips uncooked bacon
3 green peppers

Add:

1 pound fresh or a No. 2 can bean   ½ teaspoon salt
sprouts   4 whole eggs

Beat together thoroughly. Drop from a tablespoon onto a hot **oiled** grill and sauté until light brown on both sides.

Serve with soy sauce.

VARIATIONS:

Substitute 1½ cups slightly cooked chopped celery for bean sprouts.

Add 1 can sliced mushrooms or 1 cup diced cooked beef, chicken, shrimp, or fish.

Add one small can or ¼ cup peeled and sliced water chestnuts.

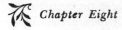

Chapter Eight

Make Your Leftovers a Treat

Many dishes such as curries, meat pies, soufflés, and casseroles call for already cooked meats and vegetables. Whenever the problem of using leftovers arises, these foods are ideal to prepare.

Leftovers have gained a bad reputation because of the necessity in the past of eating "that same old leg of lamb" on several consecutive days. With home-freezer space available, housewives can now put leftovers aside until everyone in the family is hungry for some particular food again, and the leftover can be brought out as a special treat. When freezer space permits, not only dishes containing leftovers can be made in advance, but many favorite recipes can be purposely doubled to allow some for freezing. Before being frozen, these prepared foods can be put into disposable baking dishes ready for reheating. If food is to be held only a few days, attractive casseroles made of metal, plastic, or pottery can be used in which the food may be cooked over direct heat, stored in a freezer, and later put into the oven while the contents are still frozen. Some nutritive losses do occur during reheating. Home-cooked foods, however, can be much more nutritious and carefully prepared than most commercially frozen foods.

If only a small amount of meat and vegetables remain uneaten, they can be put on an individual TV platter and wrapped, labeled, and frozen without further ado. When time to serve, reheat without thawing, and add a salad or fresh fruit to the menu. One mother I know prepares TV dinners of single servings of leftovers, and sometimes adds still frozen peas or corn to the plates before reheating them. Several such dinners accumulate, and each child gets the choice of the dinner he prefers.

Casseroles

Dozens of out-of-date recipes for casserole dishes specify cooking times as long as two hours or more. Since the fresh vegetables are customarily diced and the meat is already cooked, such long cooking is not only unnecessary but causes destruction of proteins and B vitamins, and probably the complete annihilation of vitamin C.

If a heat-resistant utensil is used, a casserole may be prepared on top of the range. Wheat germ, which makes an ideal topping, may be sprinkled over the food, the edges of the casserole wiped clean, and the browning done under the broiler, the entire process taking no more than a few minutes.

When meats are properly roasted, they retain 50 per cent or more water. If you add leftover roast meat to a cream sauce and then permit the sauce to boil, you can expect the meat to shrivel, meat juices to be squeezed out, and the sauce to become too thin. For example, after Thanksgiving many women prepare creamed turkey. Often they add the meat to the sauce too soon and wonder why the amount of meat seems to diminish and the sauce needs more thickening. After any leftover roast meat is added to a casserole, the temperature must not be allowed to go above simmering.

Increase the nutritive value of casserole dishes whenever possible by adding powdered milk and generous amounts of cheese. Since casserole dishes must depend upon the ingredients you have on hand, you should originate your own recipes for them. Prepare any cream sauce, brown sauce, or tomato sauce, or use condensed canned mushroom or tomato soup; add vegetables and leftover meat, and sprinkle with wheat germ or crumbs and cheese.

LAMB AND PEAS IN CASSEROLE

Use **leftover gravy** or prepare **2 cups medium cream sauce** (p. 135); heat and add:

1½ cups fresh or frozen peas	1 diced stalk celery with leaves
1 finely chopped onion or leek	pinch each of sage and basil

Cook **5 minutes** or until peas are tender; add:

2 diced canned pimentos (optional)	1 teaspoon Worcestershire
	1 to 2 cups diced leftover lamb

Stir well and simmer **10 minutes**; taste for salt; turn off heat; stir in **2 tablespoons chopped parsley**; wipe edges of casserole and sprinkle top with:

¼ cup wheat germ or toasted whole-wheat-bread crumbs	½ cup diced American cheese
	generous amount of paprika

Heat under broiler until cheese melts and serve immediately or freeze and reheat later.

VARIATIONS:

Prepare any cream sauce (p. 135), vinegar sauce (p. 139), tomato sauce (p. 140), or brown sauce (p. 136); add vegetables, leftover meats, cheese, and crumbs.

Instead of peas use 2 cups diced carrots, corn, cauliflower broken into flowerlets, leeks, or other vegetables; cook each vegetable only long enough for it to become tender.

Omit lamb and add 1½ cups diced leftover beef, veal, chicken, heart, or tongue, or canned tuna.

Supplement leftover meat with any canned or quick-cooking fresh meat; combine canned tuna or diced sweetbreads with leftover chicken; fresh sliced kidneys with leftover beef; sliced wieners with leftover pork; lamb liver with leftover lamb.

Use the basic recipe in preparing any casserole dish; substitute the same amounts of the following vegetables, seasonings, and meat for peas, herbs, lamb; cook vegetables only long enough to become tender.

Diced carrots, 1 chopped green pepper, diced cooked heart, chicken, tongue, or beef with dash of nutmeg, a pinch each of thyme and basil; or diced leftover veal, mutton, flaked fish, canned tuna, or shrimps with chopped fresh dill or 1 teaspoon dill seeds.

Diced leftover ham, 3 cups shredded cabbage.

Leftover diced pork or pork heart or tongue, 2 diced raw potatoes, 1 teaspoon caraway or dill seeds.

Diced cooked heart, 2 cups fresh string beans, a pinch each of basil and thyme.

A few fresh string beans, 1 diced carrot, ½ cup peas, leftover veal, chicken, or lamb, a pinch each of thyme, savory, and marjoram.

Cook 1 each diced potato, carrot, and turnip in tomato sauce (p. 140); add leftover diced tongue, Worcestershire, a pinch each of savory, basil, and marjoram. Also delicious with either brown sauce (p. 136) or cream sauce (p. 135).

Use diced carrots, 1 cup leftover brown or converted rice, meat or fish; the herbs of basic recipe.

Canned, frozen, or fresh corn, a pinch of basil, flaked fish, diced leftover ham, veal, beef, or heart; use tomato sauce instead of cream sauce.

Although croquettes are customarily cooked in deep fat, they can have an equally good flavor, fewer calories, and be prepared much more easily if sautéed.

HAM CROQUETTES

Mix together:

2 cups chopped ham
1 cup cold thick cream sauce
   (p. 135) or leftover gravy
1 egg

2 tablespoons each chopped parsley and grated onion
freshly ground black peppercorns
salt to taste

Form into oblong patties, roll in wheat germ or crumbs, and sauté in vegetable oil; or fry in deep fat at 350° F. for 5 minutes, or until brown; or freeze and cook later.

Serve with horseradish sauce (p. 137).

VARIATIONS:

If oven is being used, bake at 350° F. for 20 minutes.

Omit cream sauce and add any one of the following: 1 cup leftover rice, mashed or finely diced leftover white or sweet potatoes, or shredded and quickly sautéed raw white or sweet potatoes.

Add to basic recipe any one or more of the following: a pinch each of basil and savory; 1 tablespoon caraway seeds, catsup, or chili sauce; ¼ cup powdered milk, wheat germ, or precooked soy grits; ½ cup cooked soybeans or cooked whole wheat.

Make 2 cups thick cream sauce; use 1 cup in croquettes; dilute the remainder and prepare horseradish sauce. Use this same procedure in making sauces to serve with croquettes suggested below.

Follow the basic recipe, merely omitting ham and adding ingredients suggested.

Beef, veal, or lamb croquettes: Diced leftover beef, veal, or lamb, 1 teaspoon Worcestershire, 1 tablespoon chili sauce.

Cheese and rice croquettes: Omit cream sauce and use 1½ cups cooked rice, 1 cup shredded American or pimento cheese; add pinch of basil.

Cheese and vegetable croquettes: 1 cup shredded American cheese and 1 cup or more leftover vegetables, such as peas, corn, diced carrots, broccoli, or potatoes; or combine several leftover vegetables.

Chicken croquettes: Diced or ground chicken, ½ teaspoon paprika, a pinch of sage, 2 diced pimentos.

Crab, lobster, or oyster croquettes: 2 cups flaked crab, lobster, or chopped raw or canned oysters; add 1 tablespoon each capers and lemon juice or 2 teaspoons dill seed.

Fish croquettes: Use finely diced uncooked or flaked leftover salmon, halibut, or other cooked or canned fish. Add 1 teaspoon anise or dill seeds.

KIDNEY AND BEEF STEW

Heat **1 or 2 cups leftover brown gravy** and add:

½ to 1 cup soup stock or vegetable-cooking water (optional)
1 or 2 unpeeled potatoes cut into
quarters
2 or 3 carrots cut into quarters
lengthwise
1 quartered onion

1 or 2 quartered turnips or kohlrabi
¼ teaspoon crushed black peppercorns
pinch each of savory, marjoram,
thyme
1½ teaspoons salt

Cook until vegetables are tender; add:

diced leftover roast beef

Meanwhile remove white membrane from **1 pound beef, veal, or
lamb kidneys** and cut into ¾-inch cubes; 3 minutes before serving,
stir kidneys into stew and heat through. Taste for seasonings.

BEEF HASH

Run through meat grinder, using largest knife:

2 large unpeeled potatoes
1 small onion

enough leftover roast beef to
make 2 or 3 cups

Without covering utensil, cook over medium heat in:

2 or 3 tablespoons vegetable oil or partially hardened margarine

Turn frequently as lower portions brown. Sprinkle with:

freshly ground black peppercorns
½ teaspoon salt

¼ teaspoon celery salt (optional)
or 1 teaspoon caraway seeds

Serve as soon as potatoes are cooked through, or in about 10 or 15
minutes.

VARIATIONS:

Make into patties, roll in wheat germ or whole-wheat flour; cook slowly until brown on both sides; serve with leftover gravy seasoned with savory.

Add 2 tablespoons chives or 1 teaspoon caraway seeds.

With the roast beef, use an assortment of any leftover meats, as 1 slice liver, meat from 1 or 2 pork chops, tongue, heart, etc.

Corn-beef hash: Use leftover steamed corned beef. Prepare as in basic recipe; omit salt.

BAKED HASH

Steam in skins, then cool slightly, peel, and dice:

4 small potatoes

Combine in utensil used for cooking potatoes and heat:

½ cup red wine (optional) or liquid left from steaming potatoes	1 tablespoon soy sauce (optional)
2 cups diced or ground leftover roast beef	⅛ teaspoon each marjoram and thyme
2 tablespoons chopped parsley	diced potatoes
	½ teaspoon salt

Mix well and salt to taste. Turn into a greased casserole; sprinkle top generously with wheat germ and paprika. Wrap and freeze or bake immediately in moderate oven at 350° F. for 15 to 20 minutes.

VARIATIONS:

Use lamb or pork instead of beef; season lamb with ½ teaspoon crushed dill seeds, pork with 1 teaspoon caraway seeds.

Add 2 tablespoons or more finely diced celery or bell pepper.

Instead of herbs in basic recipe, season with rosemary, sage, or turmeric.

Although one rarely thinks of freezing soups because of limited storage space, any concentrated soup can be prepared and frozen; milk, water with bouillon cubes, canned consommé, or other liquid can be added later. Leftover vegetables can be blended in a liquefier with a little fresh and powdered milk, frozen, and made into delicious cream soups later.

Use the following procedure in preparing soups from leftovers; combine later with other fresh or leftover vegetables and rice, buckwheat, barley, millet, noodles, or spaghetti.

CONCENTRATED SCOTCH BROTH

Sauté lightly in 2 tablespoons vegetable oil, partially hardened margarine, butter, or meat drippings:

1 cup each diced carrots and   2 thinly sliced onions or leeks
   chopped celery

When onions are translucent, remove from heat and add:

1 to 2 cups diced leftover lamb   freshly ground peppercorns
½ teaspoon salt   ¼ cup chopped parsley

Add liquid and serve immediately; or cool, put into cardboard carton, label, and freeze.

For hurry-up dinner, bring to boiling in a large utensil:

1 quart soup stock or vegetable-   ½ cup hulled barley
   cooking water and 4 chicken or
   beef bouillon cubes

Simmer 10 minutes and add:

            lamb with seasonings, frozen or partly thawed

Bring to a boil, then simmer 10 minutes. Taste for salt.
Serve with whole-wheat crackers or toast.

VARIATIONS:

Add 1 pint of water to sautéed vegetables, cook barley, and then freeze.

Instead of barley, use diced fresh potatoes or leftover rice, millet, or noodles.

Omit lamb and add leftover beef, veal, chicken, or other meat.

Add ¼ teaspoon basil, rosemary, marjoram, or other herbs.

CREAMED CHICKEN

Prepare **2 cups medium cream sauce** (p. 135), using chicken stock when available instead of part of the milk; cook in sauce:

1 cup fresh or frozen peas	**1 diced carrot or leftover carrots**
2 diced canned pimentos	**pinch of sage or thyme**

Simmer 10 minutes, or until peas are barely tender. Add no earlier than 5 minutes before serving:

1½ or 2 cups diced leftover chicken

Serve over hot wheat-germ biscuits (p. 424) cut with doughnut cutter.

VARIATIONS:

Instead of 2 cups chicken, use 1 cup chicken and 1 cup or more diced hard-cooked eggs, roasted pork, veal, or lamb; or use canned tuna; or add 1 cup diced uncooked sweetbreads or brains 10 minutes before adding chicken.

Use leftover turkey, goose, or other fowl instead of chicken.

If preparing creamed chicken for a large group, steam 1 mature rabbit with every 1 or 2 chickens; if nothing is said about it, no one will know the difference. Or steam an apartment-size turkey; remove meat from bones, and cream.

Instead of cream sauce use leftover gravy. Or prepare sauce of fresh or reconstituted milk and add 2 or 3 chicken bouillon cubes or 2 teaspoons instant chicken broth. If bouillon cubes are used, salt to taste.

Add 1 small can mushrooms; use juice from mushrooms in preparing the sauce; if desired, omit sage and add 2 tablespoons sherry just before serving.

Creamed beef: Prepare **2 cups celery, curry, horseradish, mustard, olive, or onion sauce** (pp. 136–137); proceed as in basic recipe, using diced leftover beef; use or omit vegetables.

Creamed ham or pork: Prepare **2 cups caraway, curry, dill, olive, mustard, pimento, piquant, or horseradish sauce** (pp. 136–137); omit vegetables; proceed as in basic recipe, using diced leftover ham or pork. Supplement with diced wieners or hard-cooked eggs if needed.

Creamed lamb or veal: Prepare **2 cups caper, celery, curry, dill, mushroom, olive, pimento, or piquant sauce** (pp. 136–137); prepare as in basic recipe, using diced lamb or veal.

HAM CASSEROLE

Combine in a heat-resistant casserole:

¼ cup canned tomatoes or tomato   1 teaspoon Worcestershire
purée or 1 diced fresh tomato   1 cup leftover rice
½ chopped bell pepper   1½ to 2 cups diced leftover ham
1 small grated onion   ½ teaspoon salt

Cover utensil and heat to simmering. Remove from heat and stir in:

2 beaten eggs   ¼ cup sherry (optional)

Wipe edges; sprinkle over top:

½ cup wheat germ   paprika

Let sit for 10 minutes; brown top under broiler or put into oven at
350° F. for 10 minutes; or wrap, label, and freeze.

VARIATIONS:

Instead of ham, use leftover veal, beef, chicken, or other meat.
Add ½ cup chopped celery; or omit pepper and add diced canned
pimento or chili pepper.
Omit wine and season with ⅛ teaspoon basil, tarragon, or orégano;
or add 1 teaspoon caraway seeds.

JAMBALAYA

Sauté lightly in 2 tablespoons vegetable oil:

3 sliced onions   1 diced bell pepper
1 minced clove garlic

Add and bring to boiling:

1 cup soup stock or vegetable-   2 cups canned or diced fresh
cooking water   tomatoes

Stir in so slowly that boiling does not stop:

1 cup uncooked converted rice	¼ teaspoon each thyme, basil, and
dash of cayenne or Tabasco	paprika

Simmer 15 minutes, or until rice is tender; add:

2 cups diced leftover ham	¼ cup dry white wine or sherry

Serve as soon as heated through, or chill, wrap, and freeze.

VARIATIONS:

Cook brown rice first; after 35 minutes, add other ingredients and simmer 10 minutes longer, or until rice is tender.

Instead of rice use 1 cup hulled barley, millet, buckwheat, cooked unground wheat or uncooked cracked wheat.

Use leftover veal, lamb, or beef instead of ham.

Omit thyme and basil; add marjoram, rosemary, orégano, or other herbs or seeds.

LEFTOVER PORK WITH LENTILS

Bring to boiling:

2 cups soup stock or vegetable-cooking water

Add so slowly that boiling does not stop:

1 cup lentils

Simmer 30 minutes, or until lentils are tender; add:

2 cups diced fresh or canned tomatoes	3 chicken bouillon cubes
	1½ to 2 cups diced leftover roast
1 chopped or shredded onion	pork
1 minced clove garlic	¼ cup chopped parsley

Simmer 15 minutes and serve immediately; or cool, wrap, label, and freeze.

VARIATIONS:

Use leftover ham, beef, chicken, or turkey instead of pork.

Add ½ cup chopped celery or bell pepper or finely diced carrot.

Prepare in heat-resistant casserole, sprinkle generously with wheat germ and paprika, and bake at 350° F. for 15 minutes after meat is added.

Season with ⅛ teaspoon basil, marjoram, rosemary, or orégano; or add 1 teaspoon crushed dill, cumin, or caraway seeds.

SHEPHERD'S PIE

Mix together:

1 to 2 cups leftover mashed potatoes	¼ cup powdered milk

When thoroughly mixed, add and beat slightly:

1 or 2 whole eggs	sprinkling of salt

Keep out 1 cup potatoes for topping; spread any remainder over bottom of greased baking dish. Combine and heat to simmering:

2 cups leftover gravy or brown sauce	¼ cup each grated onion and finely chopped parsley
2 cups diced leftover lamb	½ cup thinly sliced celery

Pour lamb mixture into baking dish; drop mashed potatoes from spoon over lamb; sprinkle generously with **wheat germ and paprika**. Bake in a moderate oven at 350° F. for 20 minutes.

VARIATIONS:

Prepare pie without heating; wrap, label, and freeze; thaw and bake 30 minutes, or until heated through.

Instead of lamb use leftover beef, veal, ham, roast pork, or other meat.

Add ¼ cup sliced bell pepper or pimento or 1 cup shredded carrots or fresh or frozen peas.

Season meat with ⅛ teaspoon basil, rosemary, thyme, or orégano; or add chopped fresh dill or ½ teaspoon crushed dill seeds to potatoes.

STUFFED PEPPERS

Use **large red bell peppers** when available; cut in half lengthwise and remove seeds; or use **medium-sized peppers** with tops and seeds removed. Steam peppers *over* boiling water for 10 minutes. Meanwhile, combine:

2 cups cooked buckwheat groats (p. 393)

1 cup chopped canned or fresh tomatoes

¼ cup each chopped parsley and grated onion

2 teaspoons each chili powder and Worcestershire

¼ to ½ teaspoon each basil and thyme

2 cups diced or ground leftover beef

Put stuffing into peppers; pour remainder of can of tomatoes or 1 cup diced raw tomatoes into bottom of baking dish and set stuffed peppers on top; sprinkle tops of peppers with **wheat germ, Parmesan cheese, and paprika.** Refrigerate for several hours, or freeze if desired; bake in moderate oven at 350° F. for 30 minutes.

VARIATIONS:

If peppers are to be served immediately after being made, heat stuffing, pack into hot peppers, and brown under broiler. Meanwhile boil remaining tomatoes and pour over peppers.

Instead of buckwheat use leftover cooked rice, millet, hulled barley, or noodles; or use 1 cup buckwheat with 1 cup of any leftover grain.

Add ½ cup diced celery, shredded carrots, or fresh or canned mushrooms.

BEEF CREOLE

Sauté lightly in **1 tablespoon vegetable oil:**

1 large chopped onion

¼ cup each bell pepper and celery

Add:

1 teaspoon each salt, sugar, and chili powder

2 cups diced leftover beef

1 cup tomato purée

1 to 2 cups leftover gravy

Simmer 10 minutes and serve.

VARIATIONS:

Use pork, veal, chicken, turkey, or lamb instead of beef.

Vary by adding ¼ teaspoon basil, savory, orégano, or other herbs with different meats.

Add with onions ½ cup shredded carrot; or use fresh or canned chili pepper instead of bell pepper.

If no gravy is available, prepare brown sauce with water, beef bouillon cubes, and thickening; salt to taste.

VEAL GOULASH

Heat and blend together:

2 tablespoons partially hardened margarine, butter, or vegetable oil	1½ tablespoons whole-wheat-pastry flour

Add:

1 cup beef bouillon, cannned consommé, or water with 2 beef bouillon cubes	1½ teaspoons paprika
1 cup thinly sliced onions	¼ teaspoon each thyme and tarragon or basil
	¼ cup dry white wine (optional)

Simmer 10 minutes, stirring frequently; add:

2 cups diced leftover veal

Salt to taste. As soon as veal is heated, serve in a nest of buttered whole-wheat noodles, steamed unhulled barley, brown or converted rice, or steamed buckwheat. Or freeze and reheat later.

VARIATIONS:

Use leftover beef, lamb, or roast pork or other meat instead of veal.

Instead of beef bouillon, use instant chicken broth or chicken bouillon cubes.

Add ¼ cup chopped bell pepper or celery, 1 cup shredded carrots, and/or 1 clove garlic; or add leftover peas, carrots, or other vegetables only in time to reheat.

COLD MARINATED LAMB

Slice and cut into narrow strips:

2 cups leftover roast lamb

Add and stir well:

2 chopped, shredded, or grated onions	**Tabasco sauce or cayenne**
2 tablespoons chopped parsley	**freshly ground black peppercorns**
2 teaspoons chopped fresh or ⅛ teaspoon dry tarragon or savory	**¼ cup wine or cider vinegar**
	¼ cup vegetable oil
	½ teaspoon dry mustard

Put into serving dish and let stand at room temperature 3 hours; or marinate longer in the refrigerator. Serve chilled.

VARIATIONS:

Add 1 or 2 tablespoons fresh horseradish; or omit herbs and add 2 teaspoons finely chopped mint or 1 teaspoon crushed dill seeds.

Use leftover roast beef or lean pork instead of lamb; season pork with caraway seeds; omit or use herbs.

STUFFED EGGPLANT

Cut 1 large unpeeled eggplant in half lengthwise; steam in or above ½ cup water until almost tender, or about 15 to 20 minutes.

Remove center of eggplant, leaving shell ⅓ inch thick; chop pulp fine, adding water left from steaming; in utensil used for steaming sauté in vegetable oil:

1 finely chopped onion	**½ chopped bell pepper or 1 stalk celery**

Add, stir, and heat through:

1 to 2 cups diced leftover beef	**leftover diced carrots or other vegetables (optional)**
¼ teaspoon sage	**½ to 1 cup wheat germ or dry whole-wheat-bread crumbs**
1 teaspoon salt	
chopped eggplant	

Put stuffing in eggplant shells, sprinkle top with paprika, and place in shallow baking dish; bake in preheated oven at 350° F. for 10 minutes.

VARIATIONS:

Use lamb, ham, chicken, turkey, or other leftover meat instead of beef.

Omit wheat germ or dry crumbs; add 2 or 3 slices stale whole-wheat bread softened with ½ cup milk and pinched into bits.

A few minutes before serving cover top of eggplant with wheat germ and grated cheese, and brown under broiler.

Cut eggplant in half lengthwise and scoop out center with grapefruit knife before cooking; dice and sauté with onion, celery, or bell pepper, 1 minced clove garlic; add leftover meat, omitting sage and crumbs. Put filling in uncooked eggplant shells, sprinkle generously with wheat germ, Parmesan cheese, and paprika, and bake at 350° F. for 5 minutes. Or instead of leftover meat add 1 or 2 cups oysters.

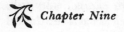 *Chapter Nine*

Meats and Meat Substitutes for Hot-Weather Dinners

The diet of most people during hot weather is often appallingly inadequate in many respects. The days are sometimes so hot that you do not enjoy cooking, and the family does not relish eating unless foods are particularly attractive and appetizing. The intake of meats, eggs, cheese, and breads may be so decreased that protein, salt, and the B vitamins become dangerously deficient. At the same time much salt and large amounts of the vitamins which dissolve in water are lost through perspiration. Iced tea sweetened with refined sugar and soft drinks frequently satisfy hunger pangs. The mother who keeps her family adequately fed during hot weather must be alert to their nutritional needs.

Why not serve your summer dinners in the delightful buffet, or smörgåsbord, style? Have your entire dinner of chilled foods, or perhaps serve one hot dish and the other foods chilled. The variety of foods which may be served cold is almost endless: appetizers and juices, jellied bouillons, sliced meats, fish, meat or fish aspics, plates of assorted sliced cheeses or a bowl of cottage cheese, chilled vegetables marinated in French dressing or other tart sauce, frozen purées, salads, and the old stand-bys, sliced tomatoes and stuffed eggs. Such foods can be prepared in the cool of the morning and kept in the refrigerator until dinnertime.

If hot-weather fatigue is to be prevented, the salt, vitamin C, and B vitamins lost in perspiration must be replaced. Add a larger amount of salt to foods than you would at other times and serve salted potato chips, perhaps spread with cheese, salty fish, ham, salted nuts, or some other well-salted food at each lunch and dinner. Vitamin C may be obtained from citrus fruits, tomatoes, and salads. See that the B vitamins are supplied by serving only dark breads, by emphasizing glandular meats in salads and cold cuts, and by serving yogurt with chilled fruits, salads, and concentrated frozen juices.

There is a prevalent idea that only a small amount of meat should be eaten during hot weather. This belief is largely a hangover from the times when refrigeration was unknown and meats spoiled too easily to be safe. If adequate protein is obtained from milk, cheese, eggs, brewers' yeast, wheat germ, and other foods, meats may be avoided without loss of health. It is difficult, however, to obtain sufficient protein from these foods without careful planning, especially during the summer when the appetite may be jaded. If you sincerely want your family to have the best health possible, you should learn the approximate protein content of foods and estimate the amount each member of your family eats daily. These figures should be so familiar that you can count protein grams as easily as the change in your purse. Unless you do such counting, it is much safer to serve meats during the summer. The quantities of food eaten need not be large or the calorie intake high.

Hot-Weather Dinners with Cold Meats

Cold meats are excellent. By varying the kinds of sauces served with cold meat, monotony can be avoided indefinitely. The sauces with a yogurt base, which are low in calories, are especially suitable during hot weather. If the meat does not slice well, the entire platter of meat may be covered with sauce and attractively garnished with parsley, radishes, and sliced eggs or stuffed olives. Many meat stuffings are delicious when cold, especially those of vegetables, grains, or fruits. Aspics of tart fruit juices and frozen purées are particularly appealing on hot summer evenings when served with meat; try purple-plum purée with cold roast beef.

Almost any vegetable can be delicious when served cold if it is first steamed, chilled, and marinated in French dressing or mayonnaise. Several vegetables of contrasting colors can be arranged on a bed of lettuce or on the same platter with the meat. The sauces made of yogurt, sour cream, or whipped evaporated milk mixed with mayonnaise can also be served with chilled vegetables.

In restaurant windows or on Swedish smörgåsbords one sometimes sees beautiful glazed meats which appear bafflingly professional. The glazing is achieved merely by brushing the chilled meat with any aspic base or jellied consommé just before it congeals. The gelatin may be dissolved in the juice left from canned fruit or peach or watermelon pickles. The glazing takes about two minutes to make and brush on, and is well worth the effort.

Following are suggestions for hot-weather menus in which cold meat serves as the entree:

See **aspic recipe** (p. 230) or **jellied consommé** (p. 300) for glazes; **meat sauces** (pp. 135–144).

Cold corned beef: Serve with horseradish sauce, marinated string beans, potato salad, watercress in tomato aspic.

Chilled liver: Steam **uncut lamb or baby beef liver;** chill, slice, and cover with **raw creole sauce.** Serve with marinated cauliflower, cottage cheese, tossed green salad, chilled raspberries with yogurt.

Chilled brains: Steam, dice, marinate in a little **French dressing;** cover with **ground pickle or cucumber sauce** and garnish with parsley. Serve with marinated broccoli, egg-celery salad, sliced tomatoes, sweet onions.

Barbecued veal: Barbecue fillet of veal; chill, slice, and put the slices together as if uncut; cover with a **glaze of jellied consommé** and serve surrounded with **diced cubes of consommé;** garnish with parsley or capers. Serve with tomato-juice appetizer, marinated parsnips, sliced cucumbers, green peppers.

Ham or shoulder: Braise or roast. Slice and serve with horseradish sauce made with yogurt, marinated turnips, sliced tomatoes, tossed salad.

Dried-beef rolls: Mix **cream cheese** generously with **horseradish and parsley;** roll inside slices of **dried beef;** surround with **assorted sliced cheeses.** Serve with marinated celery root, carrot-parsley salad.

Cold roast beef: Serve with aspic of purple plums, marinated celery and carrots, cole slaw of green cabbage, yogurt dressing.

Glazed ham: Decorate the surface with thin half slices of orange and maraschino cherries; hold in place with a glaze of ham stock left from steaming; chill the remaining glaze, dice, and arrange around the meat. Serve with mustard sauce, potato salad, applesauce mixed with toasted wheat germ, tossed greens.

Cold lamb: Serve with caper sauce; if the slices are unattractive, cover with caper sauce. Serve with apricot aspic (p. 231), marinated broccoli, assorted finger salads.

Roast lamb or mutton: Glaze with clear mint aspic (p. 231), then add coloring and make aspic cubes; serve with marinated rutabagas, sliced tomatoes and cucumbers on a bed of watercress.

Roast chicken: Stuff with rice or buckwheat stuffing (p. 132); make a glaze of stock seasoned with sage and thyme. Serve with marinated string beans, fruit salad.

Cold roast pork: Serve with frozen applesauce seasoned with red cinnamon candies, marinated onions and turnips, beet aspic (p. 231).

Cold sliced heart: After citrus-juice appetizer, serve with mustard-horseradish sauce, marinated broccoli, carrot sticks, tomato and cottage-cheese salad.

Braised shoulder of lamb: Slice and serve with pineapple-curry sauce, marinated carrots, celery stuffed with avocado, tomato-watercress salad.

Diced cold meat: Dice scraps of leftover veal, lamb, pork, or beef; fold into citron-cherry sauce. After frozen tomato-juice appetizer, serve with marinated asparagus, spiced beets, tossed salad of endive, grapefruit, and watercress.

Pork tongue: Chill and slice; drop into cold aspic seasoned with caraway seeds; put together again as if uncut; glaze and set in a bed of aspic; decorate the aspic with slices of hard-cooked egg. Serve with horseradish sauce, marinated zucchini, sliced tomatoes and leeks, mixed-fruit salad.

Fish to Be Served Chilled

Although fish salads and appetizers have become popular in America, other forms of chilled fish are used far too little. Steamed fish (p. 162), chilled, well seasoned, attractively arranged and garnished, is excellent for luncheons and hot-weather dinners.

Any of the cold sauces, whether with a base of sour cream, yogurt, whipped cream, or mayonnaise, can be served with them. In preparing nutritious lunches, summer-evening dinners, and buffets, serve chilled fish frequently.

Following are suggestions for serving fish as the entree or on buffet dinners.

See baked fish (pp. 152–154), steamed fish (p. 162), chilled sauces (p. 143).

Baked fish ring: Buy 2 whole fish or more; clean and stuff with **onion stuffing** to which is added a **generous amount of pimentos (p. 131)**; tie a string from heads to tails to form a curve and prop mouths open with toothpicks; bake with back of fish up; chill and arrange around platter with the tail of one fish in the mouth of the other, making a complete circle; fill center with **potato salad**; garnish with **tomato sections, capers, and paprika.** Serve with any chilled sauce.

Fish with beet pickles: Steam **2 pounds fillets** ½ inch thick; chill and arrange slices of **beet pickle** between layers of fillets; pour **2 to 3 table-spoons French dressing** over top and garnish with **lemon sections dipped in finely chopped parsley and/or thin slices of onion or leek.** Bony fish may be flaked and mixed with **diced tart apple and chilled sauce.**

Fish with sour cream and capers: Steam **2 pounds fillets,** chill; pour over the fillets **2 cups caper sauce** with a sour-cream base; garnish with **paprika, sliced tomatoes, lemon sections dipped in finely chopped parsley.** Vary by flaking steamed fish; stir with 1 cup sauce and pour the other cup over the top; use any variety of fish and any uncooked sauce. Garnish with **sliced radishes and stuffed olives.**

Fish with pickles, parsley, eggs: Steam small whole fish, **fillets, or steaks;** chill; arrange on platter, flaking bony or whole fish if used; cover with finely chopped **beet or dill pickles, generous layer of chopped parsley, 2 or 3 hard-cooked eggs** forced through a sieve. Garnish with **onion rings and slices of pickles and eggs.**

Fish flakes with radishes: Steam and flake 2 pounds whole fish or 1½ pounds fillets; chill; slice thin **1 bunch radishes,** add to the flaked fish, and mix with basic **yogurt or sour-cream sauce.** Put on platter and surround with **lettuce or endive;** garnish with **tomato sections.**

Fish flakes with mushrooms: Steam and flake 2 pounds fish, or use **shrimps or other sea food;** add **1 can sliced mushrooms with liquid and 3 tablespoons tart French dressing.** Chill and garnish with **strips or rings of pimento;** or serve with any sauce with base of sour cream.

Fish platter: Steam 2 pounds fillets cut into serving sizes; steam 2 un-peeled potatoes, chill, peel, and slice; place fish on serving platter, cover with sliced potatoes, 1 or 2 each sliced cucumbers and sweet onions or leeks; pour over all 1 cup French dressing; let stand 2 hours or more. Surround with celery sticks and tomato sections; garnish with parsley.

Fish with cucumber sauce: Steam 2 pounds or more fillets; put on platter and chill; pour over fish 1 cup cucumber sauce; garnish with slices of hard-cooked egg and 2 tablespoons capers.

Fish with hard-cooked eggs: Steam thin fillets; put half the fillets on a platter and cover with slices of hard-cooked eggs and leeks; add another layer of fillets; cover with sauce of sour cream to which pickle relish is added; garnish with a few slices of hard-cooked eggs and chopped parsley. Vary by covering with sliced eggs and tartar sauce diluted with vinegar and seasoned with dill and ground parsley. Vary by making alternate layers of fish and thin slices of fresh leeks or sweet onions marinated with ½ cup French dressing.

Glazed fish with aspic cubes: Stuff a whole fish with onion dressing (p. 131) and bake; use dill-seasoned aspic as a glaze (p. 225). Turn re-maining aspic into flat pan and let congeal. Dice aspic into tiny cubes and serve around glazed fish. Garnish with parsley, sliced stuffed olives, and tomato sections.

Roe with capers and olives: Steam ½ pound herring, shad, or other roe; remove the membranes and mash, mixing with 2 tablespoons each grated onion, chopped parsley, capers, and sliced stuffed olives. Chill, and garnish with paprika.

Roe with egg sauce: Mix 1 cup (½ pound) raw or steamed roe with a sauce of yogurt or sour-cream base and 2 or 3 diced hard-cooked eggs; garnish with slices of hard-cooked eggs and chopped chives and parsley.

Roe with onion sauce: Mix 1 cup (½ pound) caviar or uncooked sal-mon roe with 1 cup onion sauce; add 4 to 6 minced radishes. Serve with wheat-germ crackers.

Rolled fish fillets with pimentos: Select small fillets or cut large fillets into thin strips 2 inches wide; cut canned pimentos in half and spread over each fillet; roll and hold with toothpicks; steam quickly; chill and pyramid on platter, cover with caper or other sauce having base of sour cream or yogurt; garnish with chopped parsley and tomato sections. Vary by preparing rolls and setting in aspic (p. 225) or by spreading chopped pimentos between steamed fillets in layers in loaf pan and covering with aspic.

Spiced fish flakes: Buy 2 pounds or more of any small bony fish, such as smelts, sardines, fresh herrings, sand dabs. Steam quickly, using ¼ cup water. Flake fish, add bones to water used for steaming with ¼ cup vinegar, 4 cloves, small piece of cinnamon stick, ¼ crumbled bay leaf, ¼ teaspoon each celery and dill seeds, crushed white peppercorns; bring to a boil and let stand 20 minutes. Strain through fine-mesh strainer and pour over flaked fish; add 3 tablespoons each chives, parsley, vegetable oil; chill; garnish with slices of dill pickles.

Fish for aspics has customarily been boiled in order to season the liquid. The fish, however, should not be robbed of flavor. If the aspic is made of fillets prepared at home, the trimmings and bones may be used to flavor the stock; otherwise, a small bony fish should be purchased for making the aspic.

FISH ASPIC

Select or prepare 2 pounds or more fillets.

Chop bones left from preparing fillets or chop a small whole fish into ½-inch pieces; put bones or chopped fish into utensil to be used for steaming and add:

1¼ cups vegetable-cooking water	¼ crushed bay leaf
¼ cup vinegar	1 teaspoon dill or anise seeds (optional)
1 sliced clove garlic	
¼ teaspoon crushed peppercorns	1 teaspoon salt

Simmer seasonings 10 minutes; set rack over water and add:

2 pounds or more of fillets

Insert meat thermometer and steam 4 to 8 minutes to internal temperature of 145 to 150° F.; remove fillets to large platter.

Meanwhile soften:

1 tablespoon gelatin in   ½ cup vegetable-cooking water

Strain water used for steaming into softened gelatin; stir well, pour onto platter around the fish, chill.

When gelatin is chilled but not congealed, set in aspic around fish:

thin slices of onion and lemon   slices of stuffed olives

Chill; garnish platter with sprigs of parsley. Serve with dill or caper sauce with sour-cream base.

VARIATIONS:

If small or bony fish are to be used, steam them above 1 cup vegetable-cooking water; flake the fish and put bones, trimmings, vinegar, and seasonings into the water; simmer 10 minutes, strain into softened gelatin, cool, and add the flaked fish, 3 tablespoons sliced stuffed olives, 2 tablespoons grated onion, and ¼ cup mayonnaise; chill in an oiled ring mold or loaf pan.

Flaked fish loaf: Steam over **1 cup vegetable-cooking water** enough fish to make 2 cups when flaked; soften **1 tablespoon gelatin in ½ cup vegetable-cooking water;** stir gelatin and **2 tablespoons vinegar** into hot liquid used for steaming fish; cool, and add **½ cup chopped celery, 1 chopped green pepper, 2 tablespoons sliced olives, ½ cup mayonnaise, 1 teaspoon salt, ¼ teaspoon paprika;** chill in oiled loaf pan or a fish mold; serve on bed of **watercress with sliced cucumbers.** Canned salmon or shrimp may be used.

Whole fish in aspic: Stuff whole fish weighing 2 pounds or more with **onion or celery stuffing** (p. 131); bake (p. 152). Double the basic recipe for fish aspic, using small bony fish and adding **2 tablespoons each chopped onion and celery leaves.** Before straining add **3 crushed eggshells** to clarify the liquid. Pour 3 cups of the aspic into large loaf pan brushed with oil; when it starts to congeal, place whole fish in center of aspic with back down; chill; when gelatin has set, mix **3 tablespoons each chopped parsley and pimento** with the remaining cup of aspic and pour over fish; chill until set. Unmold on large platter and garnish with **tomato and lemon sections.** Fish prepared in this manner is strikingly beautiful.

CHICKEN LOAF

Select stewing chicken and steam (p. 54) until tender, cooking neck and wing tips in water and vinegar under rack.

Remove meat from bones and put through meat grinder with:

1 slice sweet onion or leek	1 small stalk celery with leaves
1 fresh or canned pimento	few sprigs of parsley

Evaporate the broth left from steaming to 1 cup and strain into the chicken; mix well and add:

salt to taste	freshly ground white peppercorns

Garnish top of oiled mold with slices of hard-cooked eggs and chopped parsley; press chicken firmly into mold. Chill thoroughly, unmold, slice.

VARIATIONS:

If bones are not used in preparing broth, soak 2 teaspoons gelatin in ¼ cup water and dissolve in 1 cup hot broth; season broth with pinch of sage, basil, or tarragon.

Grind with chicken 1 small can mushrooms; add liquid from mushrooms to broth.

Chicken loaf with rice or noodles: Remove bones from broth and add enough water to make 2 cups; cook in broth ½ cup **brown or converted rice or 1 cup noodles;** proceed as in basic recipe.

Pressed tongue: Use 1 veal or pork tongue, either fresh or smoked, or 1½ pounds lamb tongues. Steam over 2 tablespoons vinegar, 2 cups water, and 1 pound beef soup bones sawed into small pieces; when tender, skin tongues while hot, discard bones. Soak 2 teaspoons gelatin in ½ cup cold water and dissolve in hot broth. Proceed as in basic recipe, increasing onion or leek or adding garlic as desired. If lamb tongues are used, vary by cooking 1 teaspoon dill seeds in broth.

Veal loaf: Use 1 pound lean veal and veal knuckle sawed into ¾-inch pieces; add 2 tablespoons vinegar, 2 cups vegetable-cooking water, and steam until the veal is tender. Proceed as in basic recipe.

HAM LOAF

Soak 1 tablespoon gelatin in:

½ cup tomato juice, water, or fat-free ham stock

Dissolve in:

1 cup hot tomato juice, vegetable-cooking water, or ham stock

Cool. Meanwhile run through meat grinder:

enough leftover baked ham to make 1½ or 2 cups 1 bell pepper	several sprigs of parsley 1 small onion

Stir ham into cooled liquid; add:

¼ teaspoon paprika 1 teaspoon Worcestershire	¼ cup mayonnaise

Pour into oiled loaf pan. Chill; invert on platter and garnish with tomato sections, parsley, lettuce leaves.

VARIATIONS:

Add 1 or 2 teaspoons caraway or dill seeds to hot liquid.

Use 1 cup ham and any one of the following: 3 diced hard-cooked eggs; 1 cup shredded American cheese; ½ cup each shredded American and Swiss cheese, 1 tablespoon fresh dill; 1 cup shredded Swiss cheese; or 1 cup pimento cheese or American cheese with 3 diced pimentos.

Instead of ham, use leftover veal, tongue, heart, lamb; or 1 cup meat with 3 diced eggs or 1 cup shredded cheese; add ½ cup mayonnaise.

Cottage-cheese loaf: Soak 1 tablespoon gelatin in ½ cup pineapple juice and heat over simmer burner to dissolve; add 1 cup crushed pineapple; chill well; add 2 cups cottage cheese; mold. This is a delicious loaf.

Cheese loaf: Instead of ham in basic recipe, use 2 cups shredded American or Swiss cheese; heat 2 tablespoons chopped dill or 1 to 2 teaspoons dill seeds in vegetable-cooking water or tomato juice.

Fish loaf: Use fish stock or vegetable-cooking water; instead of ham, add 2 cups flaked fish, crab, or lobster, ½ cup mayonnaise, the other seasonings of basic recipe, ¼ teaspoon celery seeds, 2 tablespoons capers.

Mock liverwurst is one of my favorite recipes, and I hope you will also like it. Use it not only during hot weather but also for box lunches, between-meal snacks, sandwiches, and buffets throughout the year. Few foods can compare with it nutritionally. It is excellent to serve to persons who are anemic, deficient in B vitamins, or are reducing.

MOCK LIVERWURST, OR LIVER PASTE

Sauté lightly in vegetable oil without browning:

1 sliced carrot	1 sliced onion

When onion is transparent, add and steam above vegetables:

1 pound sliced lamb, veal, or baby beef liver	¼ teaspoon crushed black peppercorns

Steam liver 8 minutes. Pass liver, vegetables, and 1 clove garlic through meat grinder 2 or 3 times, using smallest knife; add and mix well:

2 teaspoons salt   ¼ teaspoon of sage
any juices left from sautéing or   smoke flavoring (optional)
grinding

Turn liver paste onto wax paper; form into a roll the size of commercial liverwurst. Chill thoroughly; cut in diagonal slices.

VARIATIONS:

Use pork liver; omit sage and add with carrot 1 teaspoon crushed caraway seeds. Or use lamb liver and season with dill seeds.

Blend with paste 2 to 4 tablespoons partially hardened margarine or butter; serve on crackers. This paste is similar to pâté de foie gras.

Add ¼ to ½ cup powdered milk.

Aside from hot-weather dinners, salads which contain meat, eggs, fish, or cheese are excellent for lunches throughout the year with nothing more than milk or yogurt, whole-grain bread, and butter. Serve this kind of salad in addition to the entree whenever the protein requirements are high, especially if you have adolescent youngsters. Meat, eggs, cheese, or fish may be added to any tossed salad (p. 266).

Although an inexperienced cook likes to have amounts of each ingredient specified, the quantities of meat and vegetables used in a salad should vary, depending on the needs of your family and the other foods you are serving at the same meal. If a salad or aspic is to be the principal protein dish, use a larger proportion of meat, fish, eggs, or cheese than of vegetables. If the salad or aspic is to be served with an entree, increase the amount of vegetables used. In making aspics, use well-seasoned soup stock rich in flavor. Have fun creating attractive designs by setting slices of hard-cooked egg, avocado, stuffed olives, and other ingredients at the sides and bottom of the mold before pouring the gelatin into it.

The average housewife has two or three salads which she serves as entrees in hot weather: usually tuna, chicken, and egg and celery salad. Often she makes little attempt to increase the variety. Actually the number of excellent meat or fish salads is almost unlimited. Such salads are splendid for using up leftovers or for introducing the nutritionally superior meats which, if not enjoyed, can be well disguised by the clever use of seasonings.

There are only two ways to prepare salads to be served as entrees. The ingredients are essentially the same whether the meat, fish, egg, or cheese salad is combined with mayonnaise and served on greens or added to an aspic; therefore I have listed the ingredients for each type of salad following the two basic recipes. Serve them in either manner you desire.

MEAT, FISH, EGG, OR CHEESE SALADS

Use the ingredients specified on pages 232 to 234.
Dice or flake:

1 to 2 cups meat or fish

Unless flavor alone is especially enjoyed, marinate with:

1 to 3 tablespoons French dressing for each cup of meat or fish

Wash the vegetables; prepare the eggs; chill all ingredients; shortly before serving combine the vegetables, meat or fish and/or cheese or eggs, seasonings, mayonnaise, boiled dressing, or other salad dressing. Add onions and/or garlic as desired, and salt to taste.

Arrange on a bed of **watercress, endive, romaine, or lettuce;** garnish with **pimento, red or green pepper rings, tomato sections, olives, or radishes.**

MEAT OR FISH ASPIC SALADS

Soak **1 tablespoon gelatin** in:

½ cup vegetable-cooking water or tomato juice

Dissolve it in:

1 cup boiling soup stock, vegetable-cooking water, or tomato juice

Add and stir well:

2 tablespoons vinegar or lemon
juice
1 teaspoon salt
⅛ teaspoon paprika

3 tablespoons finely chopped
onion
1 tablespoon Worcestershire
2 or 3 drops Tabasco

Chill, and when the gelatin starts to congeal, add:

1½ to 2 cups solid ingredients, or chopped vegetables and meat, fish,
eggs, or cheese specified on pages 232 to 234

Pour into a mold brushed with oil; chill until firm.
Unmold on a bed of **watercress, romaine, endive, or lettuce.**
Serve with mayonnaise or other salad dressing.

VARIATIONS:

Use 1 package lemon or lime gelatin; dissolve in 1¾ cups boiling
vegetable-cooking water; omit unflavored gelatin and seasonings; use as
a base for fish or cottage-cheese salad.

Decrease the amount of gelatin to 1 or 2 teaspoons if firmly jelled
soup stock is used in making aspic.

Omit vinegar or lemon juice if tart tomato juice is used.

Fruit-juice aspics: Omit the seasonings; instead of stock or vegetable-
cooking water, use apple or pineapple juice for aspics containing ham
or pork, tart plum juice for aspics of beef, grapefruit juice for lamb or
mutton. Omit vegetables and use 2 cups diced meat.

Glaze for meat or fish: Prepare the basic aspic, using cleared soup
stock or vegetable-cooking water; omit onion; when aspic starts to congeal, brush over meat or fish, applying 2 coats or more; pour any remaining aspic into shallow pan so that it is no more than ½ inch thick;
chill, dice, serve around cold meat. Glazed meats and fish are extremely
attractive and well worth the effort of preparing them.

Mint aspic for lamb or mutton: Steep ½ **cup crushed mint leaves** in
1 cup boiling water or unsweetened pineapple or grapefruit juice; cool;
strain out the leaves; reheat the juice and dissolve in it 1 tablespoon
gelatin soaked in ½ cup juice; add 2 tablespoons each sugar and lemon
juice and 1 drop green coloring. Mold and serve with roast lamb or
mutton; or add diced cold lamb before molding. Mint flavoring may be
used instead of fresh leaves.

Add the ingredients listed below to aspic recipe; or combine with mayonnaise or other dressing and serve as a salad on a bed of greens. If an aspic or salad is to be served as the entree, use a small amount of vegetables and 1½ to 2 cups eggs, meat, or fish. If either is to be served in addition to the entree, use a larger proportion of vegetables. Add a generous amount of salt when weather is hot.

Steamed brains (p. 81), parsley, American cheese, diced pickle.

Steamed brains, chopped ripe olives, pimentos, shredded carrot.

Steamed brains, chopped celery, parsley, set in tomato aspic or served on whole tomato cut petal fashion.

Cottage cheese, 1 cup or more, 2 diced hard-cooked eggs, parsley, celery, chives; serve with tomatoes or add to tomato aspic; vary aspic by adding ¼ cup mayonnaise or ½ cup sour cream.

Cottage cheese, 1 cup or more, sliced hard-cooked eggs, shrimps or flaked fish, chives, parsley; use eggs to decorate aspic mold; for a salad, arrange eggs and shrimps over tomato slices, put cheese at one side.

Sliced hard-cooked eggs, diced American cheese, chopped pimentos, celery, parsley; set in tomato aspic or add tomato wedges; use 4 or more eggs.

Chicken or turkey, celery, diced pimento, dash of nutmeg.

Chicken or turkey, parsley, fresh or canned asparagus; supplement the chicken with lean diced veal or pork.

Chicken or turkey, diced broccoli stalk, shredded carrot, pimento.

Flaked fish, such as halibut or cod, chopped cucumber, green pepper, fresh dill or crushed dill seeds.

Flaked fish, parsley, diced celery; set in tomato aspic seasoned with basil, or add tomatoes and fresh basil.

Flaked salmon or other fish, hard-cooked eggs, sliced stuffed olives, green pepper or pimento.

Flaked fish, parsley, shredded raw carrot; season boiling liquid used in aspic with 1 teaspoon anise seeds or marinate the fish in French dressing to which anise seeds are added.

Flaked fish, diced beet pickle, parsley, diced American cheese.

Flaked fish, celery, diced hard-cooked eggs or wedges of unpeeled red apple, parsley.

Flaked crab or lobster, celery, cucumbers, parsley, avocado; add ½ cup mayonnaise to aspic.

Steamed or canned shrimp, parsley, sliced stuffed olives, chopped celery; leave shrimps whole; set in tomato aspic or add sliced tomatoes.

Diced steamed shrimp, chopped celery, diced cucumbers, pimento, chips of Roquefort cheese. This is a delicious salad.

Flaked white fish, chopped mixed pickles, celery set in lime gelatin.

Flaked kippered fish, such as herring or salmon, diced beet pickles, wedges of tart raw apple, parsley.

Flaked fish, parsley, celery stalk and leaves; use thin slices of cucumber, carrot, and lemon to decorate the mold.

Diced ham, celery, green peppers, sliced hard-cooked eggs, fresh dill or crushed dill seeds.

Diced ham, parsley, green peppers; set in tomato aspic or add tomatoes to salad; season with basil or 1 teaspoon caraway seeds.

Diced lean corned beef, parsley, green peppers, 1 tablespoon each prepared mustard and ground horseradish; add tomato or celery to salad; set in well-seasoned soup stock.

Diced heart, diced cucumbers, shredded carrot.

Diced heart, shredded raw cauliflower, parsley, green peppers; add ¼ cup mayonnaise to aspic.

Diced steamed liver, parsley, celery, leeks; set in tomato aspic or add tomato sections to salad.

Diced steamed liver, green pepper, parsley, chopped green onions with tops.

Diced steamed lamb liver, 2 teaspoons crushed dill seeds, celery, parsley, chives.

Diced roast pork, celery; set in an aspic of apple juice or add diced red apples to salad.

Diced steamed sweetbreads, pimentos, celery, sliced hard-cooked eggs, parsley.

Diced steamed sweetbreads, asparagus, shredded carrot.

Diced sweetbreads, avocado wedges, chopped pimento, celery; set in a gelatin of vegetable-cooking water to which 2 tablespoons lemon juice are added.

Diced sweetbreads, diced cucumbers, sliced stuffed olives, chips of Roquefort cheese.

Diced sweetbreads, sliced canned mushrooms, pimento, celery, parsley, 2 tablespoons capers.

Steamed kidney, chopped green onions with tops, shredded raw carrot, parsley; dice kidney and marinate in tart French dressing; set in tomato aspic or add tomato sections to salad.

Diced lamb, a small amount of celery; set in mint aspic or add minced mint leaves to salad.

Diced lamb, celery, shredded raw cauliflower, pimento, fresh dill or crushed dill seeds.

Diced lamb, chopped dill pickle, green peppers, minced raw broccoli bud and chopped stalk; set in tomato aspic or add tomato to salad.

Diced tongue, green peppers, parsley, shredded carrot; set in an aspic of stock or tomato juice, or add tomatoes to salad.

Diced tongue, diced cucumbers, green onions with tops, sliced radishes, hard-cooked eggs.

Diced tongue, shredded raw cauliflower, parsley, pimento.

Diced veal, celery, parsley, chives, pickle relish.

Diced veal, shredded carrots, chopped cucumber, pimento.

Diced veal, grated Parmesan cheese, parsley, finely shredded mustard leaves or watercress.

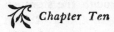 *Chapter Ten*

Serve Eggs and Cheese Daily

Eggs and cheese supply adequate protein which has an abundance of amino acids essential to health. Aside from other vitamins and minerals, cheese furnishes some calcium and vitamin B_2; eggs supply iron and vitamins A and B_2. Ideally an egg and a serving of cheese should be eaten daily, either alone or added to other foods. Although emphasis has often been put on the 1-egg cake and other ways of "economizing" on eggs, the liberal use of eggs and cheese should be looked upon as an economy which aids in preventing illnesses and saves money from medical bills.

Fertile eggs are nutritionally far superior to infertile ones and are worth additional cost when available. Natural cheeses are markedly superior to processed cheeses, and uncolored ones are to be preferred to yellow cheeses. Although all yellow cheese contains food coloring, the nutritional advantages of otherwise natural yellow cheese would appear to outweigh this disadvantage. Processed cheeses are made solid largely by the hydrogenation of the butterfat, and have the glossy surface of hydrogenated cooking fats; they cannot be recommended. Natural cheeses are solid because of the concentration of milk protein.

Contrary to popular opinion, cheese is neither "hard to digest" nor constipating; soft-cooked and raw eggs are not "easy to digest." These beliefs are based on early studies of the length of time foods stayed in the stomach; if a food left the stomach quickly, the assumption was that it was easily digested and vice versa. Later studies showed that foods pass through the stomach much as liquids pass through a funnel. Protein foods of firm texture, such as cheese and hard-cooked eggs, are held in the stomach until their proteins are digested to liquid. Extremely soft-cooked or raw eggs leave the stomach so rapidly that almost no digestion can take place; hence few nutrients from such eggs can reach the blood.

Aside from the fact that the nutrients are poorly absorbed, there are two reasons why undercooked eggs should not be eaten. Avidin, a substance in raw egg white, combines with biotin, one of the B vitamins, and prevents it from reaching the blood. Persons deficient in biotin become ill and mentally depressed, and suffer from eczema. The protein of egg white, albumen, dissolves in water or digestive juices and may pass into the blood undigested. When undigested protein reaches the blood, allergies may result. Eggs should be cooked until the white is no longer a semiliquid and the yolk is at least slightly firm. Hundreds of recipes which call for raw egg white, as in ice cream, mayonnaise, Bavarian cream, gelatin sponges, and eggnogs, have probably done much harm. If the egg is beaten and stirred into hot liquid, it cooks quickly and is safe to use.

Although eggs contain some cholesterol, they are a rich source of lecithin, which helps the body to utilize cholesterol normally. Studies with human subjects have shown that boiled or poached eggs or eggs fried or scrambled in vegetable oil have not caused the blood cholesterol to be increased. Eggs cooked in bacon drippings, lard, or hydrogenated cooking fats, however, did bring about an elevation in the blood cholesterol levels.

If you submit either eggs or cheese to high temperatures, the protein quickly becomes tough and some of its health-promoting value is destroyed. Cook both cheese and eggs gently with low heat at all times. Except when the temperature is low, as in a soufflé, cheese should be added to hot foods a few minutes before serving. Melt cheese under the broiler if you like, but avoid browning it.

Since vitamin B_2 is destroyed by light, cheese should be kept covered. Purchase cottage cheese in a carton instead of that kept in open pans at a delicatessen counter. Keep other cheeses covered with wax paper in the refrigerator; use cream cheese soon after unwrapping. During cooking, vitamin B_2 is destroyed by light so quickly that foods should be kept covered every minute possible. When eggs are fried or scrambled in an open pan, as much as 48 per cent of the vitamin is lost, whereas no loss occurs when the utensil is covered. Casserole dishes containing cheese should be kept carefully covered even when on the table.

In order to use eggs frequently in salads, sandwiches, and other foods, hard-cook a dozen at a time and keep them in the refrigerator ready to be used. Keep on hand several kinds of cheese, including grated cheese. Add generous amounts of cheese to soups, salads, egg dishes, and meat substitutes. Almost any cooked vegetable is delicious when cheese is added to it. Try to make it a rule to serve both eggs and cheese daily.

I have given methods of cooking eggs for breakfast in the basic recipes. Eggs prepared with more elaborate seasoning and served with vegetables, cheese, and other foods are intended for lunches and dinners.

SCRAMBLED EGGS

Brush grill or frying pan with **vegetable oil or partially hardened margarine;** heat to moderate temperature.

Break directly into pan:

4 to 6 eggs

Stir in thoroughly:

¼ to ½ cup evaporated or fresh milk	⅛ teaspoon ground peppercorns
	1 teaspoon salt

Cook over extremely low heat for 10 to 12 minutes, stirring 2 or 3 times. *Keep the utensil covered as much as possible.* Serve with crisp bacon.

VARIATIONS:

Add any one of the following to scrambled eggs a few minutes before serving: 1 to 2 tablespoons minced chives, leeks, fresh dill, diced pimento, or chopped parsley; ½ cup thinly diced raw or sautéed kidneys, steamed brain, or shredded or cubed American cheese; ¼ cup Parmesan cheese or shredded dried beef; 1 cup diced leftover chicken, rabbit, ham, sautéed liver, or other meat; sliced fresh or canned mushrooms; ¾ cup flaked leftover or smoked fish; or chips of drained, crisp bacon.

Use tomato purée or sauce instead of milk, or add 2 tablespoons catsup or chili sauce.

Before cooking eggs cut ¼ to ½ pound link sausages into 1-inch pieces and pan-broil until nearly done; drain fat, add eggs, and cook as in basic recipe; or cut 3 or 4 wieners into ½-inch pieces and add with milk. Vary by using any of the highly seasoned sausages.

Surround scrambled eggs with steamed or fried rice, hash-brown potatoes, or steamed kale, spinach, or other greens; top with grated cheese or cheese sauce (p. 136).

Sauté lightly before adding eggs 1 chopped or grated onion, chopped celery, and/or chopped green or red bell pepper.

Spanish-style eggs: Sauté lightly before adding eggs **1 chopped green or red bell pepper or fresh chili pepper;** or when eggs are almost done, add **1 diced pimento and 2 tablespoons chili sauce. Stir in ½ cup shredded or diced cheese.**

In order to poach eggs satisfactorily, use only fresh eggs, one to five days old. The whites of older eggs will run when dropped into water. To prevent the white from breaking apart or being uneven, the water should not be boiling or moving in any way when the egg is dropped into it; however, it should be as hot as possible without boiling. Vinegar may be added to the water to make the egg white coagulate more quickly, but the flavor is usually ruined and the acid causes the white to have a curdled, rough appearance.

When you have purchased eggs of unknown age, break one into a cup and observe the texture of the white and the contour of the membrane covering the yolk. If the white seems quite jelly-like and the yolk tends to be spherical, the egg is fresh. The white of an older egg is more liquid and the yolk is somewhat flat on top. Unless the eggs are fresh, do not try to poach them.

My pet method of cooking breakfast eggs, which can substitute for poaching, frying, or baking, is to steam them. If the utensil used holds heat, you can cover the eggs, turn off the heat, and forget about them while you have your fruit or juice; you return

to find them perfectly and evenly cooked on both top and bottom.
I heartily recommend this method to you.

POACHED EGGS

Select strictly fresh eggs; use a shallow utensil filled to the depth of
1½ inches with water; add:

1½ teaspoons salt

Bring water to boiling; turn down heat until the water is quiet;
crack an egg, hold in just above the surface of the water, and slip it in
gently; drop in other eggs, cover utensil, and simmer slowly until whites
are firm, or 8 to 10 minutes; or remove from heat and let stand 15
minutes.

Lift from liquid with pancake turner and place on **buttered whole-
wheat toast**. Sprinkle with **freshly ground black peppercorns**.

VARIATIONS:

Cover poached eggs with any cream sauce (p. 135) **or creamed fish,
lobster, crab, or shrimp** (p. 164).

Garnish with rings of green or red bell pepper, fresh pimento, or
paprika; or place pepper rings on moist grill, drop an egg inside each,
add ¼ cup water, cover, and steam eggs.

Serve covered with sautéed fresh pimentos, onions, and/or mushrooms.

Poach eggs in 2 cups medium cream sauce, such as dill, pimento, or
cheese sauce; serve sauce over eggs.

Serve poached eggs on nest of corned-beef hash or buttered chopped
spinach, chard, or beet tops.

Eggs Benedictine: Put a circular piece of **pan-broiled ham and a
poached egg** on a split, toasted English muffin; cover with **Hollandaise
sauce** (p. 138). Or use cream sauce to which is added 2 tablespoons
sherry.

Eggs with tomato sauce: Prepare 1 or 2 cups tomato sauce (p. 140);
poach eggs in sauce; serve sauce over eggs. Vary by using creole, Spanish, or other tomato sauce.

Mock poached eggs, or steamed eggs: Put ½ cup water in heated pan
or grill; drop in eggs, sprinkle with salt **and freshly ground peppercorns**, cover and steam over extremely low heat. Use poaching rings
if desired.

No egg should be so mistreated as to be fried, or actually cooked by the heat of hot fat. Almost invariably fat reaches such a high temperature that the egg white touching it becomes brown and tough; the white next to the yolk is often left uncooked. Only enough fat should be used to prevent the eggs from sticking to the grill or frying pan. The heat should be kept low at all times. Again I would recommend that a little water or milk be added to produce steam, that the utensil be covered, and that the egg be allowed to cook gently so that no part of it is tough. Eggs cooked in drippings left from pan-broiling steaks or trimmed pork chops are particularly delicious.

"FRIED" EGGS

Heat grill or shallow frying pan until moderately hot; brush lightly with **partially hardened margarine or vegetable oil;** break and drop gently into pan:

4 to 8 whole eggs

Add:

2 tablespoons top milk or water

Cover utensil and cook over extremely low heat until white is firm, or about 12 to 15 minutes; sprinkle with **salt and freshly ground black peppercorns.**

VARIATIONS:

Sauté breaded slices of eggplant (p. 341) and tomatoes; place tomatoes over eggplant and an egg on top of each serving.

Serve eggs on buttered toast and sautéed tomatoes; place crisp bacon on top.

Sprinkle ¼ cup shredded or grated cheese over top of eggs 4 minutes before serving.

"Fried" eggs baked in an oven are easily prepared. The dry heat penetrates slowly, and the eggs cook evenly from both top and bottom; almost no attention need be given them. It is usually recommended that eggs be baked in custard cups, which are a nuisance to oil, handle, and wash. Bake them in a frying pan, a baking dish, or poaching rings.

BAKED EGGS

Heat grill, frying pan, or baking dish to moderate temperature; brush lightly with **vegetable oil or partially hardened margarine** and break into it:

4 to 8 eggs

Sprinkle with **salt and freshly ground peppercorns;** place in a preheated slow oven at 325° F. and bake for 15 to 18 minutes.

VARIATIONS:

If oven is in use, add 2 or 3 tablespoons water or milk, cover utensil, and let eggs steam in the oven; substitute for frying or poaching eggs.

After egg white has set, lay slices of partly sautéed bacon across the top, or cover the eggs with ½ cup grated cheese and/or ¾ cup barbecue (p. 140) or Spanish sauce (p. 141).

Sprinkle grated American cheese over eggs and serve in indentations made in mounds of cooked spinach.

Eggs in bacon rings: Fasten partly cooked bacon into rings with toothpicks; drop an egg into each ring; bake as in basic recipe.

Eggs in meat cups: Pan-broil for 1 minute at high temperature **thin slices of bologna or any luncheon meat,** making them curl into cups; drop an egg into each cup, bake, and serve with cheese sauce (p. 136) or mustard sauce (p. 137). Vary by baking eggs **on slices of ham;** or serve ham slices on toast, **broiled tomato slices on ham,** and baked egg on top of tomato; cover with **Hollandaise (p. 138) or mock Hollandaise (p. 137), or any cream sauce** (p. 135).

Eggs with leftover meat: Combine 1½ cups ground leftover meat, ½ cup whole-wheat-bread crumbs, 1 teaspoon salt, freshly ground peppercorns, ¾ cup gravy or milk; put meat in flat baking dish, make indentations to hold eggs, sprinkle with paprika, and bake as in basic recipe.

Eggs with rice or noodles: Put **leftover rice or noodles** into oiled casserole; make depressions with tablespoon, place egg in each depression, season, and bake. Cover with **shredded cheese** or serve with cheese sauce (p. 136).

Eggs with sausage: Shape large **sausage cakes** with a hollow in the top side; pan-broil indented side until brown, turn, and drain off fat; drop eggs into hollows and bake. Or arrange partly broiled **link sausages** in circles, drop an egg into each circle, season, and bake.

Eggs with sauce: Break the eggs into baking dish; bake; prepare any cooked sauce (pp. 135–141) and pour over eggs before taking from oven.

The old expression, "She can't even boil an egg," implies that it is easy. Actually, to boil eggs perfectly at all times is extremely difficult. If you let the heat become too high for too long a period, the egg becomes tough and the sulfur compounds in the yolk break down, leaving an unappetizing green ring. If the heat is not high enough to toughen the outside, the egg white pulls apart when you remove the shell. You may enjoy a soft-cooked egg with a certain texture which you want in every egg served you. The texture of either a hard-cooked or a soft-cooked egg depends on the initial temperature of the water and the eggs, the number of eggs cooked, the amount of water used, the degree to which the utensil holds heat, the temperature to which the water is heated, and the length of time the eggs are left in it. If that is easy, I give up. The more water used, the more slowly it will heat or cool, and the longer the eggs will cook before they reach boiling and/or after the water is removed from the heat. The only way perfection can be obtained is to measure the water and to use a stop watch and a thermometer, none of which I expect a housewife to do.

BOILED EGGS

METHOD I: Use a deep utensil and bring to boiling approximately:

1 quart water

Use eggs which have been left at room temperature; slip carefully into water:

4 to 8 eggs

Cover utensil; reheat water to boiling, but let boil no longer than 5 seconds; move the utensil from heat and let stand 8 minutes for soft-cooked eggs; 25 minutes for hard-cooked ones, or until water has cooled.

METHOD II: Put cold eggs into cold water; heat to boiling, but boil no longer than 5 seconds; serve immediately for soft-cooked eggs; let stand 20 minutes for hard-cooked ones, or until water is cold.

Creamed eggs are an excellent meat substitute or extender and should be served frequently for lunches, dinners, or even late breakfasts. If the sauces used are varied, creamed eggs need never be monotonous. These dishes are especially valuable to use when one must prepare food for an invalid, a convalescent, or a small child who requires a smooth but high-protein diet. Even more powdered milk could be used in making the cream sauce than I have specified on page 135, and cheese may be added to any sauce.

CREAMED EGGS

Prepare **2 cups pimento, caper, cheese, caraway, dill, curry, mushroom, olive, onion, or piquant sauce** (pp. 136–137), using a base of cream sauce, brown sauce, leftover gravy, or tomato-cream sauce.

Stir into hot sauce:

4 to 6 hard-cooked eggs, sliced or cut in half lengthwise

As soon as eggs have heated through, or in about 5 minutes, serve over **whole-wheat toast or wheat-germ biscuits** cut with a doughnut cutter; garnish with **parsley and paprika**.

VARIATIONS:

Slice eggs in half lengthwise while hot and place on hot serving platter; pour sauce over them, garnish, and serve.

Prepare dill, mushroom, olive, onion, pimento, or cheese sauce; slice eggs over hot cooked asparagus, spinach, kale, chard, broccoli, or other green vegetable; cover with sauce.

Before adding eggs, cook in sauce 1 cup peas, diced carrots, celery, diced broccoli, or asparagus; or add leftover vegetables.

Use 4 eggs; add 1 cup diced ham or other leftover meat or ¼ pound chipped dried beef; or use dill sauce and add 1 cup diced uncooked or flaked leftover fish, shrimps, lobster, or crab; or add 1 or 2 teaspoons anise seeds to medium cream sauce, and add eggs and fish or sea food.

Instead of cream sauce prepare Spanish, Mexican, creole, or other tomato sauce (p. 140); add eggs as in basic recipe. Vary by using stuffed eggs; reheat in tomato sauce and serve with sauce over them; sprinkle with grated cheese.

STUFFED HARD-COOKED EGGS

Cut **4 hard-cooked eggs** lengthwise and remove yolks; mash yolks with fork and add:

2 tablespoons mayonnaise	dash each paprika, cayenne, freshly
½ teaspoon each mustard and	ground black peppercorns
Worcestershire	1 teaspoon salt

Fill egg whites with yolk mixture.

VARIATIONS:

Add about 2 tablespoons of any one of the following: caviar with lemon juice; minced celery, pimento, green pepper, or fresh cucumbers; nippy cheese; diced ripe or stuffed olives; chopped nuts; chives with chopped pimento, 1 or 2 drops Tabasco sauce; finely chopped chicken or other leftover meat; ground parsley and 2 or 3 minced anchovies or 2 teaspoons anchovy paste; sour or dill pickles; steamed shrimp diced with 1 teaspoon chili sauce; or add fresh dill, or dill or caraway seeds.

If a fluffy omelet is not to be tough and is to hold its shape after it is taken from the oven, it must be cooked at low temperature until the egg white is firm. A quickly cooked omelet will invariably fall and/or shrink.

FLUFFY OMELET

Use eggs which are at room temperature. Beat until smooth:

½ cup fresh milk	¼ cup powdered milk

Add and beat slightly:

4 to 6 egg yolks	¼ teaspoon freshly ground black
1 teaspoon salt	peppercorns

Beat until stiff and fold in:

4 to 6 egg whites	½ teaspoon salt

Turn into baking dish brushed with **vegetable oil or partially hard-ened margarine;** sprinkle with **paprika;** bake in preheated slow oven at 325° F. for 30 minutes.

Serve from baking dish.

VARIATIONS:

Use ¾ cup fresh milk; add and beat with yolks ½ cup toasted wheat germ or 4 tablespoons soy flour.

Add to egg yolks leftover peas, diced carrots, asparagus, broccoli, other cooked vegetables, fresh or canned mushrooms or pimentos.

At the table serve over omelet any cream sauce or tomato sauce (pp. 135–141), creamed ham, chicken livers, or sweetbreads; or creamed vegetables, such as asparagus or peas.

Bacon and bean sprouts with omelet: Add 1 cup raw or canned bean sprouts and 2 slices crisp bacon, broken to bits.

Cheese omelet: Mix with egg yolks 1 cup shredded or grated cheese; sprinkle top of omelet with cheese.

Corn omelet: Add to egg yolks 1 cup raw, canned, or leftover corn, ½ teaspoon more salt.

Creole omelet: Sauté lightly in the utensil in which omelet is to be baked 1 chopped onion, 1 diced tomato, 1 chopped green pepper; add ¼ teaspoon each salt and paprika; mix with egg yolks before folding in whites. Vary by adding pan-broiled link sausage cut into ½-inch pieces.

Fish omelet: Add 1 cup any diced raw or flaked steamed fish or canned tuna to egg yolks before folding in whites.

Mushroom omelet: Add to egg yolks before folding in whites ½ to 1 cup fresh or canned mushrooms; use liquid from canned mushrooms instead of part of the milk.

Parsley-anchovy omelet: Decrease salt in basic recipe to ½ teaspoon; add 2 teaspoons or more of anchovy paste, 4 tablespoons chopped parsley.

Rice omelet: Add ½ to 1 cup leftover rice, 1 tablespoon each cat-sup and Worcestershire, and ¼ teaspoon basil to egg yolks before folding in whites.

Tomato omelet: Add ¾ cup of any tomato sauce (p. 140) to omelet instead of fresh milk; or roll slices of tomato in whole-wheat-bread crumbs, and place on bottom of baking dish; sauté on both sides and sprinkle with salt, cayenne, and grated cheese; pour omelet over tomatoes.

QUICK EGG OMELET

Beat until smooth or blend in liquefier:

½ cup fresh milk   ¼ cup powdered milk

Add and beat slightly:

4 to 6 eggs   ¼ teaspoon freshly ground black
1½ teaspoons salt   peppercorns

Pour into heated omelet pan or frying pan brushed with **vegetable oil or partially hardened margarine;** cover and heat slowly 6 to 10 minutes; loosen the edges with spatula and fold toward center, letting any uncooked egg run to sides of pan. Again cover utensil, and heat slowly 5 to 8 minutes. Fold edges toward center and sprinkle with:

2 to 4 tablespoons chopped chives or parsley

Garnish with **paprika.**

VARIATIONS:

Mix with eggs before cooking 2 teaspoons minced fresh dill or 1 teaspoon caraway or dill seeds.

Add diced leftover meat, such as chicken or ham, to eggs before cooking.

Crab or lobster omelet: Fold omelet over **1 cup minced crab or lobster** mixed with **2 tablespoons chili sauce;** cover and serve as soon as heated.

Kidney omelet: Add **thinly sliced raw kidney;** fold omelet over kidney, cover the utensil, and heat 5 minutes before serving; or sauté the kidney 5 minutes, drain on paper, cook the omelet, place kidney in the center, fold over, and reheat.

Oyster omelet: Before folding omelet over add **1 cup chopped raw oysters;** cover utensil and heat through; or mix oysters with **½ cup thick cream sauce** (p. 135), **dash of cayenne,** and **½ teaspoon salt;** fold into omelet and heat for 5 to 8 minutes.

Spanish omelet: Sauté lightly **1 each chopped onion and green or red bell pepper or fresh chili pepper;** add eggs; cook as in basic recipe. Vary by heating **1 cup any tomato sauce** (p. 140) and serving over omelet.

THIN PANCAKES, OR PFANNKUCHEN

Sift together or mix thoroughly:

¼ cup whole-wheat-pastry flour   1 teaspoon salt
⅓ cup powdered milk

Add and beat well:

1 cup fresh milk   4 eggs

Heat a large frying pan and brush with a generous amount, of partially hardened margarine; sauté a fourth of the batter until light brown on both sides; keep hot while cooking 3 more thin omelets.

Transfer to hot serving plates; add to each 4 tablespoons grated cheese, creamed shrimp or chicken, applesauce, or fresh sweetened berries; roll, and serve while piping hot.

VARIATIONS:

Separate eggs, beat whites until stiff, and fold into other ingredients; cover utensil until time to turn.

Cut bacon strips into 2-inch lengths and pan-broil until crisp; drain and drop pieces into each omelet. Vary by adding diced ham or thin slices of boiled ham.

Swedish pancakes: Add to basic recipe 2 tablespoons partially hardened margarine; use ½ cup whole-wheat flour; bake and serve as in basic recipe.

FRENCH TOAST

Beat until smooth or blend in liquefier:

½ cup fresh milk   ½ cup powdered milk

Add and beat slightly:

2 to 4 eggs   1 teaspoon salt

Soak in mixture until soft:

6 or 8 slices stale whole-wheat, soy, wheat-germ, or rye bread

Sauté slowly in partially hardened margarine until browned on both sides.

Serve with applesauce, apricot purée, or other fruit sauce, or with fresh crushed and sweetened berries.

VARIATIONS:

Instead of fresh milk use tomato juice or tomato purée. Serve with ham or bacon.

Add to batter ½ teaspoon cinnamon, ¼ teaspoon nutmeg, and 3 or 4 tablespoons molasses or honey.

Separate eggs, beat whites stiff, and fold in after other ingredients are combined.

Cheese dishes have been so scattered throughout the book that only a few are given here. I hope that you will scatter cheese throughout your menus in the same manner. As is shown in the vegetable recipes, shredded cheese may be added to almost any vegetable in the place of butter. It may be sprinkled on the surface of many soups. Its uses are unlimited. Keep cheese on hand at all times and serve it daily.

See cheese soufflés (p. 194), chili relleno, or stuffed chili peppers (p. 192), and blintzes (p. 199).

When cottage cheese is made at home from milk which has been allowed to sour, the lactic acid causes calcium to dissolve into the whey, which is discarded. Calcium is well retained in cheese made with rennet, or junket. The cheese should not be washed to remove whey; too many vitamins and minerals are unnecessarily lost.

COTTAGE CHEESE MADE WITH RENNET

Heat to lukewarm, or 110° F.:

1 quart skimmed milk

Soak in 1 tablespoon water:

1 rennet, or junket, tablet

Add tablet to milk, stir well, and let stand until set.

Place in a large pan of hot water or over extremely low heat; fasten a cooking thermometer to edge of utensil or let dairy thermometer float on surface; stir frequently; heat to 110° F. for soft-curd cheese, 120° F. for farmer-style cheese.

Pour into a strainer lined with a clean cloth; gather corners of cloth around curds and squeeze out whey; put cheese into a dish and add:

1 teaspoon salt	½ cup sour cream or yogurt

Garnish lightly with **paprika**.

VARIATIONS:

Double or triple the quantity of milk and use 2 or 3 junket tablets.

Season occasionally with any of the following: 1 tablespoon chives, or minced fresh dill, basil, burnet, or parsley; 1 teaspoon crushed caraway, dill, celery, or mustard seeds. Let cheese stand ½ hour or longer before serving.

WELSH RAREBIT

Blend in liquefier or beat in utensil which holds heat or in top of double boiler:

¾ cup top milk or evaporated milk	1 teaspoon dry or prepared mustard
½ cup powdered milk	few grains cayenne
¼ teaspoon salt	

Heat milk to simmering, stirring frequently; *keep covered as much as possible;* remove from heat and add:

½ pound, or 2 cups, diced mild cheese

Stir well, and cover utensil; let stand 6 to 8 minutes, or until cheese is melted; stir again.

Serve over buttered toast or slices of broiled tomato or eggplant.

VARIATIONS:

Use 1 cup fresh milk and add 1 egg or 1 cup soft whole-wheat-bread cubes; add other ingredients and proceed as in basic recipe.

Use 1 cup mild American cheese combined with 1 cup Swiss, Jack, or pimento cheese or 1½ cups American and ¼ cup Roquefort cheese; add Roquefort immediately before serving.

Baked rarebit: Cut 2 or 3 slices stale whole-wheat bread into fingers 1 inch wide; place sticks over bottom and along sides of flat baking dish brushed with oil; combine ingredients of basic recipe and add 2 **egg yolks;** beat stiff and fold in 2 **egg whites;** pour into the oiled baking dish, garnish with **paprika,** and bake in a slow oven at 325° F. for 30 minutes.

Cheese fondue I: Combine 1 cup soft whole-wheat-bread cubes with 1 cup fresh milk; add ingredients of basic recipe without heating, and 2 **eggs beaten separately;** bake in slow oven at 325° F. for 25 minutes.

Cheese fondue II: Put 4 slices whole-wheat bread into oiled baking dish; sprinkle ½ to 1 cup diced cheese over them; mix 2 **eggs** with other ingredients of basic recipe, using 2½ cups milk; bake at 350° F. for 30 minutes.

Mushroom or tomato rarebit: Use 1 can condensed mushroom or tomato soup and ¼ cup each fresh milk and powdered milk; omit salt; heat, and stir in cheese.

Oyster rarebit: Heat in milk 1 minute before adding cheese 1 **cup raw oysters;** proceed as in basic recipe; omit mustard and add 1 **teaspoon dill seeds or minced fresh dill.**

Rarebit, Swiss style: Prepare as in basic recipe, using 2 cups of Swiss cheese. In center of table set bowl of rarebit with platter of dry, toasted whole-wheat or rye bread cut into 1-inch cubes. The toast is to be dipped directly into the rarebit.

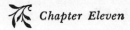 *Chapter Eleven*

Appetizers Contribute to Health

If full health for your entire family is to be your goal, appetizers should appear frequently on your menus. Appetizers play a triple role in contributing to health. They add the esthetic values of beauty and leisure to a meal. Their tartness stimulates the flow of digestive juices. They satisfy the appetite only sufficiently to decrease a desire to overeat.

An appetizer may be a glass of chilled vegetable juice or unsweetened fruit juice; fresh fruit or fresh fruits mixed with canned fruits; or almost any type of fish in catsup or chili sauce. Many delicious juices may be prepared at home by anyone who has a garden and fruit trees; a generous supply should be canned or frozen for winter use. The small amount of water left when vegetables are steamed, the vitamin C content of which is often greater than that of orange juice, can be added to vegetable-juice cocktails.

Appetizers of fruit and vegetable juices supply minerals and vitamins A and C; fish cocktails provide protein and iodine. Family needs should determine which type of appetizer is to be served.

Form the habit of serving appetizers several times each week, either in the living room or at the table. They contribute much toward making each dinner a guest meal.

TOMATO-JUICE APPETIZER

About ½ hour before serving combine in each glass:

¾ cup, or 6 ounces, tomato juice ¼ teaspoon Worcestershire
1 tablespoon lemon juice   1 teaspoon chives (optional)
1 to 3 drops Tabasco   dash of salt

Give juice a swirl with fork and set in refrigerator. Stir again just before serving; taste for salt. Garnish with sprig of watercress or parsley.

VARIATIONS:

Season with basil, orégano, marjoram, savory, or rosemary.
Add 1 teaspoon or more mild-flavored brewers' yeast.
Omit other seasonings and use ½ teaspoon freshly ground horseradish; or add crushed seeds of mustard, celery, dill, or caraway.
Tomato-grapefruit appetizer: Use equal parts of tomato juice and use fresh or canned grapefruit juice; omit Worcestershire, chives, Tabasco. Serve immediately if ingredients are chilled.
Tomato-sauerkraut appetizer: Use equal amounts of sauerkraut juice and tomato juice; season as in basic recipe. Taste before adding salt.

Any fruits or juices whose colors and flavors blend may be combined in preparing appetizers. Since few fruits supply vitamin C in generous amounts, citrus fruits or citrus juices should be served more frequently than other fruits. However, appetizers of broiled grapefruit should be discouraged; the broiling destroys vitamin C. Sea food has long been served with lemon juice, but is also delicious with tart grapefruit juice.

GRAPEFRUIT HALVES WITH OYSTERS

Cut into halves:

2 grapefruits

Remove cores and cut sections loose from fibers; put in each center:

3 raw or canned oysters or shrimps   dash each of salt and paprika
1 teaspoon freshly ground horse-   2 drops Tabasco
radish

Set in refrigerator until served.

VARIATIONS:

Instead of oysters or shrimps use small amount of flaked steamed fish; add 1 teaspoon lemon juice.

Omit oysters and seasoning; garnish grapefruit with a maraschino cherry, or a sprig of mint, or unstemmed strawberry.

ORANGE-APRICOT APPETIZER

Combine directly in each glass:

⅔ cup orange juice   ⅓ cup apricot juice or thin purée

Stir; set in refrigerator until time to serve; garnish with a sprig of mint.

VARIATIONS:

Instead of apricot juice use unsweetened pineapple juice, grapefruit juice, loganberry, strawberry, or other berry juices, a mild-flavored grape juice, or any juices light in color. Garnish with thin slices of fresh apricot or orange or grated orange rind.

ORANGE APPETIZER

Peel, dice, and remove seeds from:

2 large oranges

Put into each glass:

½ diced orange   2 tablespoons chunk pineapple

Stir, and set in refrigerator until time to serve.

VARIATIONS:

Add sliced strawberries or seeded purple grapes.

Add 1 tablespoon lime juice and slices of papaya, guava, or diced mango or kumquat.

Instead of pineapple use sliced fresh apricots, peaches, plums, or California persimmons; diced cantaloupe or Persian melon; seeded or seedless grapes; seeded black cherries and/or white cherries; grapefruit sections or wedges of unpeeled yellow pear or plum.

Orange-pear appetizer: Instead of pineapple use **sliced unpeeled pear or white seedless grapes.** Vary by adding **diced loquats or fresh guavas.**

Persimmon-grapefruit appetizer: Omit cherries and pineapple; prepare **orange and small grapefruit** sections and alternate in serving glasses with **wedges of large California persimmons.**

Melon to be used for appetizers may be cut into balls or cubes. Any melon with firm pulp may be used and served with fruit juice or mixed with assorted fruits.

CANTALOUPE-RASPBERRY APPETIZER

Mix directly in each of 4 serving glasses:

⅓ cup cantaloupe cubes or balls   ¼ cup fresh orange juice
⅓ cup fresh red raspberries

Garnish with single **fresh mint leaf.** Set in refrigerator until time to serve.

VARIATIONS:

Instead of raspberries, combine melon with diced unpeeled red apple or yellow pears; diced orange, grapefruit, or tangerine sections; diced fresh or canned pineapple; fresh whole or sliced boysenberries, youngberries, or strawberries; sliced peaches, plums, or apricots; diced fresh guavas, mango, or papaya; seeded and halved purple grapes. Cantaloupe with purple plum is especially attractive and delicious.

Omit the cantaloupe and use cubes or balls of watermelon, Persian melon, or honeydew.

Cantaloupe baskets: Cut small cantaloupes in half and remove seeds; fill the centers with **chilled unstemmed strawberries or unstemmed black or white cherries.**

Mixed-melon appetizers: Use equal parts of **cantaloupe, honeydew, and watermelon balls;** add **juice from watermelon.**

BLACK RASPBERRY-PEACH APPETIZER

Mix directly in each of 4 serving glasses:

⅓ cup black raspberries   ⅓ cup unsweetened pineapple
⅓ cup diced yellow peaches   juice

Set in refrigerator until time to serve.

VARIATIONS:

Instead of raspberries, use strawberries or other berries; unpeeled red apple or yellow pear; seeded and halved Concord grapes; or slices of purple plum.

Substitute for peaches any fresh light-colored fruit and for pineapple juice any light-colored unsweetened juice.

Apricot-grape appetizers: Combine ⅓ cup each wedges of fresh apricots and seeded halves of purple grapes, seeded black cherries, or wedges of purple plums; sweeten to taste.

Guava appetizers: Add 1 to 3 diced strawberry or pineapple guavas to any mixed-fruit cocktail; as the taste becomes familiar, cut guava into thin slices; serve sliced or diced guavas alone with orange, grapefruit, pineapple, or apple juice; add 1 tablespoon lime or lemon juice.

Loquat or papaya appetizers: Slice or dice loquats or papayas; add to any appetizers of mixed fruits; serve alone with fruit juice if the flavor is enjoyed.

Persimmon-pear appetizers: Freeze 2 large unpeeled California persimmons until solid. Just before serving, cut persimmons into ⅓-inch cubes, combine with diced unpeeled pears, and pour ⅓ cup juice over each appetizer.

Surely no more delightful appetizer could be served on a sweltering hot evening than a frozen fruit sauce or a juice chilled with frozen cubes of sauce. Frozen sauces may be served as the first course or with the entree.

FROZEN TOMATO APPETIZER, OR SHERBET

Mix in freezing tray an hour or more before time to serve:

2 cups tomato purée	1 teaspoon Worcestershire
¼ cup lemon juice	salt to taste

Set in freezing compartment; in ½ hour stir thoroughly to prevent crystals from becoming large; freeze to a firm mush. Immediately before serving stir in:

½ cup finely chopped bell pepper or parsley

Put into chilled serving glasses. Garnish with sprig of watercress.

VARIATIONS:

Vary seasonings by adding crushed celery or mustard seeds, Tabasco, dry mustard, minced fresh basil or dill, or freshly ground horseradish.

Instead of tomato purée use vegetables prepared in the liquefier, such as carrot, celery, and mixed fresh vegetables blended with tomato, pineapple, or apple juice, or vegetable-cooking water.

Frozen applesauce: Use applesauce cooked with ¼ cup small cinnamon candies; if sauce is not tart, add lime or fresh lemon juice.

Frozen apricot purée: Substitute apricot purée for tomato purée. Garnish with bits of purple plum or a light sprinkling of finely chopped mint leaves.

Frozen pear or peach purée: Purée fresh or canned fruit in liquefier with 2 to 4 tablespoons lemon or lime juice; freeze as in basic recipe.

Frozen persimmons: Freeze well-ripened California persimmons in ice tray. Immediately before serving, shred quickly without peeling. Garnish with mint leaves. Serve with lemon sections.

Frozen strawberry or youngberry purée: Instead of tomato purée use strawberry or youngberry purée prepared in liquefier; garnish with mint leaves.

When fresh juices are squeezed or canned juices opened in advance of using, loss of vitamin C occurs even if they are covered and kept in the refrigerator. The vitamin is preserved over a longer period when the juices are frozen until needed.

Cubes of frozen juices may become extremely hard and should be used only when the appetizer is to be served before dinner. Frozen cubes should be made of light-colored juices. They can be attractive and are nice for a child's party or for guests on a hot evening. If dark-colored juices are used, the entire drink becomes muddy and takes on the color of the cubes as they melt. Decorative cubes are fun to make, need take only a few minutes to prepare, and are enjoyed by old and young alike.

APPLE JUICE
WITH DECORATIVE JUICE CUBES

Fill ice tray half full of:

clear light-colored apple juice or cider

Set in freezing compartment until ice crystals form over the top.

Quickly make flower arrangements in center of each cube with fresh raspberries and tiny strawberries; bits of orange and lemon peel; tiny wedges of apricots, peaches, or red apple; halves or wedges of grapes or cherries; small mint, parsley, or watercress leaves.

Freeze until solid; add enough apple juice or cider to fill tray; complete freezing. Serve decorative cubes from ice bucket, using 2 cubes for each glass; fill glasses with chilled clear apple, grapefruit, or pineapple juice.

VARIATIONS:

Make decorative cubes of any strained, light-colored juice, as orange-juice cubes to be served in pineapple juice.

Make frozen cubes of contrasting colors by blending apricots, strawberries or peaches in liquefier, and serve in any clear juice.

Any mild-flavored and quickly steamed fish may be used for appetizers instead of crab, shrimp, and lobster which are sometimes prohibitive in price. When well seasoned, fish appetizers are thought to be made of shellfish and taste as delicious.

FISH APPETIZER

Steam ½ **pound fillets** of any white-fleshed fish (p. 162). Flake the fish and add:

½ **teaspoon salt**
2 **tablespoons lemon juice or tar-**
ragon vinegar
2 **or more tablespoons capers**

freshly ground white peppercorns
dash of celery salt and cayenne
½ **cup catsup**
1 **tablespoon fresh horseradish**

Stir, taste for seasoning, and chill.

Put into cocktail glasses and garnish with **chopped parsley or a small sprig of parsley or watercress.**

VARIATIONS:

Use barbecue or chili sauce instead of catsup.

Add 1 tablespoon or more of any one or a combination of the following: minced fresh pimento, paprika, or red or green bell pepper; chopped onions or leeks, green-onion tops, or chives, parsley or celery.

Omit capers and season with 1 to 3 teaspoons minced fresh fennel, dill, marjoram, or thyme; or add ½ teaspoon anise, dill, or celery seeds; let stand ½ hour after seasonings are added.

Instead of fish use steamed shrimp, flaked crab, lobster, or chilled uncooked or canned oysters or clams; or serve oysters or clams in half shells with sauce.

Sweetbreads and chicken livers are customarily served as canapé appetizers. You will probably agree, however, that canapés are a nuisance to make and become soggy quickly. An easier way of serving these meats as appetizers is to steam, chill, and combine them with a delightfully seasoned barbecue sauce or catsup.

SWEETBREAD APPETIZER

Steam ½ pound lamb or veal sweetbreads; chill, remove all membranes, and cut into small cubes.

Combine with sweetbreads and stir thoroughly:

¼ to ½ cup chili sauce
2 tablespoons chopped leeks, raw onion, or chives
2 tablespoons chopped pimento

2 tablespoons diced celery
salt to taste
sprinkling of ground black peppercorns

Let stand in refrigerator ½ hour before serving.

VARIATIONS:

Add 1 teaspoon minced fresh or ¼ teaspoon dried basil, savory, tarragon, or marjoram.

Appetizers of brain: Use ¼ pound lamb, veal, or beef brain; steam the brain with vinegar (p. 81); if flavor is disliked, add a generous amount of parsley, 1 or 2 diced hard-cooked eggs, 1 teaspoon chopped tarragon, dill, or other fresh herbs, or pinch of dried herbs.

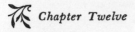

Chapter Twelve

Serve Your Salads First

A raw vegetable or a salad largely of raw fruits or vegetables should be served at almost every lunch and dinner throughout the entire year. Raw foods contribute vitamins, minerals, and bulk, and are particularly important as sources of vitamin C. Your salads need not be elaborate or take much time to prepare. A single raw vegetable will suffice: radishes, green onions, celery, carrot sticks, or strips of fresh pepper. These raw vegetables may be served with an appetizer, a soup, or the entree.

Salad dressings add nutritive value in that vegetable oils are often the only source of unsaturated fatty acids in the diet. If the oils are strictly fresh, they contain small amounts of vitamin E. Practical suggestions on the use of oils are to be found on pp. 6–7.

It is advantageous to serve a salad as the first course. Larger amounts are eaten when persons are most hungry. Salads satisfy the appetite sufficiently to decrease the danger of overeating; thus they help to maintain or reduce weight and decrease the desire for dessert.

To prevent enzyme action, only cold water should be used in washing vegetables, and they should be washed so thoroughly that they will not need to be touched by water again. Drying is essential to delicious salads and prevents nutrients and flavors from passing into the water clinging to the surface. A soft Turkish towel may be kept for drying smooth vegetables. Leafy vegetables are most easily and quickly dried in a bag, such as a cheesecloth bag about 18 inches square or an old pillow slip. When vegetables are whirled in such a bag by hand or on the final cycle of an automatic washing machine, the water is thrown from them by centrifugal force, and they are dried in a minute.

The salads most superior nutritionally are those made of green leaves. Although fruit salads are excellent, fruits are generally eaten in other ways. Unless raw green leaves are eaten in salad, they are not eaten at all. The concentration of vitamins and minerals in deep-green leaves is greater than in any other type of fresh food. Not only is vitamin A, or carotene, many times richer than in the bleached leaves, but also much richer are vitamins C, E, K, B_2, folic acid, some eight or more other B vitamins, bioflavonoids, iron, copper, magnesium, calcium, and other minerals. When leaves are bleached, they can no longer function normally as active parts of the plant; their need for vitamins and minerals is so reduced that these substances are largely removed from them. Few food habits could be of more value to health than that of eating a tossed green salad with each dinner, as do the Italians and French.

The nutritive value of salads depends on the method of handling and preparing the ingredients. In buying vegetables, purchase those which have been trimmed the least. If the roots and outside leaves or tops have been left on, the vitamin content is increased after the vegetable is gathered until wilting sets in. Except for foods which have a heavy peeling, such as oranges, bananas, pears, and apples, buy only the amount of salad fruits and vegetables which can be stored in the refrigerator. If you have a garden, gather the food just before time to chill and prepare it for the table.

Except for fruits or vegetables which bruise easily, such as berries or watercress, the following rules must be observed in preparing salad ingredients if nutritive losses are to be prevented:

Wash the vegetable or fruit carefully but quickly, using cold water; rinse and drain.

Dry thoroughly. Under no circumstances should vegetables be soaked to "freshen" them.

Unless you have a moisture-controlled refrigerator, keep all vegetables in covered refrigerator pan or plastic bags.

Chill as quickly as possible.

These recommendations have often been made, but housewives rarely follow them, largely because the nutritional reasons for such rules have not been understood.

Vitamin A and particularly vitamins C and E are destroyed by combining with oxygen. The combination of oxygen and vitamins is brought about largely by the action of enzymes which exist in all plants. During the growth period and until a fruit is ripe, these enzymes help to synthesize, or make, vitamins. When the food is overripe or after it is gathered, these same enzymes bring about the destruction of the vitamins. The saving of vitamins, therefore, means preventing enzyme action and keeping oxygen away from the food.

Since the rules for handling, preparing, and cooking foods are based on preventing enzyme action, the housewife should know certain facts about enzymes. Their action is inhibited by cold, or refrigeration. They are particularly active at room temperature. Their activity decreases as the temperature approaches boiling, or 212° F., and they are destroyed by boiling. The action of the enzyme which destroys vitamin C is inhibited by acid; the enzymes which affect B_2 are active only in the light. Leafy vegetables kept in the light and at room temperature can lose half of their vitamins B_2 and C in a day. The skin on such foods as apples, oranges, and pears largely prevents contact with oxygen; hence the vitamins they contain are not readily destroyed at room temperature.

The sweetness of most vegetables is due to three sugars: sucrose, or table sugar; glucose, or grape sugar; and fructose, or fruit sugar. Just as sugar dissolves quickly in coffee, so do these sugars speedily dissolve out during slow washing or soaking. Since vegetables contain less sugar than do fruits, their flavor is more quickly harmed. Soaking also causes loss of many aromatic oils, of minerals which give a salty tang, and of acids which give piquancy to the taste.

When foods are washed slowly or soaked, serious nutritive losses occur. Vitamins C, bioflavonoids, and all the B vitamins readily dissolve in water. For example, peas soaked for 10 minutes have been found to lose 20 to 40 per cent of the vitamin B_1 and 35 per cent of the vitamin C in the water. These vitamins and some ten or more others and all minerals except calcium dissolve out in approximately the same proportion when any vegetable is soaked. The cumulative loss of nutrients in a year's time through slow washing is tremendous.

Fresh foods should be chilled as quickly as possible and be kept chilled continuously, whether they are to be used for salads or for cooking. If food is left unnecessarily long at room temperature, the destruction of vitamins is rapidly resumed as the vegetables become warm.

Losses may occur during the preparation of salads. Contact with any equipment which contains copper brings about instant destruction of vitamin C, causing the surfaces to turn brown. When fruits or vegetables are cut, chopped, peeled, grated, or sliced, a large amount of surface is exposed to air and light, and vitamins are rapidly destroyed unless the food is so chilled that enzyme action cannot take place. Little or no loss occurs if the salad ingredients are thoroughly chilled, quickly cut or shredded with stainless-steel or well-tinned equipment, and immediately served or returned to the refrigerator.

When such foods as shredded lettuce, sliced avocado, and diced apples become brown along a cut surface, a chemical action occurs involving the destruction of vitamin C. If no copper-containing metal is allowed to touch the food, and if enzyme action is inhibited by thorough chilling and by immediately adding an acid such as lemon juice, vinegar, or French dressing, discoloration can be prevented, and nutritive value and attractiveness saved.

If you serve a properly prepared salad, you serve health in the making.

THE MOST IMPORTANT RECIPE IN THIS BOOK

If you learn nothing more from this book than a few pointers on making tossed salads (which were taught to me by a French chef), the years of work required to write it will be justified. Few foods are so sinned against as are tossed salads. Haven't you seen them mistreated to the point of being watery, wilted, tasteless, greasy, or with the vegetables so chopped that they seem already to have been chewed? The reason tossed salads are often abominably made, I believe, is that the "musts" in preparing them are so simple that they are overlooked as being unimportant. When you once get the knack of making them well and form the habit of eating them daily, all other salads seem insipid.

If a tossed salad is to be worthy of its name, the ingredients *must* be free from clinging drops of moisture; whirl them well. The salad oil *must* be added first. Previously prepared French dressing *must not* be used. The leaves *must* be so well tossed that each surface glistens with oil before lemon juice or vinegar and seasonings are added. There are sound nutritional reasons for each of these rules.

Tossing a salad consists of gently picking up the ingredients between a fork and a spoon, preferably large and wooden, lifting them 4 to 6 inches above the bowl, and whirling them slightly as they are dropped. The purpose of tossing is to allow the oil, which clings tenaciously to dry leaves, to seal the surfaces from oxygen, which can destroy vitamins, and from moisture, which can soak out vitamins, minerals, and flavor; to distribute and hold seasonings, which will adhere to the oil and give a delightful taste; and, most important, to prevent salt from drawing moisture out of the leaves, which causes them to wilt immediately and allows vitamins and minerals to be lost in the juices left in the salad bowl.

If the leaves are not well whirled, if a moist ingredient is added before the salad is tossed, or if French dressing is used so that the vinegar moistens the ingredients, oil will not adhere to the leaves; seasonings cannot be well distributed; the leaves wilt quickly; and juices carrying delicious flavors, sugars, aromatic oils, vitamins, and minerals are drawn out by the salt. The delightful crispness and the delicious taste are soon gone and can never be recaptured.

Make your tossed salad a work of art by using contrasting colors and by letting each ingredient retain its natural beauty as nearly as possible. Break rather than shred such vegetables as lettuce, endive, and Brussels sprouts. Leave the tips of watercress, New Zealand spinach, and other tender greens in attractive sprigs. Cut bell peppers, fresh pimentos, and tomatoes into strips so that their colors and textures can be seen. If foods are difficult to chew, as are carrots, rutabagas, or kohlrabi, cut them into narrow strips like shoestring potatoes, which can be easily broken with a fork, yet can add vividness and beauty. If stalks contain stringy fibers, as do celery, chard, and watercress stems, cut them across the fibers into small pieces. Mince or shred only the foods which are disliked or are unfamiliar when eaten raw, such as raw beets, cauliflower, or broccoli.

The amount of oil used and the proportion of oil to vinegar or lemon juice should depend upon your family's taste and calorie needs. A single tablespoon of oil is sufficient to cover all surfaces of the leaves in a salad for a family of four, provided the salad is well tossed. If a high-calorie diet is desired, as much as 3 or 4 tablespoons of oil may be used to 1 tablespoon of vinegar or lemon juice. I personally use 3 tablespoons of oil to 2 of vinegar in making a large salad.

The ingredients in a tossed salad should depend on the likes and dislikes of your family; therefore I have avoided giving amounts in the following recipe. When once you have captured the knack of preparing delicious tossed salads, no recipes are needed.

The recipe for tossed salad is given in great detail, but I beg you to follow it only once; after that you need never glance at it again.

Form the habit of serving a tossed salad almost daily throughout the year. If you wish to make the tossing of the salad a family ceremony carried out at the table, it can whet appetites and add graciousness to everyday living.

TOSSED SALAD

Set individual salad plates in refrigerator to chill.

Select, wash, and dry **fresh herbs** if available; cut **a clove of garlic** in half; crush well between the fingers or with a hammer; rub wooden salad bowl vigorously and thoroughly with herbs and garlic; mince and leave in bowl or discard.

Chop or dice **onions;** cut **chives and green-onion tops** with scissors; put into salad bowl.

Break **lettuce, tips of watercress, or other tender leaves** into salad bowl, leaving them in attractive pieces or sprigs.

Lay parallel on the chopping board all **leaves, stalks, and stems with stringy fibers, such as spinach, chard, broccoli, celery, or watercress** stems; shred all at the same time, cutting across the fibers; push from board into bowl.

Cut as shoestring potatoes and drop directly into bowl the raw **root vegetables, broccoli stalk, or vegetables of solid texture;** shred such vegetables as **cauliflower, broccoli bud, and beets;** slice **cucumbers and radishes.**

Add **2 tablespoons** or more of finely **chopped parsley and/or other leaves;** any leftover vegetables to which moisture clings; any diced leftover meat; flaked, steamed, or canned fish; or cubed solid cheese.

Add at the table or before serving:

1 to 3 tablespoons vegetable oil

Toss 30 times if 1 tablespoon of oil is used, 20 times for 2 tablespoons, 15 times for 3 tablespoons; do not stop until all surfaces shine with oil; not earlier than 10 minutes before serving, add:

1 to 3 tablespoons vinegar or
  lemon juice
1 to 1½ teaspoons salt
¼ teaspoon freshly ground
  peppercorns
seasonings such as Tabasco,
  Worcestershire, dry mustard,

and freshly ground horseradish
cottage cheese or crumbled cream
cheese
moist ingredients such as tomatoes,
  grapefruit, canned pineapple, or
  canned asparagus tips

Toss 10 to 12 times; taste for seasonings; add any ingredient to remain on top as a garnish, such as sliced stuffed olives, hard-cooked eggs, or chips of Roquefort cheese; or any ingredient too soft to toss, such as ripe avocado or California persimmon; sprinkle with parsley and paprika and, if needed, salt.

Serve immediately or set in refrigerator until time to serve.

VARIATIONS:

Use tarragon or wine vinegar or any herb vinegar; or use fresh lime juice instead of lemon juice.

Add any of the following seasonings with the vinegar or lemon juice: 1 or 2 tablespoons sherry, port, sauterne, or other wine; 2 or more tablespoons catsup, chili sauce, or other tomato sauce; $\frac{1}{4}$ cup yogurt, sour cream, or whipped sweet cream or evaporated milk; a dash of celery salt, paprika, or cayenne; chopped mixed pickles, anchovy paste, or chutney; 1 or 2 teaspoons curry or chili powder, or mashed caraway, cumin, dill, or celery seeds; or add the combined seasonings of your favorite French dressing.

Use as many varieties of greens as are available, such as: endive, spinach, watercress, tender dandelion greens, a few nasturtium leaves and buds, Bibb lettuce, Swiss and rhubarb chard, parsley, young beet, turnip, or radish tops, mustard greens, mustard spinach, romaine, savoy cabbage, Chinese cabbage and mustard, tarragon leaves, kale, and broccoli bud and leaves.

Occasionally use such vegetables as uncooked Brussels sprouts, raw zucchini, raw Jerusalem artichokes, uncooked fresh or unheated frozen peas, and kohlrabi. My favorites are kohlrabi cut into shoestrings and sliced water chestnuts.

FINGER SALADS

The following raw vegetables may be served alone or combined:

Large broccoli stalk, peeled and cut into sticks.
Sticks of unpeeled carrot.
Celery stalks or curls.
Cucumber fingers, peeled or unpeeled.
Peeled kohlrabi slices, sticks, or wedges.
Green onions with 4 to 5 inches of the tops.
Thin slices of large onion.

Green or red bell pepper sticks or rings.

Pimento or fresh paprika sticks or rings.

Cabbage or cauliflower stalk cut into sticks.

Unpeeled turnip slices, sticks, or wedges.

Radishes, preferably not made into "roses."

Whole cherry tomatoes with stems; the bottom half may be dipped in French dressing, then into chopped parsley or chives. Avoid if sprayed with paraffin.

Young rutabaga sticks, peeled or unpeeled.

Potato fingers should be used for winter salads when sources of vitamin C are inadequate.

FINGER SALADS WITH FRENCH DRESSING

The following raw vegetables may be soaked, or marinated, in French dressing and served by toothpick. If several are served at one time, vary the seasonings used.

Cauliflowerlets no more than ½ inch in diameter; add 1 tablespoon chopped parsley or grated orange peel for each cup of flowerlets.

Tiny clusters of broccoli buds garnished with paprika.

Raw unpeeled beets, cut into fingers slightly larger than shoestring potatoes; for each cup of beets add 3 tablespoons chives cut fine with scissors, or minced fresh thyme.

Brussels sprouts, no more than ¾ inch in diameter.

Rings of raw zucchini or small wedges of young summer squash; add to each cup 2 teaspoons minced mixed herbs or 1 clove garlic.

Unpeeled eggplant, cut into sticks ½ inch square and 2 to 3 inches long; for each cup add 2 tablespoons chives and 1 tablespoon fresh horseradish or 1 teaspoon dill seeds.

Raw potato sticks; for each cup add 1 teaspoon caraway seeds or 2 tablespoons chives cut fine with scissors; serve for winter salads when vitamin C is inadequate.

Tomato quarters; to 2 cups tomato quarters add ¼ cup chopped parsley and 1 tablespoon chopped fresh basil or 2 tablespoons chives.

Red apple wedges; cut each apple into 8 to 10 wedges; add to each cup ½ teaspoon cumin, caraway, or dill seeds.

FINGER SALADS COMBINED WITH OTHER FOODS

Stuffed celery stalks: Cut the stalks into 3- to 5-inch lengths and stuff with any of the following fillings, combined with mayonnaise:

Chopped hard-cooked egg, chives, pimento.

Equal parts of peanut butter, shredded carrot, and chopped parsley.

Mashed avocado mixed with lemon juice, Worcestershire, freshly ground white peppercorns.

Cottage cheese mixed with chopped chives or parsley.

Liver paste (p. 228) or mashed liverwurst with shredded carrot, a few drops of Tabasco.

Salmon, sardine, or anchovy, finely flaked or mashed and combined with grated onion.

Cottage, cream, pimento, shredded American, Swiss, or Roquefort cheese, mixed with chives, parsley, fresh basil, dill, or caraway seeds; add enough milk or mayonnaise to moisten.

Stuffed celery-stalk rings: Use the stalks of an entire head of celery; pull apart, wash, and dry thoroughly; save the heart for other uses; spread the inside of stalks with one or more fillings suggested above; when stalks are filled, start with center stalks and press firmly together, working from the heart outward and reconstructing the entire head; tie stalks together, chill for $\frac{1}{2}$ hour or more; cut into slices $\frac{1}{2}$ inch thick.

Cream-cheese balls: Combine cream cheese with vegetables and herbs, such as shredded carrots, raw beets; tiny fresh or frozen raw peas; finely chopped purple cabbage or celery; finely chopped parsley, chervil, or celery leaves; chives; chopped fresh sage, rosemary, or other fresh herbs; or add dill, caraway, anise, celery, or mustard seeds; make into balls.

Rainbow-cheese balls: Season cream cheese with cumin, caraway, dill, or celery seeds; make into balls of different colors by rolling them in: ground nuts; finely chopped parsley combined with fresh herbs; shredded American cheese or finely grated carrots; paprika or minced canned or fresh pimento.

Cream-cheese scrolls: Mix cream cheese with grated carrots or raw beets or finely chopped parsley, spinach, mustard greens, or other vegetables; season with 1 tablespoon fresh horseradish and roll into scrolls in chipped beef; cut into 1-inch lengths.

Stuffed cucumbers: Cut the ends of cucumbers, scoop out seeds with an apple corer; fill centers with pimento cheese, chicken salad, or any filling suggested for celery; slice crosswise and serve.

In making apple salads, generally choose red apples for salads and do not peel. Quarter, core, dice, and mix immediately with lemon juice, French dressing, or mayonnaise to prevent discoloration.

APPLE, CARROT, AND ORANGE SALAD

Quarter, core, and dice:

2 unpeeled red apples
Add:

1 or 2 shredded carrots
½ cup diced orange sections

2 tablespoons mayonnaise
dash of salt

Stir, put over bed of **watercress** on chilled, individual salad plates. Sprinkle with **coconut and paprika**.

VARIATIONS:
Serve from bowl lined with Bibb lettuce.
Instead of mayonnaise, use yogurt or French dressing.

Follow procedure of basic recipe and combine a large proportion of diced raw apple with the ingredients suggested below; mix with yogurt, mayonnaise, or French dressing and serve on a bed of watercress, endive, shredded romaine, or lettuce:

Well-drained crushed pineapple, carrot, grated orange peel, a few raisins.
Celery, carrot, ½ teaspoon dill or caraway seeds or ¼ cup diced candied ginger.
Diced or sliced banana, a few maraschino cherries, 2 to 4 minced mint leaves.
Green pepper, kohlrabi, diced ham, 1 teaspoon caraway seeds.
Shredded purple cabbage, celery, raisins.
Celery, cubes of American cheese, 1 teaspoon cumin seeds, French dressing.
Celery stalk and leaves, chopped walnuts.
Pimento, celery, parsley, green onions.
Seedless grapes, diced cantaloupe; serve with yogurt dressing.

In making avocado salad, as soon as an avocado is cut, sprinkle or brush it with vinegar, lemon or tomato juice, or French dressing to prevent discoloration.

AVOCADO AND SHRIMP SALAD

Peel and cut in half or slice over lettuce on individual salad plates:

2 small avocados

Sprinkle immediately with:

fresh or frozen lemon juice or French dressing	**dash of salt**

Combine:

1 cup steamed fresh, canned, or frozen shrimps	1 tablespoon grated onion
½ cup finely diced celery	2 tablespoons mayonnaise
	½ teaspoon salt

Mix well and put over avocado. Garnish with **strips of green pepper** or pimento and sprinkle with **paprika**.

VARIATIONS:

Instead of shrimp, use chicken, crab, or tuna salad over avocado halves or slices; or use part shrimp and part diced hard-cooked eggs.

Add diced bell pepper or shredded carrot with shrimp.

Use a large proportion of avocado combined with the following ingredients; sprinkle with salt, and serve on a bed of greens with French dressing:

Fill halves with grapefruit and orange sections; garnish with diced fresh or canned pimento.

Pile in alternate layers sliced tomato, paper-thin slices of leek or sweet onion, rings of avocado sliced crosswise; if salad is main luncheon dish, put stuffed egg on top or serve with cottage cheese.

Arrange in a circle on a flat plate orange or grapefruit slices alternating with avocado rings, thin slices of leek or sweet onion; in the center place cheese balls rolled in ground nuts.

On a bed of greens, alternate rings of avocado and unpeeled California persimmon; or cut both in wedges; if persimmons are extremely soft, freeze, slice, and serve frozen. This is a beautiful and delicious salad.

Combine grapefruit sections, wedges of avocado, and persimmon.

Alternate rings of avocado with slices of oranges; have an orange slice on top and garnish with mint leaves.

Add diced or sliced avocado to any tossed salad (p. 266).

Mix large dices of avocado with pineapple cubes and chopped ripe olives.

Slice tomatoes and avocado on a bed of endive; add ⅓ cup cottage cheese seasoned with chives to each serving; garnish with chives or parsley.

COLE SLAW

Shred very thin, then cut into 2-inch strips:

½ head of green cabbage

Add and stir well:

⅔ cup yogurt or ⅓ cup each 1 tablespoon sugar
yogurt and sour cream   ½ teaspoon salt
2 or 3 tablespoons vinegar

Garnish with **paprika.** Serve immediately or chill 1 hour or longer.

VARIATIONS:

Add ¼ teaspoon crushed celery, dill, or caraway seeds.

Combine 1 part purple cabbage with 3 parts green, or use part Chinese or savoy cabbage.

Instead of yogurt or sour cream use mayonnaise or heavy sweet cream; or omit yogurt and use only sour cream.

Combine the following ingredients with finely shredded cabbage, using part Chinese and savoy cabbage when available:

Green cabbage, chopped onion, tomato wedges, sliced cucumber, minced clove garlic; toss with oil and tarragon vinegar or mix with yogurt dressing or mayonnaise.

Shredded carrots, savoy cabbage, fresh or canned pimentos, chopped onion and parsley; stir with mayonnaise or Thousand Island dressing.

Shredded cabbage, diced apricots, orange sections, celery salt; serve with French dressing.

Finely shredded purple cabbage, diced celery stalks and leaves, young rutabaga fingers, marjoram; toss with oil and vinegar.

Shredded cabbage, quartered tomatoes, chopped green peppers, sliced cucumbers, basil; mix with yogurt or sour cream.

Shredded green cabbage, diced pineapple, apple, and/or banana, a few peanuts, 5 or 6 fresh mint leaves; stir with mayonnaise.

Shredded cabbage, chopped green pepper, grated onion or chopped chives, chopped dill pickle; stir with mayonnaise.

CARROT AND APPLE SALAD

Wash and shred:

3 or 4 small chilled unpeeled carrots

Add:

1 diced unpeeled red apple   ½ teaspoon each salt and sugar
6 or 8 sliced stuffed olives   2 or 3 tablespoons mayonnaise
⅛ teaspoon celery seeds (optional)

Stir well and serve over a bed of watercress on chilled individual plates.

VARIATIONS:

Omit olives and celery seeds and add ¼ cup raisins, dash of nutmeg. Instead of mayonnaise, use yogurt or sour cream.

Combine the following ingredients with a large proportion of chilled grated or shredded unpeeled carrots and serve on a bed of greens:

Diced cling peaches, coconut.
Drained crushed pineapple, raisins, French dressing.
Chopped bell pepper or diced red apple, 2 or 3 mint leaves, mayonnaise.
Shredded cabbage, chives or onion, chopped parsley, mayonnaise or sour cream.
Celery, onion, and chopped bell pepper and parsley.
Diced raw apple, avocado, bell pepper.

If cucumbers are tender and thinly sliced, the skins may usually be left on provided they have not been sprayed with paraffin. Cucumbers with skins lacking bitterness are now available and should be raised by persons lucky enough to have their own gardens. The habit of soaking cucumbers in vinegar should be avoided except when the juices are eaten or added to food. Chill cucumbers thoroughly before slicing them.

CUCUMBER SALAD

Arrange on chilled individual salad plates:

½ cup shredded mixed greens

Slice very thin onto greens:

cucumbers	**sweet onion or green onions with**
bell pepper, preferably red	**tops**

Garnish with:

minced leaves of fresh marjoram	**finely chopped parsley**
or sprinkling of dry leaves	

Pour over each salad:

1 or 2 tablespoons French dressing

Sprinkle with **paprika** and serve.

VARIATIONS:

Slice 1 or 2 tomatoes over greens, putting cucumbers on top.

Season with fresh basil, tarragon, or other fresh herbs; or sprinkle dry herbs mixed especially for salads over cucumbers.

See cucumber aspics, page 283.

Combine the ingredients listed below and on next page in any amounts desired; season with salt and pepper, and serve on watercress or other greens; use cucumbers as the principal ingredients:

Shoestring sticks of small cucumbers, kohlrabi, unpeeled carrots, turnips, lettuce, 4 to 6 minced basil leaves; toss with oil, vinegar, a small amount of Worcestershire.

Moisten cucumber slices with tarragon vinegar; sprinkle with salt, paprika, celery salt.

Mix cucumber, radish, and thin carrot slices with sour cream; add a few drops Tabasco; sprinkle with dill seeds.

Mix equal amounts of sliced cucumber and sweet onion; fold into 1 cup sour cream or yogurt.

Slice radishes, cucumbers, raw turnips; add 1 teaspoon dill seeds or a small amount of chopped fresh dill; serve with yogurt dressing.

Slice green onions and cut the tops with scissors; combine with sliced tomatoes, cucumbers, and a few minced leaves of basil; serve with a tart French dressing.

Sprinkle cucumbers with caraway, cumin, or dill seeds; serve with yogurt dressing.

Ripe, or red, bell peppers and fresh pimentos and paprikas are of such outstanding nutritional value that it is regrettable they are not in every market. When available, they should be added to all vegetable salads. As soon as the taste for these peppers has been cultivated, they may be served whole for salads in the same way that whole tomatoes are served, stuffed or cut in petal fashion.

Since the vitamin C content of bell peppers doubles on ripening, use red ones when available instead of green ones. Persons unaccustomed to eating ripe bell peppers often imagine them to be hot. Actually they are much sweeter and more mild than green ones. Moreover, their beautiful color is reason enough for adding them generously to salads.

STUFFED PEPPER RINGS

Remove the tops and centers from:

2 large red or green bell peppers, paprikas, or pimentos

Combine and mix well:

2 cups (1 pound) cottage cheese, beaten hoop cheese, or grated American cheese
1 small grated onion or leek or

2 tablespoons chives cut with scissors
¼ cup milk or salad dressing

Stuff cheese filling into each pepper; chill, slice crosswise, and arrange on salad greens, using 2 or more slices for each serving.

Garnish centers with parsley.

VARIATIONS:

Instead of cheese fill peppers with any fish, chicken, or meat salad.

Omit the cheese and make a filling by combining 1½ cups shredded carrots or cabbage, ½ cup drained crushed pineapple; add 2 tablespoons mayonnaise.

Fill pepper rings with any cabbage salad (p. 272).

Bell pepper-watercress salad: Combine 3 diced green or red bell peppers with 1 bunch shredded watercress, 1 grated onion, ½ cup or more yogurt dressing.

Paprika-cucumber salad: Combine 1 cup diced cucumbers and ½ sweet onion; add paprika, minced clove garlic, ½ teaspoon salt, ¼ cup tart French dressing. Serve on a bed of endive.

Most of the raw tomatoes reaching the large city markets are now sprayed with paraffin, making it necessary for them to be peeled. Sprayed cocktail tomatoes, which cannot be peeled, should be avoided; an attempt to wash off the spray with hot water ruins the fruit. If you are lucky enough to have your own garden, however, serve tomatoes unpeeled.

TOMATO PLATTER

Line platter with lettuce and slice over greens:

2 or more large tomatoes

Cut into ⅛-inch rings and put over tomatoes:

chilled green or red pepper   green onions with tops

Lay across top:

can asparagus tips

Sprinkle with:

½ teaspoon salt   ¼ cup finely chopped parsley

Pour over the entire platter:

½ cup French dressing

Marinate in refrigerator 1 hour before serving.

VARIATIONS:

Add sliced hard-cooked eggs, avocado, cucumbers, or other sliced vegetables.

If salad is main dish for lunch, serve with cottage cheese or shrimp or chicken salad.

Instead of asparagus use carrot, turnip, kohlrabi, or stalks of broccoli, chard, cabbage, or cauliflower cut into fingers.

Omit asparagus and add marinated tips of broccoli bud or cauliflowerlets.

Cut 4 whole tomatoes toward the stem end into 6 or 8 petals; set on bed of mixed greens, separate petals slightly, sprinkle generously with chopped parsley and chives, and into center of each put 1 teaspoon mayonnaise. Vary by filling centers with cottage or mashed cream cheese, chopped hard-cooked eggs, or any meat or fish salad.

Sprinkle over tomatoes 1 teaspoon minced fresh or a pinch of dried basil, tarragon, or orégano.

Add a layer of any of the following vegetables cut into paper-thin slices: raw carrots, turnips, kohlrabi, rutabagas; shredded raw cauliflower or tender buds of broccoli.

STUFFED TOMATOES

Cut ½-inch slice from stem end of:

4 large tomatoes

If tomatoes have been sprayed with paraffin, peel; remove pulp from center, chop, and combine with:

1 diced cucumber	1 tablespoon grated onion
½ cup cottage cheese or shredded Cheddar cheese	½ teaspoon salt
	¼ cup mayonnaise

Put filling into salted tomato and serve on shredded lettuce or bed of watercress.

VARIATIONS:

Add any chopped leftover vegetables to the filling.

Fill tomatoes with any meat or fish salad (p. 230).

Instead of cucumber use 1 cup shredded carrots, turnips, or kohlrabi; finely diced celery, tart apple, or green pepper; or tender buds and diced stalk of raw broccoli or cauliflower.

Make filling of ½ cup each diced celery and apple, 1 tablespoon grated onion or chopped chives, 2 tablespoons mayonnaise.

All varieties of cheese may be added to any kind of salad. The following salads are particularly advantageous for persons who need a high-protein diet. When cheese is a principal ingredient of a salad, a mild-flavored cheese should be used.

COTTAGE-CHEESE SALAD

Combine the following ingredients:

2 cups cottage cheese	1 chopped pimento (optional)
¼ cup finely chopped parsley or ½ cup shredded spinach	2 drops Tabasco
½ cup shredded carrots	½ teaspoon each salt and Worcestershire
2 tablespoons chives	

Serve on a bed of **watercress, shredded young mustard greens, or** lettuce.

Top each serving with:

1 teaspoon mayonnaise, French or Thousand Island dressing	dash of paprika

VARIATIONS:

Decrease or increase amount of parsley or spinach used or add any other finely shredded greens; or omit parsley or spinach and add ¾ cup tiny raw or frozen peas or 1 cup shredded unpeeled carrots; or add crushed pineapple with carrots and omit chives.

Use part mashed cream cheese, crumbled dry cottage cheese, or shredded American, Swiss, or Jack cheese; blend with enough milk or mayonnaise to hold together.

Mash 1 avocado, add 1 grated onion, combine with other ingredients.

Omit chives and serve salad on 1 banana cut lengthwise, 1 slice of pineapple, 2 apricot halves, or a canned or fresh peach or pear half placed on a bed of watercress.

Fruit Salads

Fruit salads should be served at lunch or at the end of the dinner course except when they are combined with a generous amount of vegetables.

Salads can be made of almost any single fruit or a combination of two or more fruits. When only canned fruit is available for salads, use individual salad plates covered with a generous quantity of shredded greens. If fresh fruits are used, place them attractively between the curved leaves of head lettuce or on a bed of romaine or crisp watercress. Following are suggestions for fruit salads to be served on individual plates.

Fresh or canned peach, apricot, or pear halves; serve with French dressing; vary by adding cottage cheese; by sprinkling with walnuts, pecans, or shredded coconut; or by serving with sour cream, yogurt, or peanut-butter dressing (p. 290).

Sliced fresh or canned peaches or sliced bananas, diced celery, ½ cup walnuts; combine with sour-cream dressing.

Cut firm peaches into bite sizes; combine with mayonnaise and any one of the following fruits: seedless grapes, diced honeydew melon, firm plums, fresh or canned apricots, sliced bananas, diced pineapple, orange sections, diced grapefruit sections, white cherries, unpeeled diced apples or pears. Instead of peaches use fresh apricots cut into sixths.

Fresh or canned apricot quarters, seeded black cherries, cream dressing.

Cut California persimmons crosswise into ½-inch slices; arrange on a bed of crisp watercress; serve with tart French dressing. This is the most beautiful salad I know of and one of the most delicious.

Firm purple plums, diced cantaloupe, honeydew, or Persian melon; serve with French or cream dressing.

Cut bananas in half lengthwise; sprinkle with chopped peanuts, walnuts, pecans, or coconut; or omit nuts and serve with cottage cheese or balls of cream cheese; use French or cream dressing; if nuts are not used, serve with peanut-butter dressing.

Cover a whole banana with cream cheese ¼ inch thick; roll in ground nuts; slice and serve with French dressing on a bed of watercress.

Slice bananas ½ inch thick; combine with cream dressing or mayonnaise and seedless grapes, white cherries, apricots, or other fruits suggested under peach salads.

Candle salad: Use individual salad plates; place 1 large slice pineapple on a bed of shredded lettuce; put ½ banana upright in the center of each slice; scoop out the tip of each banana to hold a red cherry. This salad is traditional for our Christmas Eve dinner and is sometimes used for birthday parties.

FRUIT SALAD BOWL

Line a salad bowl attractively with the leaves of:

1 head romaine lettuce

Arrange in alternate layers:

2 cups fresh or canned pineapple, diced or sliced	1 red apple cut into thin wedges
2 cups grapefruit sections	1 cup seeded or seedless grapes
	2 sliced oranges

Garnish with black or maraschino cherries and serve with mayonnaise or fruit dressing.

VARIATIONS:

Sprinkle with anise or poppy seeds.

Use equal amounts of each fruit; arrange separately on a platter over lettuce or watercress. Garnish with sprigs of fresh mint.

Omit any one fruit and add slices of chilled banana moistened with lemon juice.

Omit pineapple and grapefruit; combine grapes, apples, orange sections with fresh or canned cherries or sliced bananas, a few leaves of chopped mint or lemon balm.

Combine in layers diced unpeeled pears, red raspberries, sliced bananas.

Substitute one of the following for any fruit suggested: fresh whole strawberries; diced cantaloupe, honeydew, or Persian melon; fresh or canned apricots and/or peaches; seeded tangerine sections; firm or frozen California persimmon; fresh figs; dices of avocado.

Grapefruit salad: Combine 2 to 3 cups grapefruit sections, ½ cup chopped almonds, 1 green pepper or pimento cut into strips. Serve on a bed of endive with Roquefort-cheese dressing.

Orange salad: Cover individual salad plates with romaine lettuce; alternate on lettuce sections of orange or grapefruit, wedges of unpeeled pear, pieces of red bell pepper. Serve with mayonnaise.

Pear salad: Arrange fresh or canned unpeeled pear halves on lettuce; cover with cottage or cream cheese and cherries, strawberries, or youngberries; serve with yogurt or fruit dessing.

Stuffed-prune salad: Remove stones from steamed dried prunes or spiced prunes; stuff with cream cheese mixed with nuts, parsley, or pimento; arrange on orange slices on a bed of watercress.

MELON SALADS

Combine the following ingredients in any amounts desired and serve on individual salad plates or from salad bowl on a bed of lettuce, romaine, watercress, or endive:

Grapefruit sections, diced slices of cantaloupe or honeydew or Persian melon, topped with cottage cheese.

Unstemmed strawberries, cubes or balls of cantaloupe or Persian melon; serve with fruit dressing.

Melon balls or diced slices, white grapes, fresh peaches, sliced canned or fresh pineapple; serve with mayonnaise.

Cantaloupe and/or honeydew balls, pineapple cubes, Brazil or hazelnuts or toasted almonds.

Gelatin Salads

The liquid used in making gelatin salads should be as rich as possible in vitamins and minerals; hence I have recommended using any water left from cooking vegetables or drained from canned foods in each basic aspic recipe. The gelatin should be unflavored and unsweetened. Since both the synthetic colorings and flavorings in sweetened gelatins may be detrimental to health, they cannot be recommended. Although gelatin is a protein, it is of the poorest possible quality and should not be counted as part of the daily protein allowance.

Raw pineapple and papaya contain enzymes which quickly digest protein; hence they must not be used in a gelatin salad unless they are first heated to boiling.

ASPIC FOR VEGETABLE SALADS

Combine in a metal measuring cup:

1 tablespoon unflavored gelatin   ½ cup vegetable-cooking water

Let gelatin soften for 5 minutes and dissolve by heating over simmer burner; add:

1¼ cups vegetable-cooking water 1 tablespoon or more grated onion
  or cold fruit juice   3 tablespoons chopped parsley
¼ cup vinegar or lemon juice   1 diced bell pepper or pimento
1 teaspoon salt   ½ teaspoon freshly ground white
1 to 3 teaspoons sugar   peppercorns

Chill until gelatin starts to thicken and add any combination of vegetables and seasonings listed below.

Taste for seasonings; pour into a ring mold brushed lightly with vegetable oil. Chill and unmold by turning on edge and tapping lightly to loosen sides.

Serve on a bed of **watercress, endive, romaine, lettuce, or mixed chopped greens** with a small bowl of dressing in center.

Add to the basic recipe any of the following ingredients and seasonings:

Artichoke jellied ring: Substitute French dressing for vinegar; add 1 can of artichoke hearts, 2 diced hard-cooked eggs, ¼ cup sliced stuffed olives. Use less salt if olives are included. Serve with center filled with fish or chicken salad.

Asparagus aspic: 1 cup steamed fresh asparagus tips cut into ⅛-inch pieces, ½ cup chopped celery, ½ teaspoon mustard seed, 2 tablespoons mayonnaise.

Beet aspic: 1 cup finely shredded raw beets; use green pepper instead of pimento; tarragon or marjoram vinegar.

Cabbage aspic: 1 cup finely shredded green cabbage; increase diced pimento to ¼ cup; add ¼ cup celery, dash of cayenne, fresh dill. Vary by using ¾ cup each shredded green and purple cabbage; add 2 teaspoons crushed dill or caraway seeds.

Cabbage-cucumber aspic: ¾ cup each shredded cabbage and diced cucumbers.

Carrot aspic: 1½ cups shredded carrots; or 1 cup shredded carrot and ½ cup drained crushed pineapple; omit onion if pineapple is used.

Cucumber aspic: 1½ cups diced cucumber, ¼ cup chopped celery.

Cucumber aspic with sour cream: 1½ cups diced cucumber; use ½ cup sour cream or yogurt instead of ½ cup vegetable-cooking water; add 2 tablespoons chives.

Green-pepper aspic: Before adding vegetables pour gelatin to depth of ¼ inch in a flat mold; slice 2 eggs into gelatin and let chill; into remaining gelatin stir 2 tablespoons diced ripe olives, 1 cup chopped green peppers, ¼ cup each chopped pimentos and celery; pour into mold when gelatin holding eggs has congealed.

Mixed greens in aspic: Shred spinach, watercress, and assorted greens, making 1½ cups in all; use ¼ cup chopped onion or leek, fresh or dried basil.

Mustard greens in aspic: Select tender young mustard greens or use mustard-spinach; shred and add 1 cup with 1 cup cottage cheese.

Tomato aspic I: Instead of vegetable-cooking water use tomato juice; add 3 tablespoons chili sauce, 1 to 3 teaspoons horseradish, dried or minced fresh basil, and the other ingredients of basic recipe.

Tomato aspic II: Use tomato juice instead of vegetable-cooking water; add 1 to 3 teaspoons Worcestershire, 3 drops Tabasco, 1 teaspoon horseradish.

Watercress aspic: 1½ cups shredded leaves and diced stalk of watercress; or use ¾ cup each watercress and grapefruit sections.

For festive occasions, attractive gelatin salads can be made of two or more layers of contrasting colors. Almost any two recipes may be combined provided the colors and flavors harmonize. The mold used must be large enough to hold a quart or more, and each layer must be thoroughly chilled before the next layer is added. Such salads are easy to make if the gelatin and liquids are accurately measured.

PINEAPPLE-WATERCRESS ASPIC

Put into metal measuring cup:

1 cup cold vegetable-cooking water   2 tablespoons unflavored gelatin
or juice drained from pineapple

Soak 10 minutes and heat over the simmer burner until the gelatin
is clear; stir thoroughly.

Add exactly ½ the dissolved gelatin to:

1½ cups crushed pineapple

Stir and pour into a large mold brushed lightly with oil; chill quickly.
Combine with remaining dissolved gelatin:

1 cup vegetable-cooking water	¾ cup shredded watercress
½ cup diced cucumbers	1 teaspoon salt
1 tablespoon grated onion	¼ cup French dressing

Stir well; when pineapple layer has set, add gelatin containing watercress; chill thoroughly.

Unmold by turning on edge and tapping to loosen gelatin from the
sides of the mold; put large plate over mold, turn upside down; surround with **lettuce, romaine, or sprigs of watercress.**

VARIATIONS:

Use combinations of recipes on page 283 for layers containing pineapple and cucumbers.

Make additional layer of 2 packages of cream cheese mashed with
½ cup milk or 2 cups shredded American cheese blended with ¾ cup
milk; set with 2 teaspoons gelatin dissolved in ½ cup milk; season
with 1 teaspoon dill or caraway seeds.

Apricot-grape aspic: Proceed as in basic recipe and stir ½ cup of the
dissolved gelatin with 1¾ cups apricot purée prepared in liquefier;
pour into mold and chill; add remaining dissolved gelatin to 1¾ cups
Concord grape juice. Or use peaches instead of apricots. This salad is
both beautiful and delicious.

Carrot-cabbage aspic: Combine 1½ cups each cold vegetable-cooking
water and shredded carrots; add ¼ cup French dressing and one half

the dissolved gelatin; taste for salt, pour into a mold, chill. Combine remaining gelatin with 1½ cups each finely shredded green cabbage and vegetable-cooking water, 1 teaspoon salt, ⅓ cup mayonnaise, 3 tablespoons grated onion. When carrot gelatin is firmly set, add cabbage gelatin and chill. Substitute any other diced or shredded vegetables for carrots and cabbage.

Celery-beet aspic: Dissolve gelatin as in basic recipe; combine one half of dissolved gelatin with 1½ cups vegetable-cooking water, 1 cup finely diced celery, 1 each chopped green pepper and leek or sweet onion, ¼ cup tarragon vinegar, 1 teaspoon each sugar and salt; pour into a mold and chill. Combine remaining dissolved gelatin with 1½ cups each vegetable-cooking water and shredded raw beets, ¼ cup tart French dressing, 1 teaspoon each salt, sugar, and ground horseradish. When celery gelatin has chilled, add layer of shredded beets.

Pineapple-avocado aspic: Follow basic recipe except to omit cucumbers. Arrange slices of chilled avocado attractively in a thin layer of gelatin on oiled mold; chill; add the gelatin mixed with watercress and 1 cup diced avocado; add pineapple last.

Tomato-cucumber aspic: Prepare as in basic recipe except to use tomato aspic (p. 283) instead of pineapple. Mold cucumber and watercress gelatin first; add tomato aspic.

ASPIC FOR FRUIT SALADS

Soften for 5 minutes:

1 tablespoon unflavored gelatin in	½ cup cold pineapple, grapefruit, or apple juice

Heat slowly over simmer burner until gelatin is dissolved; add:

1 cup chilled pineapple, grapefruit, or apple juice	pinch of salt ¼ cup fresh lemon or lime juice

Stir well, and chill until gelatin starts to congeal; add any group of ingredients listed below.

Pour into a mold brushed lightly with oil. Chill and unmold by turning on edge and tapping to loosen sides; or mold in shallow pan, cut into cubes, and serve on individual salad plates on a bed of lettuce or watercress.

VARIATIONS:

Instead of juices suggested, use unsweetened apricot, orange, grape, or berry juice, or any thin fruit purée prepared in liquefier.

Apricot and prune aspic: Add 1 cup sliced fresh or drained, canned apricots, ½ cup cooked, chopped, and pitted prunes.

Banana aspic: Add 2 diced bananas mixed with lemon juice of basic recipe, ½ cup seedless grapes or sliced guavas.

Carrot-pineapple aspic: Add 1 cup grated carrots, ½ cup crushed drained pineapple.

Cheese-apricot aspic: Add ¾ cup each fresh or canned apricot wedges and cottage cheese.

Cranberry-pineapple aspic: Add 1 cup ground raw cranberries, ½ cup crushed pineapple, ¼ cup sugar, 1 teaspoon orange rind; or omit pineapple and use 1½ cups cranberries sweetened to taste.

Cucumber-pineapple aspic: Add ½ cup crushed pineapple, 1 cup diced cucumbers, 1 tablespoon chopped pimento.

Mixed fruit aspic: Dice 1½ cups of any firm fresh fruits and/or well-drained canned fruits; or use 1 cup diced fruit and ½ cup broken nuts or shredded watercress or other greens.

Watercress and grapefruit aspic: Add 1 cup each grapefruit sections and shredded watercress.

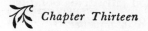 *Chapter Thirteen*

Salad Dressings

Since oils used for salads are not submitted to the sustained high temperatures of cooking, it is wiser to obtain unsaturated fatty acids from salad dressings than from cooked foods. Although some labels state that oils are cold pressed, during the extracting process all oils are more or less cooked by the heat of friction.

Such oils as safflower, soy, corn, peanut, and cottonseed appear to be nutritionally superior to olive oil. Soy, safflower, and corn oils have proved particularly satisfactory in lowering abnormally high blood cholesterol, perhaps because they have been used in experimental studies more often than have other oils. Such infrequently used oils as those pressed from sunflower seeds, sesame seeds, and wheat germ are also nutritionally excellent. Wheat germ oil contains more vitamin E than does other oils, and safflower oil is the most unsaturated.

Because oils differ in their make-up of unsaturated fatty acids, some health authorities recommend that we use a variety of them, perhaps mixing two or more. Or, after a bottle of soy oil has been used, peanut oil might be purchased, then corn oil, and so on. I usually recommend that persons use safflower or soy oil for salad dressings and a variety of the less expensive oils for cooking. If you wish to use olive oil, it is wise to combine it with an equal amount of peanut, soy, or some other more nutritious oil. Cottonseed oil has been found to be so contaminated with the poison sprays applied to destroy the boll weevil that nutritionally aware physicians have warned against its use.

It must be remembered that the need for vitamin E increases in proportion to the amount of unsaturated fatty acids obtained in the diet. Furthermore the absorption of even slightly rancid oils can cause some destruction in the blood stream of vitamins A, C, E, and several of the B vitamins. Definite rancidity can be quite toxic. Manufacturers replace the air in the top of bottled oil with an inert gas which prevents rancidity until the bottle is opened. All oils should be carefully refrigerated after the container has been opened; and any oil allowed to stand at room temperature more than a day or two should probably be discarded. Bacon dripping collected in a can on the back of a range, for example, should not be used for cooking.

No salad dressing is hydrogenated, a process which causes a liquid oil to become a semisolid or solid fat. Mayonnaise is a semisolid only because it is emulsified with egg yolk; it contains approximately 50 per cent vegetable oil.

Although the virtues of apple vinegar have been considerably overstressed, lemon juice and cider and wine vinegars are nutritionally superior for salad dressings to highly refined distilled white vinegar. Frozen lemon juice, because of its acidity, retains its original vitamin-C content; its convenience may cause it to be preferable to fresh juice for salad dressings.

FRENCH DRESSING

Combine in a pint jar:

¾ cup vegetable oil
¼ cup vinegar or lemon juice
¼ cup catsup or chili sauce
  (optional)
1 to 3 teaspoons honey or sugar

1 clove garlic cut in half
1 teaspoon salt
½ teaspoon paprika
¼ teaspoon freshly ground white
  peppercorns

Cover jar and shake until ingredients are well blended; keep in refrigerator; shake well each time before using.

VARIATIONS:

If tart dressing is desired, use ½ cup oil to ¼ cup vinegar or lemon juice.

Add any one or more of the following: 4 to 6 drops Tabasco; 1 finely chopped onion or leek; 1 teaspoon dry mustard, curry powder, or celery salt; 2 or more tablespoons chopped red or green bell pepper or pimento; 1 or 2 tablespoons chopped chives, freshly ground horseradish, or chutney; 2 tablespoons each finely chopped celery and onion; 2 tablespoons anchovy paste; 1 tablespoon Worcestershire.

Use tarragon or wine vinegar; or add 1 or 2 tablespoons minced fresh or ½ teaspoon dry basil, burnet, marjoram, orégano, or other herb or combination of herbs.

Cheese dressing: Add ¼ cup or more crumbled Roquefort cheese; omit or use catsup.

Cream dressing: Omit catsup; combine ⅓ cup each oil and cream or evaporated milk; add 2 tablespoons vinegar or lemon juice and seasonings of basic recipe. Vary by adding 1 package mashed cream cheese.

Olive dressing: To ½ cup of basic recipe add 4 tablespoons chopped ripe olives or sliced stuffed olives, 1 tablespoon chopped parsley, 1 chopped green pepper.

Nut dressing: Omit catsup and garlic; add ¼ cup or more finely chopped walnuts, pecans, other nuts, or peanut butter. Serve on fruit salads.

Salad-seasoned vinegar: Omit oil; use 1 cup vinegar, combine with other ingredients, add 6 drops Tabasco, 1 teaspoon Worcestershire, and fresh or dried herbs if desired. Keep for tossed salads.

Tomato-soup dressing: Omit catsup and use ½ cup oil; combine 1 can condensed tomato soup with other ingredients of basic recipe; add 1 tablespoon Worcestershire, 1 teaspoon dry mustard, 1 tablespoon grated onion; increase vinegar or lemon juice if tart dressing is desired. Salt to taste.

MAYONNAISE

Combine and beat well or blend in liquefier:

2 egg yolks	1 to 3 teaspoons sugar
1 teaspoon salt	¼ to 1 teaspoon dry mustard
4 tablespoons vinegar or lemon juice	¼ teaspoon freshly ground peppercorns

Add slowly, beating constantly:

1½ to 2 cups salad oil

Add more oil if thicker texture is desired. Store in refrigerator.

VARIATIONS:

To 1 cup mayonnaise add one of the following: ½ cup whipped evaporated milk or whipped cream; ½ cup chili sauce and 2 tablespoons chopped green or red bell pepper; ¼ cup chopped sour or dill pickle and 2 tablespoons chopped onion; 2 tablespoons each chopped pickle, sliced stuffed olives, capers, parsley; 1 teaspoon paprika and ¼ cup tomato catsup; ½ cup chopped cucumber; 2 to 4 tablespoons grated horseradish.

Cheese dressing: To 1 cup mayonnaise add 2 teaspoons Worcestershire, ¼ cup grated American or crumbled Roquefort cheese or 1 package mashed cream cheese.

Peanut butter and banana dressing: Stir into ½ cup mayonnaise 1 banana mashed with 1 tablespoon lemon juice, 4 tablespoons peanut butter, ¼ cup cream or evaporated milk. Serve with fruit salads.

Thousand Island dressing: To 1 cup mayonnaise add ¼ cup each chopped mixed pickles and chili sauce, 2 diced hard-cooked eggs, 2 tablespoons each chopped pimentos and onion.

YOGURT, OR LOW CALORIE, DRESSING

Mix well:

1 cup, or an 8-ounce jar, yogurt	½ teaspoon salt
2 tablespoons lemon juice or tarragon or wine vinegar	½ to 1 teaspoon paprika
	1 minced clove garlic
¼ to ½ teaspoon dry mustard	1 finely chopped or grated onion

Let stand in refrigerator 15 minutes or longer before using.
Serve on head lettuce or any mixed-vegetable salad.

VARIATIONS:

Add one or more of the following: 1 teaspoon minced fresh or ¼ teaspoon dried basil, marjoram, burnet, or savory; 1 tablespoon mayonnaise or vegetable oil; 1 teaspoon Worcestershire; 3 drops Tabasco; 1 tablespoon catsup or chili sauce; ½ to 1 teaspoon curry powder; 1 teaspoon caraway, cumin, or dill seeds.

Omit garlic and onion; serve on fruit salads.

Substitute 1 cup condensed tomato soup for yogurt; add seasonings of basic recipe, 1 tablespoon vegetable oil, ¼ cup vinegar.

Cheese dressing: Add to basic recipe or to yogurt only 4 tablespoons shredded American cheese or crumbled Roquefort cheese.

"Cream" dressing: Whip ½ cup chilled evaporated milk until thick; add seasonings and ¼ cup vinegar or lemon juice. Use for reducing diets; this dressing is even lower in calories than yogurt.

SOUR-CREAM DRESSING

Mix well:

1 cup sour cream	2 to 4 tablespoons Roquefort or
¼ teaspoon paprika	bleu cheese

Chill thoroughly and serve over mixed greens or fruit salad.

VARIATIONS:

Omit cheese and add 1 or 2 tablespoons honey, ¼ cup drained crushed pineapple or juice from sweet canned or spiced fruit; serve on fruit salads.

Use yogurt instead of sour cream.

Add any seasonings suggested for French dressings or mayonnaise.

COOKED SALAD DRESSING

Mix in a saucepan:

1 tablespoon whole-wheat-pastry flour	2 tablespoons partially hardened margarine or vegetable oil
1 teaspoon salt	1 clove garlic
1 to 3 teaspoons sugar	1 cup fresh milk or evaporated milk
2 eggs	

Stir continually while simmering until thick; use cooking thermometer and heat only to 185° F.; *do not boil;* cool, and beat in:

⅓ cup vinegar or lemon juice	1 teaspoon dry mustard

Store in covered jar in refrigerator.

VARIATIONS:

Vary by using tarragon or wine vinegar or any vinegar seasoned with herbs; or use ¼ cup vinegar or lemon juice and add 2 tablespoons sherry.

Add any of the following: 1 chopped cucumber and/or 2 tablespoons each chopped onion and parsley; green or red bell pepper or pimento or ¼ cup chopped celery; if to be used on fruit salad, omit garlic and add ¼ cup non-hydrogenated peanut butter.

Cream dressing: Omit garlic; use 1 or 2 tablespoons sugar; add ½ cup whipped evaporated milk or whipped cream. Serve on fruit salads.

Fruit dressing: Use lemon juice; omit garlic; instead of milk use grapefruit, pineapple, or orange juice with 1 teaspoon grated orange or lemon rind.

Sour-cream dressing: When cold, add 1 cup whipped sour cream, few grains of cayenne.

Thousand Island dressing: Add 3 or more tablespoons each chopped sour or dill pickle, parsley, chili sauce; 1 chopped hard-cooked egg.

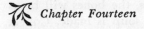 *Chapter Fourteen*

Soups Are Fun to Make

Except for cream soups, little can be said in favor of soups as they are usually made; the flavor of the bones is incompletely extracted and the vegetables are generally watery and overcooked. Delicious soups rich in vitamins and minerals can be made by imitating the thrifty French, famous for their soups. Before fresh vegetables are added, stock rich in flavor should be prepared. Soup stock may be defined as an extract of bones, meat scraps, and vegetables. The more vegetables and bones you use in making stock, the more delicious the soup will be.

If you want excellent soup, go on a salvage drive and save vegetable parings: tomato trimmings, provided the fruit has not been sprayed with paraffin; pea hulls, washed before hulling; wilted stalks of celery and asparagus, tops of green onions, turnips, radishes, beets, and young carrots not eaten as greens or used in salads; wilted or outer leaves of lettuce, cabbage, spinach, chard, kale, parsley, and other greens; the peelings of squash, carrots, beets, turnips, cucumbers, rutabagas, kohlrabi, and any vegetable so shriveled or tough as to require peeling; unused stalks of cauliflower, cabbage, broccoli, and lettuce; and the seeds and stems of peppers. Keep all the vegetable parings and trimmings in a large plastic bag in the refrigerator until it is bulging.

Housewives who are not squeamish have told me that they add to the soup bag the bones and meat scraps left on the plates after meals. Since pasteurization temperature is 140° F. and the stock will be boiled at 212° F. for several hours, the bones will be as sterile as surgical gauze by the time the soup is made. Collect every variety of bones: pork, veal, lamb, beef, chicken, turkey, rabbit, and game. As the small bones and meat scraps accumulate, put them into another bag and keep them next to the freezing unit; whenever you have a large bone, such as a ham bone or a turkey carcass, make soup stock the following day.

Third, if you are Scotch and not squeamish, save leftovers which are usually thrown away: vegetable salad remaining in the bowl and on the plates; cooked vegetables still on the plates; and any leftovers which cannot be used in other ways. These scraps will also be thoroughly sterilized. Before washing dishes, put these leftovers into a large covered pan low enough to go into the refrigerator. Also throw into it any cooking water you have not used. When parings, bones, meat scraps, and leftovers have accumulated, it is time to make stock. Although only a small per cent of women will actually prepare stock week after week, dozens of housewives have written me that the soups they have made from stocks thus prepared have been foods for the gods. Even if you have no desire to make soup, the stock, used instead of water for general cooking, can add immeasurably to the flavor of foods and the enrichment of the diet by supplying minerals and heat-stable vitamins.

The minerals in bones are held in a base of connective tissue, like a solid bed of gristle. The purpose in making soup is to break down the connective tissue in the bones and thereby extract minerals, flavor, and unrefined gelatin. Although the customary method of making soup is to simmer it at 185°F., a higher temperature is preferable; bones contain no vitamins. Delicious soup stock can be made in half an hour by cooking the bones in a pressure cooker.

All well-made soup stock should be rich in calcium, which can be dissolved from the bones by adding vinegar. Acid also hastens the breakdown of connective tissue and thus shortens the cooking time. Since salt attracts, or draws out, juices, it is important that salt be added with the water and vinegar. As the stock is boiled, calcium combines with acid and the taste of vinegar disappears. If any odor of it remains, the lid of the utensil may be removed and the vinegar quickly evaporated off by rapid boiling before the vegetable parings are put in.

The vegetable scraps and parings used in making soup stock should be cooked only a short time. Their flavor must be retained; little vitamin C should be destroyed; and the sulfur compounds, which give a strong flavor to overcooked vegetables of the cabbage family, must not be allowed to break down. The more thoroughly the vegetables are chopped, however, the more flavor and nutritive value pass into the stock. An understanding of the quantities of nutrients gained from vegetable parings will serve a dual purpose of emphasizing the nutritive value of scraps which are usually thrown away and of showing the tremendous harm done when vegetables are washed slowly, soaked, or boiled.

Of the known vitamins, the bioflavonoids, vitamins B_1, B_2, B_6, C, niacin, pantothenic acid, para-aminobenzoic acid, folic acid, cholin, inositol, and biotin dissolve in water as readily as does sugar. Of these, only folic acid and vitamin C are harmed at boiling temperature. Unless submitted to heat for a long period, vitamin B_1 is destroyed only by a temperature above boiling. Vitamins A, or carotene, E, and K do not dissolve in water; but when vegetables are chopped or are cooked until the cell walls soften and break down, these vitamins are spilled into the cooking water. If vegetables are thoroughly chopped and quickly cooked in soup stock, the larger amount of all of these vitamins passes into the stock.

The minerals lost when vegetables are soaked or boiled are those gained in making soups. Studies have shown that vegetables boiled only 4 minutes, even though they are not chopped, lose an average of 50 per cent of their phosphorus, sodium, magnesium, potassium, iron, and manganese into the cooking water. These minerals occur in the form of salts as easily dissolved in water as is table salt. Other studies have shown that when vegetables are boiled until the cell walls are soft and then are allowed to stand for a half hour, as cooked vegetables often do in restaurants, as much as 90 per cent of their total minerals may pass into the water. If vegetable parings and leftovers are boiled slowly for 15 minutes, the greater part of their minerals is extracted into the stock, although further soaking is advantageous.

When bones are not otherwise available, they should be purchased for making stock. Bones of young animals contain more connective tissue than do those of older animals. It is for this reason that veal bones are usually recommended for making jellied bouillons. The meat of veal, however, lacks flavor and makes less delicious soup than ribs, backbones, shoulder blades, and other bones trimmed from mature young beef when rolled roasts are prepared. These bones are excellent for making soups as well as jellied bouillons, consommés, and aspics provided about ⅛ inch of meat is left on them. Since they are not customarily used for soup, they can be obtained from the butcher at almost no cost. I have made as much as a gallon of delicious and stiffly jellied stock from 10 cents' worth of such bones. When the flavor of the stock is to be obtained largely from meat rather than bones, beef shank and oxtails are best to use.

Brown stock and consommé are customarily made by first searing the bones and meat. Since such high temperature may cause the meat fat to become carcinogenic, this procedure is not recommended.

Soup stock may be used in preparing dozens of dishes other than soup. Rice, macaroni, noodles, gravies, sauces, stews, casserole dishes, and many others are far more delicious when cooked with stock than with water. A single pint of stock can be made to equal a quart or more of milk in calcium content. Delicious jellied bouillons, aspics, and jellied meats and fish prepared with well-made stock should be served far more often than they customarily are.

Although a large amount of stock may be prepared at one time, the soup itself should usually be prepared for only one meal. Fresh vegetables to be eaten in the soup should be cooked for the shortest time possible. Instead of cooking the vegetables in the soup, a far more delightful flavor can be obtained by sautéing them in a little fat taken from the stock; the flavor thus remains in the vegetables and they do not become watery and soggy.

The seasoned stock should be added only a few minutes before the soup is served.

It is sometimes desirable to cook meat with soup, but such meat usually becomes stringy and lacks flavor. The full nutritive value of the meat is retained and freshness of flavor is achieved if the meat is ground and added to the soup just before it is served. Since the pieces of ground meat are small, heat can penetrate and cook them almost instantly. When leftover meat is to be eaten in soup, it should be added only in time to heat through.

The nutritive value of soups can be greatly increased with almost no cost by adding soy flour to them; it thickens the soup only slightly, and if used in moderate amounts, does not alter the taste. Cream soups are made creamier and more delicious as well as more nutritious by the addition of powdered milk. It is especially important to use these products when the budget is limited, when the protein requirements are high, or when meat substitutes or meats low in protein are served at the same meal with soup.

Since vegetable parings usually accumulate more quickly than do bones, and since their vitamin and mineral content is far too great to be wasted, their nutrients should be extracted and the water used in general cooking. I have given the name vegetable-cooking water to such extract and have included it in hundreds of recipes throughout this book. Any water left from steaming vegetables should also be added to it.

The woman who prepares delicious soups realizes that persons who use only canned soups miss a great deal of fun. If friends drop in on a cold evening or your husband gives a poker party, onions can be quickly sautéed, seasonings and rich stock added, and the soup served piping hot generously sprinkled with cheese; in less than 10 minutes you can have a delicious soup. Neither the soup nor the praise will be soon forgotten.

It is easy to get into a rut by serving two or three kinds of soup without varying the seasonings or ingredients. I hope you will try each recipe before preparing a particular one the second time. Although measurements of vegetables are given in cups, they are intended to be only approximate; they should be measured with the eye, and the quantities varied with your family's food likes and needs. Make it a rule to serve soup once or twice each week, often having it as the main dish of the meal.

Soup Garnishes and Accompaniments

Soup should be made appealing by the aroma of herbs and other seasonings, by attractive garnishes, and by interesting accompaniments. Garnishes and accompaniments need take only a few minutes to prepare, and the effect is an added "something" which makes the cook into an artist. Try each of the following garnishes and accompaniments.

Almonds, toasted and chopped: Sprinkle on bouillons or a bland cream soup, such as cream of asparagus soup.

Apple: Cut unpeeled red apple into tiny wedges, sprinkle on the surface of any soup where tartness or color is needed; delicious with chicken bouillon.

Bread sticks: Cut stale whole-wheat, wheat-germ, or rye bread into sticks without removing the crust; serve heated, lightly toasted, fried with garlic, or topped with cheese which is then melted and garnished with paprika or chopped parsley.

Bacon bits: Pan-broil until crisp; break into bits and sprinkle over thick soups before serving.

Caraway, cumin, and dill seeds: Sprinkle lightly on vegetable and meat soups; use caraway or dill seeds on cream of potato soup.

Cheese: Sprinkle grated Parmesan, Swiss, or shredded American cheese on any variety of soup; use chips of Roquefort on a bland cream soup, such as cream of celery or asparagus.

Cheese puffs: Make cheese puffs (p. 427) no more than 1 or 2 inches in diameter. Fill with cream cheese or shredded American cheese. Serve hot.

Chili sauce and catsup: Put a single teaspoon of chili sauce or catsup in the center of each serving if color and seasoning are needed.

Crackers: Serve wheat-germ, soy, rye, or whole-wheat crackers. They may be sprinkled with cheese and reheated.

Eggs: Slice or grate hard-cooked eggs and use on any vegetable or cream soup. If protein is needed, a hard-cooked egg may be cut in half lengthwise and used for each serving.

Finger salads: When a low-calorie diet is desired, serve instead of crackers or breadstuffs.

Grated orange or lemon rind: Add a light sprinkling of orange rind to cream soups; add lemon rind to vegetable soups and fish bisques.

Lemon slices: Cut extremely thin and float 1 slice on the surface of bouillons or cream soups; top with a single mint leaf or a tiny sprig of parsley, or dust lightly with paprika.

Nutmeg, mace, or ground clove: Add a faint suggestion rather than a sprinkling to any vegetable or cream soup; add nutmeg to cream of spinach or chicken soup.

Nuts: Serve with one-dish-meal soups to supply additional protein; reheat roasted peanuts, almonds, soy nuts (p. 531), or other nuts.

Orange slices: Use a small orange, slice thin, float on the center of cream soups.

Popcorn: Heat with a small amount of partially hardened margarine; add salt if needed; or roll in or sprinkle with grated cheese and serve piping hot.

Potato chips: Freshen in oven or under broiler. Sprinkle with grated Parmesan or American cheese. Serve hot garnished with paprika.

Peppers: Dice uncooked red or green bell peppers and use as a garnish.

Soup dumplings: Prepare dumplings (p. 73), using half the recipe; season with basil, orégano, or marjoram; drop from a teaspoon into boiling soup, bouillon, or consommé; cover utensil; boil slowly 10 minutes without removing lid and serve.

Sour cream: Float 1 tablespoon on the surface of spinach soup or borsch.

Toast cubes, or croutons: Make of whole-wheat, wheat-germ, or rye bread and serve as both a garnish and an accompaniment to any soup.

"Buttered" toast cubes: Sauté bread cubes in partially hardened margarine; sprinkle lightly with parsley or minced chives or fresh herbs.

Cheese croutons: Sauté bread cubes quickly and while hot sprinkle generously with grated cheese.

Garlic croutons: Sauté gently 1 clove garlic in partially hardened margarine; discard garlic and sauté bread cubes.

SOUP STOCK

Select large soup kettle with flat base and tight-fitting lid; put over heat and add:

accumulated bones, meat trim-   ¼ cup vinegar
mings, and/or fresh bones   2 teaspoons salt
2 quarts water

Cover kettle and simmer 3 to 4 hours or cook 30 minutes in a pressure cooker. If odor of vinegar can be detected at the end of this period, uncover kettle and boil vigorously for a few minutes until vinegar has evaporated; add:

chopped parings and leftovers   1 whole cayenne or chili tepine
¼ to ½ teaspoon crushed black   2 or 3 crumbled bay leaves
or white peppercorns

Force the chopped vegetables down into stock and cover utensil; reduce heat and boil slowly 15 minutes.

Remove stock from heat; if convenient, let soak overnight; strain stock through colander and discard bones and parings.

If stock is not to be used immediately, pour it into a jar and chill; remove fat. Freeze if desired.

Use stock for sauces, jellied meats, soups, bouillons, consommés, and for general cooking.

VARIATIONS:

Cook in stock heart or tongue to be served cold, reheated, or added to soup.

If the odor of vinegar does not disappear quickly, add 2 or more crushed eggshells.

Beef stock for jellied bouillons, consommés, aspics: Purchase 2 pounds or more of ribs, backbones, or any bones from young but matured beef. Prepare as in basic recipe. If stock is not a firm jelly when chilled, reheat and add 2 to 4 teaspoons gelatin soaked in ½ cup water.

Chicken stock: Purchase 2 pounds or more chicken feet. Wash and chop bones into 1-inch pieces; proceed as in basic recipe. Delicious stock which costs almost nothing can be made from chicken feet. Stilbestrol is injected into the necks of most commercially grown chickens; therefore do not make stock from chicken necks.

Clear soup stock: To clear stock for making jellied meats, reheat strained stock and add several shells from raw eggs or the uncooked white of 1 egg; stir well, simmer 5 minutes, and strain. Small particles stick to raw egg white and are held fast as soon as it cooks.

Dark soup stock: Include ½ pound or more of soup meat, preferably heel of the round; dredge with whole-wheat flour; brown well before adding water and bones.

Light soup stock: Use fresh veal or lamb bones, chicken legs, or leftover chicken, turkey, rabbit, veal, and pork bones; omit any vegetable scraps which may give a dark color.

Stock of uncooked meat and fresh bones: Purchase beef shank or oxtail; ask butcher to saw shank into 1-inch pieces. When meat is almost tender, add vegetable parings, cook and strain. Squeeze juices from parings and discard bones, returning meat to soup.

Vegetable-cooking water: Use or omit bones; put vegetable parings, salad and vegetable scraps, and leftovers to be discarded into large utensil; add 1 or 2 teaspoons salt and enough water to cover when cooked. Boil slowly for 15 minutes. Shred any leafy vegetable after cooking, and let stand 4 hours or overnight; strain through colander. Use for general cooking, decreasing the amount of salt called for in the recipes. Using this extract instead of water can add immeasurably to health, especially when vegetables are free of sprays and grown on composted soil.

Bouillons and consommés are merely variations of seasoned soup stock. A bouillon is usually made of brown stock and delicately seasoned. A consommé is made from one or more kinds of bones and highly seasoned. Both are customarily served clear. Their delightful odors and meat extracts stimulate the flow of the digestive juices. When they are properly made, their virtue lies in the fact that they supply vitamins and minerals without calories.

BEEF CONSOMMÉ

Remove fat from 1 quart stock made from assorted beef bones; heat and add:

pinch each of marjoram, thyme, and basil	1 to 2 tablespoons minced chives or tops of green onions
1 small clove garlic (optional)	1 to 3 drops Tabasco

Stir well and simmer 10 minutes. Taste for seasoning and discard garlic; garnish with extremely thin slices of lemon topped with a dash of paprika. Serve with wheat-germ crackers.

VARIATIONS:

If stock is not clear, add with seasonings 1 to 3 crushed shells of uncooked eggs; pour directly into soup plates by passing through fine strainer; add chives or onion tops after straining.

If more calories are desired, cook soup dumplings (p. 299) in consommé.

Add any diced leftover meat.

Beef bouillon: Omit garlic, Tabasco, and two herbs.

Chicken bouillon: Season chicken stock with a pinch of thyme or sage. Serve with puffs filled with melted cheese and garnish with nutmeg or tiny wedges of red apple. Vary by serving with dumplings (p. 299) or by seasoning each serving with grated lemon rind or Parmesan cheese.

Consommé with egg: Omit chives and garlic; remove from heat and add 2 well-beaten eggs; stir, cover utensil, and let stand 5 minutes; garnish with minced canned pimento.

Jellied bouillon with chicken: Omit herbs and garlic; clear chicken stock with eggshells and season with a pinch of sage, chervil, basil, or thyme; strain into molds or flat pan to chill; when it starts to set, add a small amount of leftover chicken. Serve with lemon sections and soy crackers.

Jellied consommé: Clear consommé with eggshells, strain into shallow pan, chill, cut into small cubes before serving. Vary by pouring into molds over slices of lemon or hard-cooked egg. Garnish lightly with parsley and Parmesan cheese; serve with rye crackers.

Onion soup: Sauté until transparent in 2 tablespoons fat from soup stock 4 to 6 thinly sliced onions; do not brown; add ½ teaspoon salt and 1 quart stock; make 1 slice toast for each person, cover with grated Parmesan cheese, melt under broiler; put toast into soup plate and pour soup over it. Garnish with paprika.

Tomato jellied bouillon: Prepare stock for jellied bouillon, using 1 quart tomato juice instead of water; season with basil, Tabasco, white peppercorns. Pour into molds or a shallow pan, chill, and unmold or cut into cubes. Garnish with chives and serve with toasted almonds or peanuts.

Soups of meat and vegetables may be served when the entree is low in protein. What more could one want for dinner, how-

ever, than a delicious, piping-hot soup with enough for second
and third helpings, a green salad tossed while the soup is heating,
fresh bread, butter, and milk? Perhaps the most nutritious and
to many the most delicious of these soups is that made of ground
meat, cooked only by the heat of the soup itself. This soup is
also excellent to make when no stock is available and time is
limited. Compared to the overcooked varieties, one taste is con-
vincing evidence of the soundness of cooking vegetables and
meat a short time only. Long cooking should be used only for
soup stocks.

Some years ago, I served a man and his wife a dinner which
consisted of nothing more than the following soup. Although it
received considerable praise, when I invited the couple to dinner
again, the husband exclaimed, "For heaven's sake, don't have
that same soup."

"You said you liked it," I answered, considerably surprised.

"We did, but my wife's served it every night since."

Because the following soups are planned to be served as one-
dish meals, each recipe makes 2½ quarts.

GROUND MEAT AND VEGETABLE SOUP

Combine in soup kettle:

1 can tomato purée	1 chilled unpeeled diced potato
1 minced clove garlic	1 to 2 teaspoons salt
1 or 2 chopped onions	¼ crushed bay leaf
2 chopped stalks celery	pinch of marjoram, thyme, or
2 chilled unpeeled diced carrots	savory

Cover utensil and simmer until vegetables are almost tender, or about
10 minutes; add and heat quickly:

2 quarts soup stock or	½ teaspoon freshly ground pep-
2 cans consommé with vegetable-	percorns
cooking water	

Pinch to bits and add, stirring rapidly:

1 pound lean ground beef

Taste for seasoning. Reheat to simmering and serve immediately.

Garnish with parsley and accompany with hot soy crackers sprinkled with grated American cheese.

VARIATIONS:

Omit tomato purée and 2 cups soup stock; use 2 cups canned or diced fresh tomatoes.

If no stock or consommé is available, use vegetable-cooking water with 4 beef bouillon cubes; salt to taste.

Season with basil, orégano, or other herbs.

Mix with small amount of stock and add ¼ cup soy flour, ½ cup soy grits, or ¼ to ½ cup instant tiger's milk.

Instead of the ground beef use cooked and diced veal, lamb, pork, or beef heart, or any diced leftover meat; or add diced meat left from making stock.

Substitute the following vegetables for any vegetable in basic recipe: turnips, kohlrabi, celery root, green pepper, tomatoes, corn, rutabagas, string beans, broccoli, cabbage, beets, green peas, a few shredded leaves of any greens; cook all vegetables the shortest time possible to make them tender.

Chicken gumbo: Select a stewing chicken, disjoint, dredge with whole-wheat flour, and brown well; add 3 cups each water and fresh or canned tomatoes, 1 tablespoon salt, 3 tablespoons vinegar; simmer 2 hours; add ½ cup brown rice, ½ teaspoon crushed white peppercorns; simmer ½ hour; add 3 cups sliced okra, 1 thinly sliced onion; simmer 10 to 12 minutes. Serve with hot wheat-germ crackers.

Chicken or turkey soup: Use stock prepared from chicken feet, bony parts of stewing chicken, or turkey carcass; strain; cook in stock ½ cup brown or converted rice; proceed as in basic recipe, adding celery, carrots, onion, parsley, pinch of sage; omit other herbs and vegetables. Add 1 or 2 cups diced chicken or turkey when available.

Clam chowder made with tomatoes: Dice 2 slices bacon with scissors, pan-broil in soup kettle, drain off most of the fat; add and sauté carrots, celery, onion and potato, omitting garlic and herbs; add crushed white peppercorns, salt, 2 cups tomato purée, 5 cups soup stock or vegetable-cooking water; immediately before serving add 2 cups or more minced fresh or canned clams and 2 tablespoons chopped parsley. Vary by adding 1 cup fresh or frozen corn with clams.

Heart or tongue soup: Cook beef, veal, lamb, or pork heart or tongue in soup stock while stock is being prepared; remove, skin the tongue, and dice 1 or 2 cups of meat; prepare soup as in basic recipe or any variation; add 2 cups diced heart or tongue before serving.

Italian meat soup: Prepare stock of shank or oxtail; when meat is almost tender, add crushed black peppercorns, herbs, garlic, and onions; instead of vegetables of basic recipe add 1 cup fresh peas, 1 or 2 diced zucchini, 1 chopped leek or onion; 4 shredded leaves curly or green cabbage; cook about 10 minutes. Serve as soon as vegetables are tender; sprinkle generously with **Parmesan cheese.**

Pepper-pot soup: Cook 1 or 2 pounds tripe while preparing stock; remove when tender, and cut with scissors into narrow strips; brown thoroughly 2 or 3 slices diced salt pork; drain off melted fat; add stock, tripe, vegetables and seasonings of basic recipe, and 2 diced green peppers.

Soup with meat balls: Use half the recipe for **meat loaf;** mix well, mold into balls 1½ inches in diameter; prepare soup as in basic recipe and drop in meat balls 8 minutes before serving.

Vegetable purées are soups thickened by the bulk of the vegetables themselves. The conventional method of preparing them is to overcook the vegetables until they are mushy and colorless, and to pass them through a colander, a technique so tedious and so destructive of flavor, to say nothing of nutritive value, that they are rarely served except to sick persons. If the fresh chilled vegetables are quickly shredded or blended in a liquefier, then shortcooked in well-seasoned stock, the resulting soup is worth adding to the menu. Since these soups are designed for light lunches or the first course of a dinner, the recipes are on the basis of approximately 5 cups.

MIXED-VEGETABLE PURÉE

Blend in liquefier with 1 cup water or stock the following chilled vegetables:

1 each carrot, onion, turnip, green pepper, pimento
2 stalks celery with leaves

several sprigs of parsley
few leaves of cabbage, spinach, mustard (optional)

Add vegetables to:

1 quart rapidly boiling soup stock

Boil 1 minute, reduce heat, add:

pinch each of basil, savory, marjoram

1 teaspoon Worcestershire
1 teaspoon salt

Simmer no longer than 8 minutes; taste for seasoning. Serve with wheat-germ crackers.

VARIATIONS:

When no liquefier is available, shred or chop vegetables or pass them through food grinder together with any leftover vegetables or meat and add to stock and seasonings.

If no soup stock is available, use 1 quart vegetable-cooking water; before salting add 2 or more beef or chicken bouillon cubes or 2 teaspoons meat extract; or use canned consommé. Salt to taste.

Add ¼ to ½ cup soy grits or ¼ cup instant tiger's milk to any purée.

Make purées of any of the following vegetables alone or combined: onions, spinach, carrots, peas, green peppers, celery, celery root, tomatoes, leeks, zucchini, pimentos. Add chopped parsley to all purées just before serving.

Buckwheat-tomato purée: Add to 3 cups boiling stock ½ cup whole unwashed buckwheat; simmer 5 minutes; add 2 cups tomato juice or purée, 1 each chopped or ground onion, green pepper, and carrot; pinch of basil; simmer 10 more minutes. Whole unpolished barley, millet, or converted or brown rice may be substituted for buckwheat.

Spinach purée: Boil 1 bunch shredded spinach and 1 shredded onion 3 minutes in 1 quart beef stock; add 1 teaspoon salt and 1 cup tomato purée or Spanish-style tomato sauce; serve as soon as heated through. Cut hard-cooked eggs lengthwise and put two halves into each soup plate before serving. Garnish with 2 tablespoons sour cream or yogurt topped with dash of paprika.

VEGETABLE SOUPS WITHOUT MEAT

Dice, shred, or cut into fingers the following chilled vegetables and sauté in fat from stock:

2 unpeeled carrots	2 or 3 stalks celery
1 or 2 onions or leeks	1 unpeeled potato

Add:

¼ teaspoon crushed black peppercorns	pinch each of basil, marjoram, and savory
1 crushed bay leaf	

Cover utensil, keep heat moderate, and do not brown; when vegetables are tender, add and heat quickly:

1 quart soup stock or vegetable-cooking water

¼ cup soy flour shaken with a small amount of stock

1 teaspoon salt

2 tablespoons parsley

any leftover vegetables, as peas, chopped broccoli, etc.

As soon as soup is hot, serve with cheese popcorn or hot roasted peanuts.

VARIATIONS:

If no stock is available, use vegetable-cooking water and before salting add 2 beef bouillon cubes or 2 teaspoons beef extract. Or use canned consommé.

Instead of any of the vegetables in basic recipe add one or more of the following diced or shredded vegetables: string beans, turnips, rutabagas, kohlrabi, cauliflower, zucchini, broccoli; fresh or frozen peas or corn; fresh or canned tomatoes. Add vegetables only in time to cook tender.

Add ½ cup soy grits to basic recipe or any variation.

Borsch, or Russian beet soup: Sauté in fat from soup stock 1 cup each unpeeled beets and carrots cut into thin fingers, ½ cup diced onion; cook 10 minutes; add 2 cups shredded green cabbage; cook 8 minutes longer; add 1½ teaspoons salt, 1 quart soup stock or vegetable-cooking water, 1 cup tomato purée; bring to boiling and serve immediately before beets lose color. If borsch must stand before being served, add 2 tablespoons lemon juice, ½ teaspoon sugar. Put 2 tablespoons sour cream or yogurt into each soup bowl.

Corn soup: Pan-broil 2 slices bacon and remove when crisp; pour off most of fat; add and sauté vegetables of basic recipe, omitting herbs; add 1 cup tomatoes, 2 cups stock or vegetable-cooking water, 2 cups fresh, frozen, or canned corn, 1 diced pimento, diced crisp bacon, parsley. Serve as soon as heated.

Okra soup: Sauté with other vegetables of basic recipe 2 cups diced okra, 1 chopped green pepper; add 1 cup fresh or canned tomatoes or purée.

Rice-tomato soup: Cook ½ cup brown or converted rice in 4 cups boiling vegetable-cooking water or soup stock; add salt, crushed peppercorns, soy flour, 1 cup tomatoes, pinch each of basil and savory, and vegetables of basic recipe except potatoes. Vary by substituting for rice whole buckwheat, unground wheat, or unpolished whole barley.

Cream soups are excellent served at lunch, as a first course for dinner, or as a one-dish meal provided additional protein is supplied by other foods. These soups are easy to make and require only about 10 minutes of working time. Powdered milk added to cream soups improves flavor and richness as well as nutritive value. Cream soup should not be boiled, particularly after powdered milk is added.

CREAM OF CHICKEN SOUP

Combine and heat to boiling:

1 quart chicken stock

pinch each of sage and thyme

¼ teaspoon crushed peppercorns

1 teaspoon salt

Add and cook 8 minutes:

½ cup chopped celery

1 cup fresh or frozen peas

1 or 2 diced carrots

2 diced pimentos (optional)

Shake, beat, or blend in liquefier until smooth and add:

1 cup chicken stock or fresh milk

½ cup powdered milk

3 tablespoons whole-wheat-pastry flour (optional)

Cover and simmer 10 minutes; *do not boil;* taste for seasoning, garnish with **nutmeg or paprika.**

VARIATIONS:

When available, add 1 or more cups diced chicken.

Omit flour; add leftover mashed potatoes, or beat 1 or 2 whole eggs with powdered milk; add to basic recipe or any variation.

Substitute 1 can chicken soup for chicken stock and prepare half the recipe; or omit stock and before salting add with other ingredients 2 or more chicken bouillon cubes or 1 to 2 tablespoons instant chicken broth with 1 quart fresh or reconstituted milk.

Add to vegetables in basic recipe, or substitute for one or more, any of the following: shredded string beans, chopped onion or leek, diced cucumber, diced celery root, diced zucchini or summer squash, chopped green or red bell pepper.

Chicken-cucumber soup: Omit vegetables of basic recipe; cook 5 minutes in chicken stock 2 sliced or diced cucumbers; proceed and season as in basic recipe. Garnish with **thin slices of orange.** Serve with toasted almonds.

Chicken-mushroom soup: Before adding other ingredients sauté fresh chopped mushrooms in fat taken from stock or add 1 can sliced mushrooms to soup; or omit salt and substitute 1 can condensed mushroom soup for flour and 1 cup fresh milk. Omit or include vegetables of basic recipe.

Clam chowder made with milk: Blend in soup kettle 3 tablespoons each whole-wheat-pastry flour and melted partially hardened margarine or butter; add slowly and heat 1 quart whole or reconstituted milk; simmer 10 minutes and add the powdered milk, salt, paprika, and peppercorns of basic recipe, 2 cups or more minced fresh or canned clams; omit the other ingredients of basic recipe. Serve as soon as heated to simmering; garnish with **parsley.** Serve with whole-wheat-bread sticks sprinkled with cheese.

Turkey soup: Prepare as in the basic recipe, using stock from turkey carcass.

Cream vegetable soups need be thickened only with powdered milk and the bulk of the vegetables themselves. Instead of overcooking the vegetables and then puréeing them, shred, chop, or liquefy the chilled vegetables and sauté them or cook them in milk. Cream soups prepared in this manner have a delightful freshness and need only to be heated before being ready to serve. If the soup is to be served as the principal dish of the meal, double the following recipes.

CREAM OF VEGETABLE SOUP

Use utensil for making soup and sauté in **partially hardened margarine or butter:**

1 chopped onion or leek

When onion is transparent, add, *cover utensil,* and heat to simmering:

3 cups fresh milk	1 teaspoon Worcestershire
¼ teaspoon freshly ground black peppercorns	1½ teaspoons salt
	1 to 4 drops Tabasco

When milk is hot, add the following and simmer 3 to 6 minutes:

1 to 2 cups shredded, liquefied, or grated vegetable	1 or 2 diced pimentos if color is needed

Keep utensil covered as much as possible. Blend in liquefier until smooth and add 5 minutes before serving:

1 cup fresh milk   ⅓ to ½ cup powdered milk

Serve as soon as heated through; *do not boil;* taste for seasoning, stir in 2 tablespoons chopped parsley, and garnish with **paprika or chives.**

VARIATIONS:

Make soup with reconstituted milk, using 2 cups instant powdered milk dissolved in 1 quart water.

Add ½ cup soy grits to any cream soup.

Beat ¼ to ½ cup soy flour or 1 or 2 whole eggs with fresh and powdered milk.

Add 1 or 2 cups of any of the following chilled and shredded, liquefied, or grated vegetables: carrots, celery, celery root, corn, fresh or leftover lima beans, onions, spinach or equal parts of parsley and spinach, mustard greens, mustard-spinach, or other greens or mixed greens. Vary by adding bits of crisp bacon to spinach soup or soups of other greens.

Season any cream soup with one or more of the following: a generous dash of nutmeg or mace; 1 minced clove garlic sautéed with onion; mustard, celery, or dill seeds; a few leaves of fresh or a pinch of dried basil, tarragon, or thyme.

If soup is to be the principal dish of the meal, double recipe; slice 1 hard-cooked egg into each bowl.

Avocado soup: Prepare as in basic recipe, using **white peppercorns;** add ½ cup **diced ham or chicken** if available. Just before serving add 2 **mashed ripe avocados.** Garnish with **thin orange slices.** Serve with whole-wheat cheese wafers.

Clam chowder made with potatoes: Pan-broil 3 **slices salt pork** cut into bits with scissors; drain; add and sauté with onion of the basic recipe 2 **cups diced unpeeled potatoes;** when vegetables are almost tender, add ½ to 1 teaspoon rosemary and the milk, salt, peppercorns, and powdered milk as in basic recipe; add 1 **pint canned or minced fresh clams** and serve as soon as heated through. Garnish with **parsley.**

Corn chowder: Pan-broil 4 slices diced bacon; drain off most of the fat; sauté with onion 1 or 2 diced unpeeled potatoes; proceed and season as in basic recipe, adding 2 **cups canned, frozen, or fresh corn;** heat only to simmering; just before serving add slowly 2 **cups thick tomato purée.** *Do not boil.* Serve as a one-dish meal with cheese croutons.

Cream of leek and potato soup: Sauté lightly 2 **chopped leeks or sweet onions** and 4 **diced potatoes;** proceed as in basic recipe; **add 1 to**

2 teaspoons caraway or dill seeds; beat ¼ teaspoon paprika and 2 egg yolks with fresh and powdered milk. Serve with hot rye-bread cubes rolled in grated cheese. This is one of my favorite soups.

Cream of mock-oyster soup: Liquefy 2 cups salsify or oyster plant; prepare and season as in basic recipe, adding ¼ teaspoon crushed dill or celery seeds or paprika.

Cream of mushroom soup: Omit onion of basic recipe; sauté lightly 2 cups sliced fresh mushrooms; proceed as in basic recipe. Garnish with dash of mace or nutmeg.

Cream of oyster soup: Drain liquid from 1 pint oysters into 3 cups whole milk; heat; add salt, white peppercorns, 2 tablespoons each grated onion and partially hardened margarine or butter; chop the oysters or leave whole and add with powdered milk. Serve with whole-wheat crackers.

Oyster chowder: Sauté 2 diced potatoes, 1 stalk celery, 1 leek or sweet onion; add milk and proceed as in cream of oyster soup.

Cream of potato soup: Proceed and season as in basic recipe, cooking 4 or 5 diced potatoes in hot milk; add 1 teaspoon chopped dill or 1 or 2 teaspoons dill or caraway seeds. Vary by seasoning with celery salt. Do not liquefy raw potatoes; the starch quickly thickens into a wallpaper paste.

Cream soup of mixed vegetables: Shred and sauté for 5 minutes 1 each carrot, stalk celery, small onion, green pepper, turnip, potato; proceed and season as in basic recipe; garnish with dash of nutmeg.

Cream of pea soup: Liquefy with the fresh and powdered milk 2 cups fresh chilled or frozen and thawed peas; proceed and season as in basic recipe; cook peas only 3 minutes. Garnish with slice of orange.

Cream of pea soup made of split peas: Simmer 1 cup dried split peas in 3 cups vegetable-cooking water until almost tender, or about 1 hour; add crushed white peppercorns, 2 teaspoons salt, 1 or 2 chopped onions; when onions are tender, add fresh and powdered milk, 3 tablespoons partially hardened margarine or butter, Worcestershire. Garnish with grated lemon or orange rind.

Cream of tomato soup: Add to sautéed onion 1 pint tomato purée or diced fresh or canned tomatoes, 2 whole cloves, peppercorns and salt, 1 or 2 teaspoons sugar, pinch of basil; in separate utensil heat to simmering the fresh milk and stir in powdered milk; just before serving add tomatoes to hot milk so slowly that protein can neutralize acid and prevent curdling. If no powdered milk is available, mix 1 cup fresh milk with ½ cup soy flour before adding tomatoes. *Do not add* soda. Garnish with parsley.

Cream of watercress soup: Liquefy with the fresh and powdered milk 1 bunch watercress; prepare and season as in the basic recipe; add ⅛ teaspoon nutmeg.

Delicious bisques, or rich soups thick with vegetables, can be made of almost every variety of fish and are often enjoyed even more than the popular chowders. They take only a few moments to prepare. When one tastes soup of fish which is seasoned with onions, celery, garlic, tomatoes, and herbs without being over-cooked, one realizes that fish bisques are a treat already missed overlong. The collars of large fish, or the portion directly behind the gills which is left from cutting steaks, may be purchased at little cost and are excellent for making bisques. If ⅓ pound sea food or fish is allowed per person, these soups become excellent for one-dish meals.

FISH BISQUE

Purchase 1½ or 2 pounds of collars from red snapper, salmon, halibut, or other fish.

Wash and drop into:

1 quart boiling vegetable-cooking water

Time carefully and simmer 2 to 3 minutes for each inch of thickness; remove and flake the meat; drop bones and skin, including scales, into water used for cooking; add:

¼ teaspoon ground peppercorns	2 teaspoons salt
1 crushed bay leaf	1 tablespoon vinegar

Boil slowly about 15 to 20 minutes.

Meanwhile pan-broil in utensil to be used for making soup:

2 slices bacon, cut into bits

Dice fine or shred the following chilled vegetables and cook with bacon:

2 each carrots and onions	1 minced clove garlic
2 stalks celery and leaves	1 teaspoon crushed anise or dill
1 green or red bell pepper	seeds

When vegetables are almost tender, strain boiling fish stock directly over them; add:

2 cups vegetable-cooking water

Immediately before serving add:

flaked fish

Taste for salt; garnish with parsley and **thin slices of lemon** sprinkled with paprika. Serve with rye or soy crackers.

VARIATIONS:

Prepare the recipe with flounder, barracuda, fresh cod, tuna, or any favorite fish.

If no skin or bones are available for making stock, add seasonings, 1 tablespoon lemon juice, and vegetable-cooking water to bacon and vegetables; add diced raw or flaked canned fish just before serving. If canned tuna is used, drain the oil before adding to bisque.

Add $\frac{1}{4}$ to $\frac{1}{2}$ cup soy grits or $\frac{1}{4}$ cup soy flour to basic recipe or any variation.

Make bisques with the following combinations of vegetables, using any amounts desired: celery, carrots, potatoes with fresh dill; onions, peas, carrots; cabbage, carrots, celery, potatoes; tomatoes, celery, corn; string beans, carrots, pimentos; leeks, carrots, potatoes.

Bisque of canned salmon: Sauté vegetables; add seasonings, 1 quart vegetable-cooking water or any stock, 2 cups fresh or canned tomatoes; immediately before serving add 2 cups flaked canned salmon. Serve with cheese popcorn.

Bisque with mushrooms: Omit garlic, onions, and green pepper; sauté 1 cup fresh or canned mushrooms with other vegetables; proceed as in basic recipe. Garnish with **thin lemon slices or chopped parsley.** Serve with whole-wheat crackers.

Bisque of shellfish: Use 2 cups fresh or canned shrimp, crab, lobster, or fresh oysters; instead of fish stock use **vegetable-cooking water.** Proceed and season as in basic recipe or any variation. Serve with toasted cheese sticks.

Tomato bisque: Instead of 2 cups vegetable-cooking water use **2 cups** tomato purée or canned tomatoes; season with **orégano or basil.**

Since legumes are rich in protein, split-pea, bean, and lentil soups should be served frequently, especially if the budget is limited. The proteins they contain lack some of the essential amino acids; therefore when these soups are served as the principal dish of the meal, meat or other adequate protein should be added to them.

Although bean, lentil, and split-pea soups are customarily prepared with ham bone, delicious soups can be prepared with accumulated bones or without bones. If the skin from cured ham or bacon is cooked with the soup, or if smoke-flavoring is used, the popular ham flavor is added. Vinegar causes legumes to become tough; hence calcium cannot be extracted from the bones unless previously prepared stock is used.

NAVY-BEAN SOUP

Use bone and skin left from **baked or steamed ham or cured shoulder** or purchase a **ham hock**.

If cooked ham is used, trim off edible meat scraps and save.

Pour over bones and skin and bring to boiling:

2 quarts water

Wash quickly, drain, and add without soaking:

2 cups white navy beans

Cover utensil, lower heat, and simmer 2 hours; add:

¼ to ½ teaspoon crushed black peppercorns
½ cup soy flour shaken with 1 cup water
1 crushed bay leaf

⅛ teaspoon marjoram, **savory,** and/or basil
1 or 2 chopped onions
1 small cayenne pepper **or chili** tepine, pierced with **toothpick**

Simmer 20 minutes longer, or until beans are tender; mash about half the beans; taste for salt and add more if needed.

Discard bones, cartilage, skin, cayenne or chili pepper; add **ham scraps,** if any, and garnish lightly with **chives.** Serve with garlic croutons.

VARIATIONS:

Add ½ cup soy grits to any bean, lentil, or split-pea soup.

Vary by adding any one of the following seasonings when beans are almost tender: 2 teaspoons Worcestershire; ½ teaspoon paprika, curry powder, dry mustard, or celery or caraway seeds; 1 chopped bell pepper or chili pepper; 3 drops Tabasco; 1 minced clove garlic; 1 or 2 thinly sliced carrots or kohlrabi, 1 chopped stalk celery.

Bean soup without bones: Cook beans in **vegetable-cooking water** with skin from cured pork; or when beans are almost tender, add **diced bacon or ham or bacon drippings and/or smoke-flavoring;** season as in basic recipe.

Black-bean soup: Substitute 2 cups **black beans** for the navy beans; proceed as in basic recipe; season with ¼ **teaspoon savory.**

Chili soup: Prepare as for **chili with meat** (p. 179), adding soup stock to give the consistency desired. Serve with toasted bread sticks or tortillas.

Kidney-bean soup: Prepare as in basic recipe; season with **pinch each of basil, thyme,** and **savory,** 1 teaspoon each **Worcestershire** and **dry mustard,** 1 chopped onion, 1 minced clove garlic. Add ½ pound **sliced wieners.** Garnish with **green-onion tops** cut with scissors.

Leftover boiled bean soup: Pan-broil ½ **pound bulk pork sausage** or 2 slices **bacon or ham;** remove ham or bacon, but let sausage remain in utensil; drain, leaving 2 or 3 tablespoons fat; sauté lightly **1 chopped onion, 1 stalk celery, 1 diced carrot;** mash beans and add to vegetables; add 1 cup **tomato purée** and enough **stock or vegetable-cooking water** to give the consistency desired; add **smoke-flavoring** to taste, **4 or 5 drops Tabasco, diced bacon or ham** if used. Taste for **salt;** serve with 1 tablespoon **chili sauce** in center of each serving.

Lentil soup: Cook 2 cups lentils in 1 quart stock 30 minutes, or until tender; pan-broil ½ **pound pork sausage;** drain off part of the fat and sauté lightly with sausage 1 minced clove garlic, 1 finely diced carrot, 2 chopped onions; add **salt, peppercorns, bay leaf,** 1 teaspoon each **Worcestershire** and **caraway seeds;** add sausage and 1 quart stock to lentils and simmer 10 minutes. Serve with whole-wheat crackers. Vary lentil soup by preparing and seasoning like any bean soup; by adding sliced **wieners or other sausage, or 1 to 2 cups tomato purée;** or by seasoning with 1 **teaspoon curry powder.**

Lima-bean soup: Prepare as in basic recipe or any variation; use **2 cups dried lima beans.** If assorted bones are used, pan-broil 1 or 2 slices **ham or bacon;** remove; sauté onions, 2 each **finely chopped stalks celery and carrots;** dice ham or bacon and add to soup with vegetables and 1 cup **tomatoes.** Season as in the basic recipe; garnish with **nutmeg and/or chives.**

Minestrone, or Italian soup: Cook 2 cups black-eyed beans as in basic recipe, using fresh beef shank; when beans are almost tender, add 1 cup tomatoes, 2 teaspoons salt, 2 teaspoons fresh or ½ teaspoon dried basil, 1 cup broken spaghetti, 1 chopped onion or 4 to 6 green onions with tops, 2 cloves garlic, 2 sliced summer squash or zucchini, 12 to 15 thinly sliced string beans, ½ to 1 cup green peas. Before serving sprinkle generously with parsley and grated Parmesan cheese.

Pinto-bean soup: Cook beans until tender in stock made from assorted bones; when beans are almost tender, dice and brown 2 slices salt pork; add seasonings of basic recipe, 2 cups tomato purée, smoke-flavoring to taste, pinch of orégano, and/or 1 teaspoon cumin seeds. Garnish with orange slices. Serve with rye crackers.

Split-pea soup I: Follow basic recipe or any variation, using split peas instead of beans. Cook 40 minutes before seasoning. Add 1 teaspoon Worcestershire. Garnish with thin slices of orange or lemon sprinkled with paprika. Serve with wheat-germ crackers. Vary recipe by adding 2 chopped stalks celery and/or pimentos; or omit other herbs and season with 2 or 3 teaspoons dill or caraway seeds. For me, caraway seeds added to bean, lentil, or split-pea soup make the difference between mediocrity and sheer delight.

Split-pea soup II: Cook 2 cups peas in vegetable-cooking water for 40 minutes; add 2 or 3 diced carrots, 1 chopped onion or leek, 3 tablespoons bacon drippings, 2 teaspoons salt, generous amount of cayenne, ¼ teaspoon thyme. Simmer 10 minutes longer; mash the peas thoroughly. Vary by adding 6 to 8 sliced wieners 5 minutes before serving.

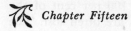

Chapter Fifteen

Keep the Flavor and Nutritive Value
in Your Vegetables

The principal weakness in American cooking lies in the preparation of vegetables. As they are customarily cooked, much of their flavor and 50 to 90 per cent of many nutrients are lost before they reach the table. These losses are largely avoidable. Surely the stoical eating of waterlogged, tasteless boiled vegetables is proof that Americans have character.

Vegetables to be cooked should be handled in the same manner as salad vegetables. Ideally they should be gathered immediately before being cooked. If you must purchase them, try to reach the market in the morning and choose vegetables which are trimmed the least. With a few exceptions, such as potatoes, dry onions, and corn on the cob, wash and dry them immediately. Chill and put them into a dark place as quickly as possible to stop enzyme action. If they are left at room temperature and in the light, much folic acid, vitamin B_2, and 50 per cent or more of the vitamin C in most fresh vegetables can be lost in a few hours.

The greatest culinary crime is soaking. Boiling, or soaking as vegetables are softened, is a form of soaking at its worst. Vitamin C and the many B vitamins pass out of the vegetables and dissolve in water as quickly as sugar dissolves in coffee. Studies have shown that when whole vegetables are boiled (soaked) only 4 minutes, 20 to 45 per cent of the total mineral content and 75 per cent of the sugars they contain pass into the water. Since vegetables are frequently soaked both before and during cooking

317

for much longer periods, as much as 75 to 100 per cent of the sugars, minerals, and water-soluble vitamins are often lost. The color of the water left after beets are washed slowly or boiled indicates how easily and quickly substances can pass out of vegetables, even though unpeeled. The losses are accelerated when vegetables are soaked after being peeled, chopped, sliced, or shredded, and particularly after the cell walls are softened by cooking.

During World War II, scurvy, resulting from a total lack of vitamin C, appeared in English communities where cabbage, a rich source of this vitamin, was a principal food. Part of the vitamin had been destroyed needlessly; the remainder had been discarded in the cooking water. The cumulative loss of vitamins and minerals brought about by soaking and boiling is unquestionably a causative factor in numerous illnesses and diseases. From the point of view of nutrition, the chief purpose in recommending vegetables is to supply vitamins and minerals; any form of soaking largely defeats this purpose. It is nothing less than disgraceful in a country where animals have been fed scientifically for more than half a century that people are served vegetables which have been carelessly soaked before and during cooking.

When nutritive value is lost, flavor is also lost. All vegetables contain aromatic oils which give them their characteristic odor and flavor; since they are not true oils, they readily dissolve in water. Minerals add a certain saltiness to the taste. Vegetables also contain sugars which cause them to be sweet if they are properly prepared and cooked. If you want your vegetables to be delicious, do not let them soak during slow washing or by letting water cling to them after they are washed; cook them by any other method than boiling.

The next greatest nutritive loss is caused by peeling vegetables. In root vegetables, the minerals, which are concentrated under the skin, are discarded when the vegetable is peeled. In sautéed parsnips, steamed eggplant, and French-fried potatoes, for example, the peeling adds flavor. If a vegetable is chopped, shredded, or diced, the only person who knows whether or not it is peeled is the one who has done the work. In case you spend

20 minutes daily peeling vegetables, in the course of a year you will have spent 121 hours, or 15 entire working days—an astounding waste of time. The waste of food value is even more startling. The average family throws away annually potato parings alone equivalent in iron to 500 eggs, in protein to 60 steaks, and in vitamin C to 95 glasses of orange juice. *Make it a rule to peel vegetables only when the skin is tough, bitter, or too uneven to be thoroughly cleaned.*

Provided vegetables are not soaked, the saving of vitamins C and B_2 during preparation and cooking depends largely on preventing enzyme action and excluding oxygen and light. Enzymes are inactive when cold and are destroyed by heat. Vitamin C is destroyed only in the presence of oxygen, and vitamin B_2 only in light. Prepare chilled vegetables so quickly that they will not reach room temperature. If such vegetables as fresh corn and peas are left at room temperature, the sugars they contain are quickly changed by enzyme action into starch, and their sweetness and delightful flavor are lost. When you must prepare vegetables before time to cook them, put them back into the refrigerator. Unless they are chilled, cut them as little as possible. The peel, if left on, can prevent contact with oxygen and hence preserve vitamin C. In order to destroy the enzymes rapidly, heat all vegetables as quickly as possible. Preheat the oven or the utensil to be used, have the utensil filled with steam, which displaces oxygen, and try not to lift the lid during cooking.

After the enzymes are made inactive by heat, destruction of vitamin C continues slowly unless there is contact with alkali. Minerals in hard water harm vitamin C during cooking; the addition of soda destroys it rapidly; and contact with iron and copper-containing utensils causes instant and complete destruction. Although vitamin A in yellow and green vegetables and fruits is usually not harmed in cooking, the vitamin A in butter and margarine is quickly destroyed by heat; if these fats are used for seasoning, they should be added after the vegetables are cooked. The destruction of vitamin B_1 is slow unless the vegetables are cooked at a temperature above boiling, like those which are fried or cooked under pressure; the shorter the cooking time, the less the loss of vitamins B_1 and C. Vitamin B_2 is harmed during cooking only when glass utensils are used or the vegetable is cooked without being covered. Folic acid, the anti-pernicious anemia vitamin, is quickly destroyed by heat; yet the other B vitamins, unless at a temperature above boiling, and vitamins E, K, and the bioflavonoids appear not to be harmed.

Many of the aromatic oils which give vegetables their delightful taste volatilize and are lost in proportion to the cooking time. If the best flavor and the most nutrients are to be retained, cook vegetables for the shortest time necessary to make them tender. Since chopping, shredding, and dicing shorten the cooking time, these procedures are recommended provided the vegetable is chilled, is not soaked, or is not ruined in appearance.

Frozen vegetables retain their nutritive value during freezing and storage, although 50 per cent of the vitamin C may be lost before they are frozen. After they are thawed, losses occur more quickly than in fresh vegetables; these vegetables should be put on to cook while still frozen. They cook in approximately half the time required for fresh vegetables.

Salt attracts moisture, and when a vegetable is salted at the beginning of cooking, its juices, which carry vitamins, minerals, sugars, and flavors, are drawn out. Studies have shown, for example, that spinach salted during cooking loses 47 per cent of its iron content but when unsalted only 19 per cent. Except when vegetables are cooked in a sauce, they should be salted just before being served.

If vegetables are properly prepared and cooked, their natural colors are preserved. Discoloration before cooking can be prevented by keeping them thoroughly chilled and by avoiding all contact with copper-containing equipment. Green vegetables contain plant acids which react chemically during cooking with the coloring matter, changing it to olive-gray. If the vegetable is cooked quickly and overcooking is avoided, little acid is freed, and the bright color is preserved. The white and red vegetables, such as turnips, cauliflower, celery root, purple cabbage, and red onions, discolor or turn dark upon contact with alkali. The minerals in hard water quickly destroy the attractiveness of such vegetables. If you must use hard water in cooking, add a drop or two of vinegar to it. Proteins have the capacity of combining with both acids and alkalies; hence discoloration can be prevented and the natural colors be intensified by cooking vegetables in milk or with any protein.

All liquids in which vegetables have been cooked should be used, regardless of the amount. The less liquid left from cooking them, the more concentrated are the nutrients in it. When cooked vegetables are soft in texture and only a little water has been used in cooking them, this water, carrying nutrients and flavor, is usually absorbed back into them. If vegetables are not absorbent and all the water is evaporated, the nutrients are dried to the pan and are lost; in this case, a tablespoon of liquid should be added before serving.

If a meal is delayed after the vegetables are ready to serve, they should be quickly chilled and reheated later, thus preventing continued loss of vitamin C. Women have been warned repeatedly that serious nutritive losses occur when foods are reheated; not infrequently leftover vegetables are thrown away because "all the vitamins are destroyed by reheating." Although reheating should be avoided whenever possible, little loss need occur if the vegetable is quickly reheated in only a small amount of liquid, if the temperature is kept low, if oxygen is replaced by steam, and if light is excluded. Canned vegetables should be reheated in the liquid in which they are canned and all the liquid should be used.

The recipes advising that vegetables be purposely and unnecessarily cooked twice should be largely avoided. When two processes are used in cooking a vegetable, the second is permissible only if no cooking liquid from the first process is discarded and if longer cooking is necessary to make a vegetable sufficiently tender to be palatable.

Make it a rule to cook vegetables in the shortest time possible, guarding carefully against overcooking. The shorter the cooking time, the more delicious the flavor of the vegetables. In order to prevent overcooking and to have the family ready to eat dinner the minute the vegetables are done, serve a first course of salad, soup, or appetizers. With a few exceptions, the vegetables can be put on to cook immediately before the first course is eaten.

Your ability as a cook is shown not by the desserts you make, but by the quantity and variety of vegetables your family demands.

Methods of Cooking Vegetables

It has often been pointed out that there is no objection to boiling vegetables, or cooking them covered with water, if the water is rapidly boiling before the vegetable is dropped into it; if it is quickly reheated to boiling; if the vegetable is not overcooked; and if *all* the cooking liquid is used. Such a statement is true, but the catch is that all the liquid is not used. For twenty-five years housewives have been urged to save the water left from boiling vegetables, and many have tried; yet probably not one housewife out of the millions in the entire country has actually done it. Since the nutritive losses are so great when the cooking water is discarded, vegetables should be cooked by any other method than boiling.

If health is to be produced and nutritive losses are to be kept to a minimum, a good cooking method should meet the following requirements: to destroy enzymes quickly, the initial heating must be rapid; to prevent loss of vitamin C, contact with oxygen should be avoided by leaving the vegetable unpeeled, by covering cut surfaces with oil, or by displacing the oxygen in the utensil with steam; the vegetable should be cooked the shortest time necessary to develop tenderness; every drop of liquid which touches the vegetable should be used. If these rules are observed and any vegetable to be cut is first thoroughly chilled, probably 95 per cent of all nutrients can be retained.

Perhaps the best method of cooking vegetables is the so-called waterless method. All fresh vegetables contain 70 to 95 per cent water, which is sufficient for cooking them if the heat is controlled so that no steam escapes. The utensil used must have a tight-fitting lid and must distribute heat evenly to the sides and the lid; thus the vegetable cooks by heat coming from all directions. Although vegetables may be cooked without any added water, a tablespoon or two should usually be put into the preheated utensil in order to replace oxygen by steam and thus protect vitamin C. The success of the method depends upon keeping the heat so low after the first few minutes that no steam escapes. Since the vegetables can be cooked largely over a simmer burner, waterless-cooking equipment pays for itself in saving fuel; it pays for itself many times over in promoting health.

Steaming in a pressure cooker is excellent provided the cooking time is checked with stop-watch precision. Since directions are included with the equipment, I have not given them in the recipes. Only a few tablespoons of water need be used, and it should be brought to boiling before the vegetable is put into the utensil. As soon as the cooking time has expired, the utensil should be cooled immediately. All liquid used should be served with the vegetable or added to soup stock. During steaming, moisture continually condenses on the surface of the vegetable; since sugars, minerals, vitamin C, and the B vitamins can dissolve into the moisture, considerable nutritive loss occurs unless the liquid is used, especially if the vegetable is diced or otherwise cut. The disadvantage of the method is that vegetables overcook quickly. In this case a large proportion of vitamins C, B_1, B_2, and niacin can be destroyed; the sulfur compounds in the strong-flavored vegetables break down; if the vegetables contain protein, its health-building value is harmed; aromatic oils are driven off quickly and flavor is lost.

If steaming is done without pressure, the vegetables should be left uncut and unpeeled whenever possible so that a minimum of surface is exposed to moisture. Since steam held above boiling water is exactly the same temperature as the water, the vegetables cook in the same time required for boiling. When no cooking liquid is discarded, the vegetables need not be placed on a rack above the water.

Vegetables can be cooked with little nutritive loss in the top of a double boiler if no equipment is available for waterless cooking. A few tablespoons of water are put into the utensil and brought to a rolling boil; the vegetables are added and steamed over high direct heat until the enzymes are destroyed, the oxygen is replaced by steam, and most or all of the water has evaporated. The vegetables are then placed over boiling water to finish cooking. Since they cannot burn, they need no watching. The temperature in the top of the double boiler ranges from 206° to 210 °F., at which vegetables cook as quickly as at boiling temperature after they are once heated through.

Fat used to season vegetables should preferably be added at the end of cooking; thus the vitamin A in butter and margarine is preserved, and less oxygen can combine with the unsaturated fatty acids in vegetable oil. Housewives who have no waterless cooking utensils usually own a frying pan, and therefore sautéing in oil is a practical method of cooking vegetables largely in their own juices. No more than 2 tablespoons of oil need be used. The vegetable should be stirred thoroughly with the hot oil so that all cut surfaces can be sealed from oxygen, juices can be held in, and direct contact with moisture can be prevented. It is important that no drops of water cling to the vegetable; otherwise the fat will not adhere to it. When contact with moisture and air is prevented, the natural colors are preserved or even intensified. The frying pan should be covered with a tight-fitting lid and the heat reduced as soon as the vegetable is heated through. If the heat is controlled, the vegetable will cook without shriveling or browning. This method is a variation of waterless cooking rather than of frying.

Another excellent method of cooking vegetables is to simmer them in milk. The nutrients in vegetables dissolve less readily into milk than into water. If the vegetable is thoroughly stirred with the milk, protein coats the surfaces and neutralizes the acids or alkalies which cause discoloration; thus the color is preserved and often intensified. Vegetables cooked in milk are milder and sweeter than those cooked in water. The milk itself is so delicious that there is little danger of its being discarded. Cooking should be done at a simmering temperature, or about 200° F., which destroys the enzymes quickly and cooks the vegetable in approximately the time required for boiling. If a simmering temperature is maintained, the milk will not boil over, scorch, or curdle.

When the temperature cannot be controlled, a double boiler can be used; the vegetable should be heated quickly over direct heat and then cooked over boiling water. Only ½ cup milk is needed if the utensil holds in steam, but if a tight-fitting lid is not available, the vegetable may be covered with milk. The milk should be saved and used again, made into cream soup, or thickening added and a cream sauce prepared.

Broiling is an excellent method of cooking vegetables but is used far too little. The initial heating is rapid, the vegetables cook quickly, and no moisture need touch them. Unless the cooking time is extremely short, the vegetable should be brushed or tossed with oil to prevent contact with oxygen and unnecessary loss of vitamin C. The success of the method lies in keeping the heat moderate or low after the vegetable is once heated through; otherwise it shrivels and becomes unattractive.

Apart from the extra calories it provides and the oxidation of oil, frying meets the requirements of an excellent method provided the vegetables are first thoroughly chilled. The initial heating is rapid, the cooking time is short, and the vegetable cooks in its own juices. Contact with oxygen is prevented by fat and steam. If the heat is kept moderate so that shriveling is prevented, carrots, beets, parsnips, turnips, and many other vegetables can be delicious when fried.

Although baking is far superior to boiling as a method of cooking vegetables, vitamin C is largely destroyed because of slow initial heating, long cooking, and exposure to oxygen if the vegetables are peeled. Wrapping food to be baked in aluminum foil slows the initial heating even more, hence increases the vitamin C destruction. The loss can be minimized but not prevented if peeled vegetables are oiled and put into a preheated oven. Whenever possible, whole vegetables to be baked should first be steamed until they are heated through and the enzymes are destroyed; then they may be transferred to the preheated oven. If vegetables are to be sliced and baked in a casserole, the liquid used should be hot, the casserole and the oven preheated, and, to prevent contact with oxygen, the casserole tightly covered to hold in steam; otherwise sufficient liquid should be used to cover the vegetables.

Shredding chilled unpeeled vegetables and then steaming or sautéing them quickly or cooking them with a small amount of milk is still another excellent cooking method, especially when preparing food for small children, persons on smooth diets, or those who cannot chew well. Vegetables prepared in this manner are unusually sweet; since they cook in a few minutes, almost no flavor or nutritive value is lost. Persons who dislike beets, for example, usually enjoy them when they are shredded and cooked quickly.

With so many excellent methods of cooking vegetables available, to cook them by boiling is to be indifferent to health.

Most of the vegetables obtainable are of extremely poor quality; their flavor can be improved by sprinkling them not only with salt but also with ½ teaspoon of sugar just before serving.

Research has shown that it is wiser to season steamed vegetables with a small amount of oil rather than with butter or margarine. To keep oxidation to the minimum, the oil should be added immediately before the vegetable is served. The Italians have seasoned their vegetables with oil for centuries and consider them delicious. Mayonnaise stirred into hot vegetables can also add a delightful flavor as well as help keep the blood cholesterol within normal bounds.

If it is desirable to serve a vegetable in a cream sauce, the vegetable should be cooked in milk and thickening added at least 10 minutes before the vegetable becomes tender enough to serve. When a vegetable to be creamed cooks quickly, as do frozen peas or fresh or frozen corn, the sauce should be prepared first. The proportions of flour to liquid for cream sauce should be memorized: 2 tablespoons of flour to 1 cup of milk or cream. Mix the flour with a little milk until smooth, dilute it to a thin paste, and stir it into the remaining hot but not boiling milk.

At the end of a meal, vegetables and meats left uneaten may be attractively arranged on individual tins and wrapped, labeled, and frozen; thus TV dinners, nutritionally superior to commercial ones, are available at no extra cost.

GLOBE ARTICHOKES

Cut off inedible tips of:

4 large chilled artichokes

Tuck into each:

¼ crushed bay leaf   **bits of minced garlic**
pinch of basil

Put petal end down into:

½ cup boiling water

Cover utensil and steam 20 to 30 minutes, or until tender; drain and save liquid; sprinkle artichokes with salt. Serve hot with melted butter or chilled with mayonnaise.

VARIATIONS:

If utensil does not distribute heat, steam on a rack above water.

Before cooking, tuck into the artichoke leaves chopped parsley, onion or green-onion tops, celery leaves, chives, or crushed black peppercorns.

Cook artichokes in soup stock or juices around a pot roast or Swiss steak.

Steam without seasoning; serve with Hollandaise sauce or remove leaves from center of whole steamed artichoke and serve hot filled with cheese sauce (p. 136) or creamed chicken, crab, or lobster; or chill, fill with shrimp or chicken or fish salad and serve as a luncheon dish.

Cut into halves, cook in ½ cup hot milk or enough milk to cover; drain off milk and use for cooking other vegetables.

French-fried artichokes: Use cooked or canned artichoke hearts; dip in batter (p. 158) and French-fry at 350° F. until brown.

Jerusalem artichokes, tubers of the sunflower family, are so similar in appearance and taste to new potatoes that most persons quickly learn to enjoy them. These artichokes are rich in sugar and must be washed rapidly if their delightful taste is to be retained. They become tough if cooked at high temperature or overcooked. Raw Jerusalem artichokes, which have the texture of cabbage stalk, are particularly delicious in salads.

JERUSALEM ARTICHOKES SIMMERED
IN MILK

Slice, dice, or cut into halves:

1 pound chilled unpeeled artichokes

Drop into:

½ cup hot milk

Stir to cover all surfaces with milk protein; cover utensil and simmer 6 to 10 minutes; add:

1 teaspoon salt   **2 tablespoons chopped parsley**

Garnish with **paprika.**

VARIATIONS:

Steam whole unpeeled artichokes in waterless-cooking utensil; serve unpeeled or remove peeling when tender; or peel before cooking and simmer in enough milk to cover.

Add 1 small chopped onion and/or 1 clove garlic before steaming; discard garlic; or add chives or green-onion tops cut with scissors.

Remove from heat and add ½ cup diced American cheese; cover utensil until cheese is melted; stir; garnish with parsley.

Steam with any vegetable which cooks in the same time, such as fresh or frozen peas or diced carrots or turnips.

Cook in 1 cup top milk and thicken to make cream sauce; add 1 diced pimento, few grains of cayenne, or after removing from heat add ½ cup diced American cheese.

Broiled Jerusalem artichokes: Cut unpeeled artichokes into fingers, mix with **1 tablespoon vegetable oil,** and put on oiled baking sheet; keep heat high until browning starts, or about 2 minutes; turn with pancake turner, brown the other side, lower heat, and cook 6 or 8 minutes.

Fried Jerusalem artichokes: Slice unpeeled artichokes and fry 8 to 10 minutes in preheated vegetable oil; turn 2 or 3 times during cooking; or sauté without browning in **1 tablespoon each fat and water.**

ASPARAGUS COOKED IN MILK

Allow 1/3 pound asparagus per serving.

Break off ends where stalks snap easily; tie stalks into bunches for individual servings or keep parallel in utensil.

Drop chilled asparagus into:

2 cups hot milk, or enough to cover

Cover utensil, and simmer 8 to 10 minutes, or until tender; pour off milk and use for cream soup made of tough ends of stalks.

Add:

1 or 2 tablespoons oil, partially   **1/2 teaspoon salt**
hardened margarine, or butter

VARIATIONS:

Dice asparagus and cook in 1/2 cup milk.

Put asparagus on hot serving platter or plates, sprinkle with shredded American or Parmesan cheese, and garnish with paprika.

Steam asparagus in or above 1/4 cup boiling water; or stand stalks in small amount of water in top of double boiler and steam.

Asparagus patties: Follow recipe for zucchini patties (p. 354); cut asparagus into 1/4-inch pieces.

Asparagus soufflé: Add 2 cups ground raw asparagus to plain or cheese soufflé (p. 194).

Creamed asparagus: Cook in 1 cup milk; thicken by adding 2 tablespoons whole-wheat flour mixed with 1/4 cup cold milk; cut asparagus into 1/2-inch pieces if lengths and sizes are irregular.

With cheese: Cook asparagus in heat-resistant baking dish; wipe edges of dish after making cream sauce; cover top with **wheat germ or toasted whole-wheat-bread crumbs and 1/2 cup shredded American cheese**; cover utensil until cheese is melted.

Sautéed asparagus: Heat 1 tablespoon **partially hardened margarine or oil** in frying pan; add asparagus stalks, a few tablespoons of water; cover utensil and steam 12 to 15 minutes; keep heat low to prevent shriveling.

The bean sprouts most often sold, or the sprouts of the mung bean, should be little more than heated through. If they are overcooked even a few minutes, the water they contain dries out and they become shriveled and tasteless. If soybean sprouts are used, they should be cooked about 5 minutes longer than the mung sprouts.

STEAMED BEAN SPROUTS

Wash, drain, and shake or whirl dry:

2 cups beans sprouts

Add to:

3 tablespoons boiling water

Steam only long enough to heat through, or about 4 minutes. Season with **½ teaspoon salt** and **dash of paprika**.

VARIATIONS:

Steam in ¼ cup milk; add chopped parsley, diced pimento, or dash of nutmeg.

Bean sprouts with tomatoes: Pan-broil 1 slice bacon and drain on paper; add 1 diced fresh or ½ cup canned tomatoes, 2 tablespoons chopped onion, ½ diced bell pepper, crushed peppercorns, ½ teaspoon salt; simmer 5 to 8 minutes; add and heat bean sprouts; break bacon into small pieces and add with 1 teaspoon soy sauce just before serving.

CRISP SHREDDED BEETS

Wash thoroughly, trim, and shred:

4 to 6 chilled unpeeled beets

Put into preheated frying pan with:

1 tablespoon water and lemon juice or vinegar   **2 teaspoons partially hardened margarine or oil**

Stir, cover utensil, and cook over moderate heat for 5 minutes. Add and stir:

½ teaspoon salt

Serve piping hot but crisp.

VARIATIONS:

Put beets into casserole brushed with oil; cook for 7 minutes in hot oven at 400° F.

Omit fat and cook beets in ¼ cup milk.

Baked beets: Put beets over boiling water, and heat rapidly for 10 minutes; transfer to moderate oven, at 350° F., and cook until tender, or about 30 minutes; cut petal-fashion and sprinkle with **salt, paprika, and butter or partially hardened margarine.**

Beets cooked with tops: See page 362.

Beets simmered in milk: Dice 4 to 6 medium unpeeled beets in ¼-inch cubes or cut into fingers; put into utensil with **¼ cup hot milk and ¼ teaspoon crushed black peppercorns;** stir beets to moisten all surfaces with milk protein; cover utensil, lower heat, and simmer 8 to 12 minutes; sprinkle with ½ teaspoon salt.

With herbs: Add **1 tablespoon chopped mint, dill, chives, fresh basil, chervil, or 2 tablespoons parsley.**

With sour cream: Just before removing from heat add **½ cup sour cream or yogurt.**

Sautéed beets: Slice **6 to 8 unpeeled beets;** sprinkle lightly with **lemon juice or vinegar;** put into heated frying pan with **2 tablespoons partially hardened margarine or oil;** except for initial heating, keep heat low; turn with pancake turner occasionally; cover utensil and cook 10 to 15 minutes, or until tender; sprinkle with **salt and pepper;** or cook in **2 teaspoons fat and 2 tablespoons water; cover and steam.**

Spiced beets: Cut **6 beets** into fourths, fingers, or cubes; put into hot utensil with **4 tablespoons boiling water, 1 tablespoon vinegar, 3 cloves and 1-inch piece of cinnamon stick;** cover and steam 12 to 18 minutes; add **2 tablespoons sugar, 1 teaspoon salt;** or cook all seasonings with water and add diced beets steamed without being peeled.

With herbs: Omit spices and steam beets with **vinegar, water, 1 tablespoon oil, ¼ crushed bay leaf, 1 minced clove garlic;** or just before serving add molasses and salt to taste, **1 teaspoon chopped fresh mint, tarragon, or savory leaves.**

Bell peppers should be eaten as frequently as possible because of their content of vitamins A and C. Since the vitamin C content doubles as the pepper becomes red, use ripe ones when available.

SAUTÉED BELL PEPPERS

Dice into bite size:

4 to 6 bell peppers, preferably red
Put into:
2 tablespoons heated vegetable oil

Stir well, cover utensil, keep heat moderate, and cook 8 to 10 minutes; sprinkle with salt and pepper. Serve while still slightly crisp.

VARIATIONS:

Simmer peppers in ¼ cup milk or ½ cup medium cream sauce; add ½ cup cubed cheese before serving.

Sauté peppers with an equal amount of sliced onions and 1 clove garlic; discard garlic before serving.

SAUTÉED CARROTS

Cut into fingers or slice crosswise:

6 to 8 chilled unpeeled carrots
Put into:
1 or 2 tablespoons partially hardened margarine or butter

Stir well and add:

1 tablespoon water

Cover utensil, heat quickly, and reduce temperature; turn occasionally and brown only slightly; cook for 10 to 15 minutes.

Season with:

½ teaspoon salt   freshly ground black peppercorns

VARIATIONS:

If waterless cooking utensil is available, steam carrots in their own juice and add fat just before serving.

Dice carrots; sauté without browning; add 1 teaspoon dark molasses or brown sugar.

Sauté with carrots 2 diced unpeeled apples or 1 or 2 sliced onions or raw potatoes.

To prepare carrots to be served with a roast, slice in half lengthwise and sauté in fat dipped from dripping pan; sauté with carrots small whole onions and potatoes cut in half lengthwise; allow about 20 minutes for cooking.

Sautéed mixed vegetables: Slice 1 onion, 1 green or red bell pepper or pimento, 1 or 2 each unpeeled carrots, turnips, potatoes; sauté together, turning frequently; sprinkle with salt and pepper. At college, a group of us used to live on this dish when we were broke; we called it "fried stew."

BAKED CARROTS AND APPLES

Slice in alternate layers into a heat-resistant casserole:

4 or 5 chilled unpeeled carrots, cut into quarters lengthwise   1 to 3 unpeeled apples, quartered and then sliced

Top with bits of partially hardened margarine or butter; sprinkle with:

1 teaspoon salt   3 tablespoons hot water
1 teaspoon grated lemon rind

Cover casserole, steam 5 to 10 minutes, then bake in hot oven at 400° F. for 15 to 20 minutes, or until tender; or cook until tender over direct heat.

VARIATIONS:

Omit lemon rind; top with wheat germ or whole-wheat-bread crumbs; bake until tender, and sprinkle with ½ cup grated or cubed American cheese; garnish with paprika; leave uncovered in oven until cheese melts.

STEAMED CARROTS

Use waterless-cooking utensil. Put:

6 chilled unpeeled carrots

Into:

¼ cup boiling water

Cover utensil, heat quickly, then simmer about 15 minutes, or until tender; cut in halves or quarters lengthwise. Add:

½ teaspoon salt   2 teaspoons oil or mayonnaise

Serve at once.

VARIATIONS:

Season with lemon juice and chopped parsley.

Add ¼ teaspoon minced mint leaves after cooking 10 minutes.

Dice carrots and cook with diced celery, chopped or grated onion, or fresh or frozen peas.

When carrots are barely tender, put on chopping board and cut into ⅛-inch rounds; reheat with 1 tablespoon oil, 2 tablespoons chopped parsley, and 3 or 4 diced green onions.

Cook in ½ cup soup stock, milk, or cream sauce; at the beginning of cooking add crushed white peppercorns and pinch of thyme.

Steam whole unpeeled carrots on rack above boiling water; season with vegetable oil, butter, or partially hardened margarine and 2 table-spoons parsley; or transfer to flat baking dish, sprinkle with ¾ cup shredded cheese; melt under broiler; or chill, cut into fingers, mix with French dressing or mayonnaise, serve cold.

Broiled carrots: Cut carrots into fingers ⅓ inch thick and toss with 1 tablespoon vegetable oil; place on baking sheet and broil at moderate heat until browning starts, or about 4 minutes; turn with pancake turner; lower heat, cook until tender, or about 10 minutes; season with salt and pepper.

Carrots simmered in milk: Cut carrots in half and drop into enough hot milk to cover, or about 2 cups; simmer 10 to 15 minutes; drain off milk and save or make into cream sauce; season carrots with salt, pepper, paprika.

Deviled carrots: Just before serving add 2 tablespoons each oil and brown sugar, 2 teaspoons dry mustard, dash cayenne, ½ teaspoon salt. Cut carrots lengthwise and mix well with seasonings.

Shredded carrots: Shred unpeeled carrots; cook 5 minutes in small amount of milk, water, or 1 tablespoon French dressing or vegetable oil; or bake in preheated oiled casserole; ¼ cup or more shredded cheese may be added.

GREEN CELERY WITH LEAVES

Use outer green celery stalks and leaves; dice stalks into ¾-inch pieces and shred leaves.

Add approximately:

2 cups diced stalks to ½ cup simmering milk

Stir well to cover all surfaces with milk protein.

Cover utensil, heat quickly, and simmer 8 to 10 minutes; add:

shredded celery leaves

Stir well and cook 2 minutes longer. Season with:

½ teaspoon salt   **dash of cayenne**

Garnish with strips of canned pimento.

VARIATIONS:

When celery is tender, remove from heat and add ½ cup cubed American cheese or 2 tablespoons Parmesan cheese; serve as soon as cheese melts.

Broiled celery: Dice celery into ½-inch pieces and toss with 1 tablespoon vegetable oil; broil on baking sheet at high temperature 2 minutes, turn, and cook 2 minutes longer before lowering heat; broil until tender, or about 12 minutes; add salt and paprika.

Celery cooked in soup stock: Cut in half lengthwise the bases of 2 small bunches of celery, leaving the stalks about 5 inches long; drop into ¾ cup boiling soup stock; cover utensil and cook 12 to 15 minutes, or until tender; remove to serving platter, thicken stock by adding a paste of 2 tablespoons whole-wheat flour and water; simmer 10 minutes, and pour over celery.

Celery with cheese: Cut in half lengthwise the bases of 2 bunches of celery. Steam in vegetable-cooking water; put into flat baking dish, add salt, and cover with 1 cup grated cheese; sprinkle with paprika; melt cheese under broiler without browning it.

Celery with tomatoes: Sauté lightly 1 each chopped onion and bell pepper; add 1 cup canned tomatoes, pinch of basil, ¾ teaspoon salt, crushed black peppercorns; heat to boiling; cut in half lengthwise the bases of 2 small bunches of celery, leaving stalks 4 to 6 inches long; wash, drop into hot tomatoes, and cook until tender, or about 15 minutes.

Creamed celery: Cook diced celery in 1 cup milk thickened with 2 tablespoons whole-wheat flour mixed smooth with top milk; add ½ cup American cheese if desired; garnish with paprika.

Marinated celery: Cut in half lengthwise the bases of 2 small bunches of celery; steam, chill, and marinate in French dressing; serve chilled.

Sautéed celery: Cut into 1-inch pieces; sauté slowly in bacon drippings, partially hardened margarine, or butter; sprinkle with paprika.

Celery root, or celeriac, is a bulbous root 4 to 6 inches in diameter covered with rough skin. Since it cannot be cleaned thoroughly, it must be peeled. The texture of cooked celery root is similar to that of potatoes; its taste resembles that of celery, but it is milder and sweeter. The stalk and leaves, which are stronger in flavor than celery, are excellent for seasoning. Celery root discolors easily; consequently it should be chilled thoroughly and dropped into hot liquid immediately after being peeled and cut. When quickly prepared and simmered in milk, it is snowy white and so delicious that people usually enjoy its taste the first time they eat it.

CELERY ROOT

Heat to simmering:

½ cup milk

Peel, cut into fingers ½ inch thick, add, and stir:

1 or 2 celery roots, or about 2 cups
¼ teaspoon crushed white peppercorns

Cover utensil, heat rapidly, and simmer over direct heat or in double boiler 12 to 15 minutes; add:

½ teaspoon salt

Garnish with paprika.

VARIATIONS:

Add 2 tablespoons chopped parsley or chives.

Increase milk to ¾ cup; thicken with cream sauce; add a few diced pimentos, chopped parsley, or a dash of nutmeg.

Baked celery root: When oven is being used, cut small celery roots in half without peeling them; brush the cut surface with oil; bake until tender, or 20 to 25 minutes, and remove skin; salt and garnish with paprika; or steam until hot, then bake.

Chilled celery root: Cut into halves and steam until tender; chill, peel, dice, and marinate with ¼ cup French dressing or mayonnaise.

Mashed celery root: Cook as in basic recipe until tender; pass through hot ricer or mash; add salt, butter, and milk left from steaming.

Sautéed celery root: Peel and slice celery root crosswise; moisten with 1 tablespoon lemon juice; sauté over low heat in **vegetable oil or bacon drippings**; sprinkle with **salt and paprika**.

Steamed celery root: Steam whole unpeeled celery root until tender; pierce with fork, peel while hot, dice or quarter, and serve with oil, mayonnaise, butter, or partially hardened margarine and paprika.

Chayote is a variety of squash with pale-green meat and a soft edible seed. Small tubers, which taste much like sweet potatoes, grow on the roots; they can be cooked like sweet potatoes or served in salads. The tender leaves and raw young fruit are also excellent in salads.

SAUTÉED CHAYOTE

Pan-broil until crisp:

1 to 3 slices bacon

Meanwhile cut **1 to 2 chilled chayotes** lengthwise into quarters without removing seed; if peel is tender, leave unpeeled; hold quarters together and slice crosswise in ¼-inch pieces.

Remove bacon to paper; put chayote into:

1 tablespoon hot bacon drippings

Keep heat high until chayote is heated through; leave utensil uncovered to allow moisture to evaporate, turn frequently, and serve while still slightly crisp, or in about 8 minutes.

Season with:

½ teaspoon salt	freshly ground black peppercorns
crushed bacon	

VARIATIONS:

Sauté with chayote chopped or sliced onion, bell pepper, pimento, or celery.

Slice chayote crosswise ½ inch thick; dip in egg stirred with 2 tablespoons milk and in wheat germ or whole-wheat-bread crumbs; fry in shallow or deep fat; season with salt and freshly ground peppercorns.

Cut into wedges lengthwise; steam with small amount of water or cook in waterless-cooking utensil or in top of double boiler; season with salt, oil or mayonnaise, and paprika.

Baked chayote: Cut chayotes into halves lengthwise, brush all surfaces with oil, and bake in a moderate oven for 20 to 30 minutes, or until tender; season with **salt and pepper;** garnish with **parsley;** or steam until hot, then bake.

Broiled chayote: Cut chayotes into ½-inch slices crosswise, brush with oil, broil on baking sheet 10 to 12 minutes; season with **salt and pepper.**

Chayote with cheese: Add ½ **cup cubed American cheese** to chayote steamed in its own juices, in milk, or in cream sauce; garnish with **parsley and paprika.**

Creamed chayote: Prepare 1 cup **medium cream sauce,** add sliced chayotes, cook until tender; **salt.**

EDIBLE-POD PEAS SIMMERED IN MILK

Remove ends and strings from:

1 pound chilled edible-pod peas

Put into:

½ cup hot milk

Stir well, heat quickly to simmering, cook 8 to 10 minutes; add:

½ teaspoon salt

Serve at once.

VARIATIONS:

Cut carrots into thin sticks and cook with edible-pod peas; season with salt and paprika.

About 8 minutes before serving add and cook peas with vegetable stew or in gravy around Swiss steak.

Creamed edible-pod peas: Prepare 1 **cup or more cream sauce;** stir in chilled peas and simmer 12 minutes.

Steamed edible-pod peas: Steam the peas above ¼ cup water; or cook by waterless method or in top of double boiler with 1 tablespoon boiling water. Serve hot; or chill, mix with French dressing, and serve on a bed of lettuce.

EGGPLANT WITH ONION

Cut into ½-inch slices or 1-inch cubes:

1 chilled unpeeled eggplant

Use utensil for waterless cooking; put eggplant into:

2 tablespoons boiling water   **1 teaspoon vinegar**

Cover utensil, heat quickly, and simmer 15 minutes; add:

1 grated onion

Leave eggplant whole or chop to any desired texture; season to taste with salt, freshly ground peppercorns, cayenne. Garnish with chopped parsley. Serve hot, or chilled as a relish.

VARIATIONS:

Season with finely chopped celery, pimento, or bell pepper; or add 1 or 2 tablespoons oil, mayonnaise, or French dressing.

Add onion and cook with eggplant cut into 1-inch cubes.

Omit onion and season with oil, fresh lemon juice, salt, and chopped parsley.

Season eggplant with 2 tablespoons tomato catsup or ¼ teaspoon onion or celery salt, or a dash of nutmeg.

Mash after steaming and serve with partially hardened margarine or butter.

After removing from heat add ¾ cup cubed American cheese; stir, cover utensil, and serve as soon as cheese is melted.

Baked eggplant: Put diced eggplant into preheated casserole with ½ cup boiling soup stock, ¼ teaspoon crushed black peppercorns, pinch of savory, ½ teaspoon salt; stir, cover, and bake 20 minutes at 350° F.

Chilled eggplant: Cut into cubes or leave in slices; steam and chill; add seasonings of basic recipe and ¼ cup French dressing; serve for hot-weather dinners.

Eggplant with bacon: Pan-broil 1 strip bacon and cook with it 1 clove garlic; remove bacon, discard garlic, and sauté cubed eggplant; cover utensil, heat rapidly, and cook until tender, or about 10 minutes; add bacon broken into bits, 2 tablespoons each chopped pimentos and chopped parsley. Vary by cooking with **2 or 3 link sausages** cut into ½-inch pieces.

Leftover eggplant: Put in flat baking dish, cover with **cheese**, and heat in oven; or marinate with **French dressing** and serve chilled; or add **1 tablespoon whole-wheat flour and 1 egg** to 1 cup eggplant, stir well, and fry as patties.

Steamed eggplant: Steam small whole unpeeled eggplants above ½ cup water until tender, or about 20 minutes; split lengthwise, fluff pulp with a fork, and season with **butter or partially hardened margarine, salt, paprika,** and **chives or parsley.** If oven is being used, bake whole unpeeled eggplant until tender.

Eggplant casserole with clams: Omit onion; use heat-resistant casserole and cook diced peeled eggplant in ¾ cup of milk. When almost tender, add and beat in **2 eggs, 1 cup or 1 small can clams with juice, ¾ teaspoon salt,** freshly ground peppercorns. Sprinkle generously with **wheat germ, Parmesan cheese,** and **paprika.** Brown in oven 10 minutes at 300° F.

EGGPLANT CREOLE

Pan-broil until crisp:

2 slices bacon

Remove bacon, drain off part of the fat, and sauté lightly:

1 chopped onion   **1 diced green or red bell pepper**

Add and heat to boiling:

2 peeled diced or 1 cup canned tomatoes

Meanwhile cut into 1-inch cubes:

1 large or 2 small chilled unpeeled eggplants

Add eggplant to other vegetables, stir well, heat quickly, and simmer 12 to 15 minutes; add:

bacon cut in small pieces   **1 teaspoon salt**

Serve at once.

VARIATIONS:

Omit bacon and green pepper; just before serving add ½ cup diced American cheese.

Eggplant in casserole: Prepare as in basic recipe, using heat-resistant casserole; when tender, sprinkle with ½ cup toasted wheat germ or whole-wheat-bread crumbs, ¾ cup cubed American cheese, paprika; cover utensil until cheese is melted.

Eggplant with rice: Omit bacon; cook ½ cup converted or brown rice in bacon drippings and 1 cup tomato juice or soup stock; simmer until almost tender before adding eggplant and other ingredients; or add 1 cup leftover steamed rice to basic recipe.

SAUTÉED EGGPLANT

Cut 1 chilled unpeeled eggplant in ¾-inch slices; dip in:

**1 egg stirred with
2 tablespoons milk or white wine**

Roll in:

Parmesan cheese mixed with wheat germ or whole-wheat-bread crumbs

Let dry for 10 minutes or more; sauté in:

1 tablespoon preheated vegetable oil

Cover utensil; turn once, and cook until golden brown on both sides. Sprinkle with:

**salt   chopped parsley
freshly ground peppercorns**

VARIATIONS:

Cut eggplant lengthwise into 1-inch sticks; sauté as in basic recipe until well browned; sprinkle generously with lemon juice and chopped parsley or nippy cheese and paprika; or serve cheese, sautéed onions, fried tomato slices, or diced leftover meat between matching slices of sautéed eggplant.

Broiled eggplant: Cut eggplant crosswise into slices ½ inch thick;

dip in **egg and wheat germ or crumbs** or brush with **oil** and sprinkle with **paprika**; put on oiled baking sheet and broil at moderate heat until browned, or about 6 to 8 minutes; turn and brown the other side; if slices are not tender, lower heat to finish cooking; sprinkle with **salt and grated cheese.**

Eggplant grill: Brown both surfaces of eggplant slices quickly at high heat; place **1 slice tomato** and **½ strip bacon** on top of each slice; lower heat and broil slowly until bacon is crisp; sprinkle with **salt and chopped parsley.**

GREEN STRING BEANS

String and shred lengthwise:

1 to 1½ pounds chilled green beans

Drop into:

¼ cup boiling water

Stir well; cook over low heat for 10 to 15 minutes, or until just tender; stir in:

½ teaspoon each salt and sugar   **2 tablespoons vegetable oil**
freshly ground peppercorns   **2 tablespoons chopped parsley**

Serve immediately.

VARIATIONS:

Season beans with chives or 1 finely chopped onion or leek, ¼ teaspoon mustard or celery seeds, or pinch of basil.

Steam beans and season just before serving with 1 or 2 tablespoons French dressing or mayonnaise. Or occasionally add 1 or 2 tablespoons lemon juice or vinegar.

Cook beans in 2 tablespoons each water and oil; season with celery salt, smoke-flavoring, garlic, or 2 or 3 strips crumbled sautéed bacon; or brown slivered almonds in same pan and sprinkle over beans.

Put uncooked beans on chopping board and cut into ½-inch lengths; steam 20 minutes; just before serving add ½ cup cubed American or pimento cheese or 2 tablespoons each parsley and oil.

Season with crisp sautéed bacon, 2 diced pimentos, 1 tablespoon Worcestershire, dash of cayenne.

Chilled string beans: Cook as in basic recipe; chill and marinate in ¼ cup French dressing, mayonnaise, Thousand Island dressing, or any sauce of yogurt or sour cream (p. 143). Serve on bed of lettuce.

Creamed string beans: Cook beans in ¾ cup top milk; when almost tender, add salt and thickening for cream sauce; season with paprika, dash of celery salt, nutmeg, or chopped pimentos; or add ½ cup cubed or shredded American cheese just before serving.

String beans simmered in milk: Shred beans, add to ½ cup hot milk, and heat to simmering; stir to cover surfaces with milk protein; simmer 12 to 15 minutes; add ½ teaspoon salt; or simmer in enough milk to cover; drain milk and save.

String beans with sour cream: Cook as in basic recipe until tender; add 3 tablespoons canned mushrooms and ½ cup sour cream or yogurt.

String beans with tomatoes and cheese: Prepare beans as in basic recipe; cook with beans 1 chopped onion and add ½ cup canned or fresh, peeled, and diced tomatoes; after removing from heat add ½ cup diced or shredded cheese.

Succotash: Prepare 1 pound beans as in basic recipe; when almost tender, add 1 to 2 cups fresh, canned, or frozen corn; serve as soon as corn is heated through.

Sweet-sour beans: Steam beans cut into 1-inch lengths; season with salt, freshly ground black peppercorns, 2 or 3 tablespoons each oil and vinegar, ¼ cup sugar. Serve hot or cold. Add grated onion if desired.

Kohlrabi, a rich source of vitamin C, is somewhat similar to turnip in appearance except that the bulb grows above the ground. Its meat is sweet and has the delightful crispness of raw cabbage stalk, making it a "must" for salads; the crispness may be retained by short-cooking. The taste is similar to that of young sweet cabbage and turnips. It is unfortunate that kohlrabi is not grown in every garden.

The skin of kohlrabi is so tough that it must be peeled. Since it discolors quickly, it is most attractive when steamed with milk.

KOHLRABI

Peel and dice 5 to 7 chilled young kohlrabi bulbs; put immediately into:

½ cup simmering milk

Stir to coat all surfaces with milk protein; cover utensil and simmer 8 to 10 minutes. Add:

½ teaspoon salt

Serve while still slightly crisp.

VARIATIONS:

Steam or bake whole unpeeled kohlrabies; peel before serving; cut petal-fashion; serve with salt, paprika, and partially hardened margarine or butter.

Broiled kohlrabi: Peel kohlrabies and cut into ¼-inch fingers; toss with 1 tablespoon oil and put on baking sheet; broil at moderate heat until browning starts, or about 5 minutes; turn with pancake turner, lower heat to finish cooking.

Chilled kohlrabi: Cut peeled kohlrabies into fingers, steam in small amount of water; chill quickly; marinate in **French dressing** for 2 or 3 hours before serving.

Kohlrabi with cheese sauce: Cut peeled kohlrabies into halves or wedges; simmer until tender in **top milk**; remove from heat, add ½ cup cubed American cheese, ¼ teaspoon salt; stir; garnish with parsley and paprika.

Kohlrabi with tomatoes: Sauté lightly in vegetable oil 1 minced clove garlic, 1 chopped onion, 2 cups sliced kohlrabi; add 1 cup canned or diced fresh tomatoes, ¼ teaspoon crushed black peppercorns, ¼ teaspoon salt; cook until kohlrabi is tender, or 10 to 12 minutes. Vary by adding 1 chopped ripe bell pepper or pimento, a pinch of basil.

Sautéed kohlrabi: Slice kohlrabies and sauté in 1 or 2 tablespoons vegetable oil or bacon drippings; turn occasionally; keep heat moderate to prevent shriveling.

Steamed kohlrabi: Cut kohlrabies into fingers and steam in small amount of water and ¼ teaspoon vinegar; stir well to prevent discoloring; season with salt and paprika. Vary by adding ½ cup cubed cheese or 1 tablespoon mayonnaise or French dressing.

SAUTÉED MUSHROOMS

Unless mushrooms are sandy, try to keep water from touching them. Go over them carefully with a damp cloth, as if washing a baby's face.

To prevent drying out and shriveling, toss mushrooms with oil. Put into a heated utensil, cover, and cook no longer than 3 to 5 minutes. Sprinkle lightly with:

salt   paprika

Serve at once.

VARIATIONS:

Add and reheat with mushrooms any leftover meat, such as diced turkey, ham, beef, or chicken.

Toss with oil, bake uncovered in flat baking dish 10 minutes at 300° F.; or cook in covered casserole with **1 tablespoon vegetable oil**; sprinkle with **salt and freshly ground white peppercorns.**

SAUTÉED OKRA

Slice crosswise:

2 cups chilled okra

Add to:

2 tablespoons boiling water

Cover utensil, heat rapidly, and simmer until tender, or about 10 minutes; add and stir:

½ teaspoon salt   1 tablespoon chopped parsley
generous dash of paprika   1 tablespoon vegetable oil

VARIATIONS:

Cut okra crosswise into ½-inch pieces; toss on wax paper with ½ cup yellow corn meal; fry until golden in ¼ cup oil or bacon drippings.

Sauté okra with ½ cup finely diced celery, 1 chopped onion, green or red bell pepper, or fresh or canned pimento.

Just before serving add 2 tablespoons chopped chives or green onion with tops, 1 teaspoon mixed fresh herbs, or 1 tablespoon mayonnaise.

Okra with tomatoes: Sauté lightly 1 chopped onion, 2 diced stalks celery; add 1 cup canned or diced fresh tomatoes or purée, 2 cups sliced okra, 1 teaspoon salt, ¼ teaspoon crushed black peppercorns, pinch of basil; simmer 10 minutes. Before serving, ½ cup cubed cheese may be added.

Oyster plant, or salsify, is a slender root somewhat like a parsnip. The tender leafy tops may be chopped and added to tossed salads, used in making soup stocks, or quickly cooked with other greens. The root may be cooked with carrots, parsnips, turnips, and other vegetables until its bland taste is enjoyed.

OYSTER PLANT WITH TOMATOES

Cut 6 to 8 chilled scraped oyster-plant roots into fourths, then into fingers 2½ inches long. Put immediately into:

1 cup boiling tomatoes	¼ teaspoon crushed black pepper-corns

Stir well to coat all surfaces with acid from tomatoes; cover utensil and steam until tender, or about 10 to 15 minutes.
Add:

½ teaspoon salt	dash of cayenne

Taste for seasonings and serve.

VARIATIONS:

Add chopped onion, celery, and/or green or red bell pepper.

Omit tomatoes and cook in ¼ cup vegetable-cooking water to which is added 1 teaspoon vinegar; evaporate most of the water before serving.

Just before serving stir in 2 tablespoons chopped parsley or ½ cup cubed or grated nippy cheese; cover utensil until cheese melts.

Dice or cut into ¼-inch slices and cook with 1 tablespoon hot water in waterless-cooking utcnsil or top of double boiler; season with ½ teaspoon salt and 1 tablespoon chopped parsley or chives.

Chilled oyster plant: Steam with small amount of water, chill quickly, and marinate with French dressing or any sauce of sour-cream or yogurt base. Serve on bed of lettuce.

Creamed oyster plant: Cut oyster plants into fingers and cook in 1 cup cream sauce; add salt, pepper, pinch of basil, 1 teaspoon Worcestershire, or ¼ cup cubed American cheese; or omit cream sauce, cook in milk, and season with salt and cayenne.

Mock oysters: Steam unpeeled oyster plant until almost tender; peel and cut into ¾-inch pieces; dip in batter (p. 158) and fry in shallow fat or in deep fat at 350° F. until golden.

Sautéed oyster plant: Slice chilled scraped oyster plant crosswise or cut into fingers; sauté in 1 tablespoon each hot fat and water; cover utensil, heat quickly, then cook slowly until tender, or about 10 minutes. Salt.

Parsnips are often disliked largely because of the abominable method of cooking them in water, which they soak up like a sponge. They are most delicious if not touched with water after they are thoroughly washed. Even when they are steamed, sugar quickly dissolves out; if overcooked only a few minutes, the pulp becomes waterlogged and mushy. Parsnips cook quickly; hence recipes which advise cooking them twice should be avoided. Since the sugar in parsnips burns easily, the heat should be kept low after they have been heated through.

SAUTÉED PARSNIPS

Cut 4 to 6 chilled unpeeled parsnips into fingers ¼-inch thick and about 2 inches long; drop into:

2 tablespoons hot vegetable oil

Stir well, cover, and heat rapidly; lower heat and cook very slowly 10 to 12 minutes; stir 2 or 3 times and let brown only slightly.
Season with:

½ teaspoon salt

VARIATIONS:

A few minutes before serving add 1 to 3 teaspoons dark molasses; stir well.

Cut small parsnips in half lengthwise; sauté with 2 tablespoons each oil and water, keeping heat extremely low.

Baked parsnips: Cut unpeeled parsnips into fingers and put into preheated oiled casserole; add ½ teaspoon salt and 1 tablespoon hot water;

cover and bake in preheated oven at 350° F. for 15 minutes, or until tender. If sweet parsnips are enjoyed, add **1 tablespoon each lemon juice and brown sugar or dark molasses** before baking. Or select thick short parsnips; leave whole and unpeeled; brush with oil and bake slowly in moderate oven until tender, or about 30 minutes.

With cheese: Cut parsnips lengthwise into halves or fourths; bake in covered casserole until almost tender; remove cover to finish cooking; salt, and sprinkle generously with **cheese and paprika.**

Broiled parsnips: Dice or cut into fingers, toss with oil, place on oiled baking sheet; broil under moderate heat until browning starts, turn with pancake turner, brown other side slightly; lower heat to finsh cooking; after initial heating keep heat low to prevent shriveling.

Chilled parsnips: Cut unpeeled parsnips into fingers; cook in water-less-cooking utensil or top of double boiler; or steam whole parsnips on rack above water. Chill quickly, dice if whole, and marinate in **French dressing;** garnish with **paprika.**

Fried parsnips: Slice parsnips across and fry like raw fried potatoes in 2 tablespoons fat; keep heat low, turning frequently to prevent burning; cover and cook only until tender, or about 10 minutes; season with **salt and serve.**

Peas should be quickly washed in a sieve under running water and not touched again with water unless absolutely necessary. When peas are kept at room temperature, enzymes quickly change sugar into starch, thereby causing loss of sweetness and flavor; if they cannot be cooked immediately, they should be chilled quickly or frozen. Be particularly careful not to overcook them.

PEAS SIMMERED IN MILK

Add 2 cups chilled or frozen peas to:

¼ cup hot milk

Stir well to cover surfaces with milk protein; cover utensil, and simmer until tender, or about 2 to 5 minutes for frozen peas, 7 minutes for fresh peas.

Season with:

½ teaspoon salt	**1 or 2 tablespoons partially hard-ened margarine or butter**

If peas are not of good quality, stir in ½ teaspoon sugar.

VARIATIONS:

Steam in water and season with 1 tablespoon oil or mayonnaise.

Season with 2 teaspoons chopped parsley, ¼ teaspoon minced mint leaves, or 1 diced canned pimento.

Cook in 1 tablespoon hot water in waterless cooker or top of double boiler.

Creamed peas: Cook in **1 cup medium cream sauce; salt to taste.**

Peas with other vegetables: Simmer peas in **milk or cream sauce** with one of the following vegetables: **chopped celery, leeks, or pimentos; diced celery root, turnips, kohlrabi, summer squash, or carrots.** If the other vegetable takes longer to cook, add peas 5 minutes before serving.

Soufflé of fresh peas: Add 1 or more cups uncooked fresh or frozen peas to soufflé (p. 194).

Zucchini or vegetable marrow may be used instead of summer squash in any of the following recipes.

SUMMER SQUASH WITH CHEESE

Slice or cut into 1-inch pieces:

6 to 8 chilled unpeeled summer squash

Sauté squash in **2 tablespoons partially hardened margarine or vegetable oil** with:

1 minced clove garlic	pinch of savory or basil
1 chopped onion	crushed black peppercorns

Stir well, cover utensil, heat quickly, then simmer 10 minutes. Remove from heat, and add:

1 teaspoon salt	½ cup diced American cheese

Stir well and put into serving dish.

In the utensil used for squash, heat quickly:

¾ cup canned or diced fresh	¼ teaspoon salt
tomatoes	½ teaspoon sugar

Pour tomatoes over squash.

VARIATIONS:

Instead of summer squash use small crookneck squash or zucchini in the preceding or following recipes.

Season steamed squash with 1 tablespoon mayonnaise or 1 tablespoon each oil and wine vinegar, chopped green onions with tops; 1 chopped chilled bell pepper or 1 small stalk celery diced; ½ cup tomatoes or tomato sauce; or add ½ cup sour cream or yogurt instead of cheese and omit tomatoes.

Instead of savory or basil season with sage, chives, marjoram, or mixed herbs, or a few coriander or dill seeds.

Omit other ingredients and steam squash with 1 tablespoon water, using waterless-cooking utensil or top of double boiler; or steam with diced onion, celery, or pimento; season with salt and paprika.

Baked summer squash: Split unpeeled summer squash petal-fashion into 6 parts, cutting toward the stem end; put into a low baking dish and brush surfaces with **vegetable oil;** set in preheated oven at 400° F. and bake 10 to 15 minutes; sprinkle with **salt and Parmesan cheese;** garnish with **chopped chives or parsley and paprika.**

With sauce: Bake squash and serve covered with **cheese sauce** (p. 136) or **tomato sauce** (p. 140).

Broiled summer squash: Choose large summer squash and cut cross-wise ¼ inch thick, saving smaller parts for tossed salad; brush slices with oil, dip in **wheat germ or whole-wheat-bread crumbs,** and put on oiled baking sheet; broil under moderate heat until brown on both sides; sprinkle each slice with **grated cheese** and put a **slice of small tomato** on top; broil tomato 3 to 6 minutes without turning.

Creamed summer squash: Cut 1½ pounds squash into 1-inch wedges; cook in **1 cup hot cream sauce;** simmer 10 to 12 minutes; add **1 teaspoon salt.** Vary by adding ½ cup **cubed American cheese** and 2 tablespoons **diced canned pimentos;** cover until cheese melts; or omit cream sauce and simmer in ½ cup **milk; season with partially hardened margarine or butter.**

Sautéed summer squash: Quarter squash and slice; add **2 cups squash** to 1 tablespoon oil or bacon drippings; add pinch of **thyme or dash of celery salt, crushed white peppercorns;** stir well, cover the utensil, lower heat when squash is heated through, and simmer 8 to 10 minutes; salt.

With other vegetables: Sauté 1 cup each squash and one of the following vegetables: **chopped onions, green pepper, sliced carrots, kohlrabi, turnips, or potatoes.**

Sautéed with bacon: Pan-broil **1 strip bacon** with **1 clove garlic;** remove bacon when crisp and discard garlic; sauté sliced squash until tender; add bacon cut into small pieces, ½ teaspoon salt.

Steamed summer squash: Steam whole unpeeled squash; cut petal-fashion, serve with salt, paprika, partially hardened margarine or butter; or cut into wedges, steam in a small amount of water until tender.

Summer squash in batter: Cut squash into small wedges; stir 1 to 2 cups wedges into a batter of 1 egg, 2 tablespoons milk, ½ teaspoon salt, ¼ teaspoon celery or 1 teaspoon dill seeds, ¼ cup each soy grits and wheat germ or whole-wheat-bread crumbs; allow to stand in refrigerator at least 10 minutes; pour from tablespoon onto hot oiled grill and sauté at moderate temperature until well browned.

With crumbs: Cut large squash into ¼-inch rounds; dip into 3 table-spoons milk mixed with ½ teaspoon salt, then into **wheat germ or whole-wheat-bread crumbs**; sauté until golden brown; serve garnished with **thin slice of leek or sweet onion.**

With tomatoes: Dip large slices of squash into **milk and crumbs;** sauté, **salt,** and put on serving platter; use same utensil to sauté **tomatoes** rolled in **crumbs or wheat germ;** put **thin slices of leeks or sweet onions** on slices of squash and cover with **tomatoes.**

The following recipe was used by our great, great grand-mothers. Although stewed tomatoes are rarely served these days, they are far too delicious for the recipe to go out of circulation. My husband's favorite vegetable is a stewed-tomatoes-and-corn combination which he recommends so heartily that he has re-peatedly asked, "Have you put it in your cookbook?"

STEWED TOMATOES

Use 2 cups canned or 3 to 5 peeled and diced fresh tomatoes; cook fresh tomatoes until tender, or about 10 minutes; bring canned ones to boiling; add:

1 tablespoon sugar	1 tablespoon partially hardened
½ teaspoon salt	margarine or butter
crushed black peppercorns	

Crumble or cube 2 slices of stale **whole-wheat bread** and put into serving bowl. Pour boiling tomatoes over bread.

VARIATIONS:

Add pinch of basil, orégano, or marjoram or ½ teaspoon dill or caraway seeds.

Stewed tomatoes with corn: Omit bread; add 1 to 2 cups fresh, canned, or frozen corn; cook no more than 3 minutes longer, or only enough to heat.

TOMATOES WITH GREEN ONIONS

Loosen skin on 4 or 5 fresh tomatoes by piercing with large fork and holding over high heat; peel, dice, and put into heat-resistant casserole. Cook over direct heat 5 minutes and add:

8 to 10 green onions cut into ½-inch pieces	pinch of basil or orégano
¼ teaspoon crushed black pepper-corns	1 to 3 teaspoons dark molasses or sugar
	½ teaspoon salt

Simmer 5 to 8 minutes; move lid to one side to let juice evaporate; remove from heat and sprinkle surface with:

¼ cup toasted wheat germ or whole-wheat-bread crumbs	½ cup cubed American cheese

Serve as soon as cheese melts.

VARIATIONS:

Instead of fresh tomatoes use 2 cups canned tomatoes and 1 or 2 chopped leeks or dry onions; or omit onions.

Add with onions chopped ripe bell pepper or pimento, celery, okra, eggplant, corn, kohlrabi, or mixed vegetables.

Slice tomatoes; put into hot oiled casserole and sprinkle with crumbs and seasonings of basic recipe; add **grated cheese and paprika**; bake at 350° F. for 10 to 12 minutes.

Broiled tomatoes: Peel 2 or 3 firm tomatoes and cut into ¾-inch slices; sprinkle slices with **bits of raw diced bacon**; broil on oiled baking sheet under moderate heat until tender, or about 8 to 10 minutes; or omit bacon and sprinkle with **grated Parmesan cheese**; garnish with **chopped parsley.** Vary by rolling in 4 tablespoons wheat germ or whole-wheat-bread crumbs mixed with ½ teaspoon salt, freshly ground black peppercorns, and a pinch of basil; dot top with butter or partially hardened margarine.

Sautéed tomatoes: Cut 3 or 4 firm ripe or green tomatoes into ½-inch slices; dip in whole-wheat-bread crumbs or wheat germ mixed with ½ teaspoon each salt and cumin or caraway seeds; sauté in 2 tablespoons vegetable oil 8 to 10 minutes, or until golden brown on both surfaces. Vary by marinating sliced tomatoes with 2 tablespoons French dressing for ½ hour; dip in seasoned crumbs and sauté; put tomatoes on platter, heat juices drawn out by marinating, and serve over tomatoes.

BAKED TOMATOES

Cut in half and place in low heat-resistant serving dish:

2 or 3 large tomatoes

Mix together and pat over tomatoes:

¼ cup each finely chopped   ¼ teaspoon basil
   parsley and onions or olives   3 tablespoons mayonnaise
⅓ cup wheat germ

Sprinkle with:

paprika

Bake in moderate oven at 350° F. for 8 to 10 minutes.

VARIATIONS:

Cut into ¾-inch slices and sprinkle with diced green onions, wheat germ, Parmesan cheese, and paprika. Bake only 8 minutes.

Use canned tomatoes; drain off most of the juice and sprinkle wheat germ and seasoning over top; omit mayonnaise and add ½ to 1 cup shredded Cheddar-type cheese.

Baked stuffed tomatoes: Peel, remove centers, and salt whole tomatoes; mix diced pulp with 1 cup wheat germ or crumbs, 1 tablespoon vegetable oil, ¼ cup chopped parsley, 1 minced clove garlic, dash of salt and ground peppercorns; stuff into tomatoes and pat over top; sprinkle with Parmesan cheese and paprika. Bake at 300° F. for 15 to

20 minutes. Vary stuffing by adding fresh or canned corn, leftover chopped vegetables, macaroni, steamed rice, leftover diced meat or flaked fish, chopped green pepper or onion, basil and/or tarragon.

Vegetable marrow is a member of the squash family which resembles summer squash. Prepare vegetable marrow, young crookneck squash, and zucchini by recipes given for summer squash (pp. 349–351). Since these squashes contain a large amount of moisture, the flavor is more delightful if part of the juices is allowed to evaporate before the vegetable is served.

ZUCCHINI PATTIES

Chop in chopping bowl:

4 chilled unpeeled zucchini	4 green onions or 1 dry onion

Add and stir:

2 eggs	¼ cup wheat germ or whole-wheat-
1 teaspoon salt	bread crumbs
freshly ground black peppercorns	dash cayenne

Drop from tablespoon onto oiled grill or frying pan. Brown on both sides; cover and sauté 5 to 8 minutes.

VARIATIONS:

Use summer or crookneck squash instead of zucchini.

Add to patties any one of the following: 1 tablespoon catsup; 1 teaspoon Worcestershire; 1 diced pimento, green pepper, or celery stalk; 2 tablespoons chopped parsley or powdered milk.

Add to zucchini diced leftover meat or vegetables or a small amount of any unfamiliar vegetable, such as kohlrabi, Jerusalem artichoke, vegetable marrow, okra, oyster plant.

STUFFED BAKED ZUCCHINI

Cut lengthwise:

2 large zucchini

Scoop out pulp, leaving shells no thicker than ¼ inch; make dressing by chopping together:

squash pulp   **2 stalks celery**
1 onion

Sauté the chopped vegetables with oil until onion is transparent; add and mix well:

2 tablespoons chopped parsley **¼ cup wheat germ, soy grits, or**
pinch of savory or basil   **whole-wheat-bread crumbs**
½ teaspoon salt

Stuff dressing into zucchini shells; put into baking dish with **2 tablespoons water**; place **strips of bacon** on top and place in moderate oven at 350° F. for 15 minutes, or until bacon is browned.

VARIATIONS:

Add to stuffing any diced leftover meat or vegetables.

Use medium-size zucchini; leave whole, remove centers with an apple corer, stuff, and bake.

Serve Intensely Green Vegetables Often

Intensely green leaves, which offer the greatest concentration and the widest variety of vitamins and minerals of all the vegetables, should be eaten frequently or even daily. A half cup of cooked beet or turnip tops, for example, supplies approximately 19,000 units of vitamin A, or carotene, whereas the roots contain none. If handled carefully before cooking, heated rapidly to destroy enzymes, and quick-cooked in their own juices, green leaves lose little nutritive value in cooking. Although the greens may be eaten daily in tossed salads, cooking causes the nutrients to be so concentrated that a small serving equals an amount impossible to eat raw; hence the value obtained from cooked leaves may be many times greater than from raw ones.

Leafy vegetables are often disliked because of the texture rather than the taste. Except for extremely tender or small leaves, such as New Zealand spinach and watercress, or those containing almost no stringy parts, such as mustard-spinach, it is wise to shred all leaves and especially all stalks before or while cooking them. Mature greens, such as large beet and turnip tops, can be cooked palatably provided they are carefully shredded.

The flavor of greens can be controlled largely by the method of cooking. Plant acids cause many of the more mature greens to have a pungent and sometimes bitter flavor. The flavor becomes mild when these acids are neutralized by proteins. If you wish to change a pungent flavor into a mild one, cook the greens in milk, cream sauce, batter, or a soufflé. The milder the taste desired or the stronger the flavor to start with, the greater is the amount of protein which should be used in cooking. If this procedure is followed, very mature and bitter greens can become delicious.

As much as ½ cup or more of water may cling to greens after they are washed. If carelessly allowed to remain on the leaves, this water quickly dissolves out sugars, iron, vitamin C, and many other nutrients; the water also dissolves out oxalic and phytic acids which cause the green to change to an unappetizing olive-gray and which leave the teeth-on-edge feeling experienced after eating improperly cooked spinach. Immediately after being washed, greens should be whirled dry. When greens are allowed to cook in their own juices, the heat should be kept low and they should be stirred frequently until steam is formed.

During cooking, the oxalic acid in spinach combines with calcium in the vegetable cells, forming calcium oxalate. This salt does not dissolve in the digestive juices and therefore cannot enter the blood. Although no thought need be given to extracting it, spinach must not be relied upon as a source of calcium. Whenever possible, cook spinach in milk or cream sauce.

The recipes for cooking green leafy vegetables can be used interchangeably; any greens may be substituted for those in the basic recipes. I urge you to prepare your favorite greens by each of these recipes, then gradually combine the less familiar leafy vegetables with old favorites until you have cooked each of the green leafy vegetables in the following list.

beet tops*
broccoli leaves*
Brussels sprout leaves
cabbage, outer green leaves
cauliflower leaves, young outer or tender inside leaves
celery leaves
celtuce
chicory, or witloof
Chinese cabbage*
Chinese celery*
Chinese mustard
dandelion, thick-leafed cultivated variety*
endive, or escarole*
kale*

lettuce, Bibb or dark-leafed *
mustard greens*
mustard-spinach*
 New Zealand spinach*
parsley*
radish tops*
rhubarb chard,** green leaves*
rhubarb chard, red leaves†
savoy cabbage, loose outer leaves*
sorrel *
spinach
Swiss chard *
tampala*‡
turnip tops*
watercress*
wild greens*

* Greens of outstanding nutritive value.
** Except for its red stems, this is the same as Swiss chard.
† May be prepared by any recipe given for purple cabbage (pp. 368–369).
‡ Similar to spinach in texture, but more tender and sweet; the flavor of the celery-like stalks resembles that of artichoke.

CREAMED RHUBARB CHARD

Prepare:

1 to 1½ cups thick cream sauce (p. 135)

Meanwhile cut into ¼-inch shreds:

1 or 2 bunches of well-whirled rhubarb chard and stalks

When available, use part green and part red leaves.

Add chard to cream sauce, stirring until all leaves are covered with sauce; simmer 6 to 8 minutes, stirring occasionally.

If juices from chard have not thinned cream sauce to desired consistency, add a small amount of milk; before serving add:

½ teaspoon salt

Garnish with **paprika.**

VARIATIONS:

Add a dash of nutmeg or mace or 1 small grated onion or leek.

Instead of plain cream sauce prepare caraway, celery, cheese, dill, egg, mock Hollandaise, olive, pimento, or piquant sauce (p. 137), using thick cream sauce as base instead of medium cream sauce; cook chard in sauce.

Combine any of the following vegetables with chard: 1 cup or more shredded green, purple, Chinese, or savoy cabbage or shredded greens of any kind.

Instead of chard use any greens listed on page 357 or any combination of greens.

Remove from heat, stir in ½ cup cubed or grated cheese; cover utensil until cheese melts; or garnish with sliced or sieved hard-cooked eggs.

Prepare in baking dish over direct heat; when vegetable is heated through, sprinkle top with wheat germ or whole-wheat-bread crumbs and grated cheese; finish cooking in oven.

MUSTARD GREENS WITH SALT PORK

Dice with scissors:

1 or 2 slices salt pork

Pan-broil until crisp. Drain off most of the drippings. Cut into ¼-inch shreds:

1 to 2 bunches chilled mustard greens

Put into hot fat; stir well; keep heat moderate and turn frequently until mustard has wilted; lower heat and steam 4 to 6 minutes. Taste for salt. Sprinkle with **freshly ground peppercorns.**

VARIATIONS:

Instead of mustard greens use any greens or any combination of greens listed on page 357.

Cook greens with 2 tablespoons bacon drippings instead of salt pork; or pan-broil 1 or 2 slices bacon; remove when crisp and cook greens; add ½ teaspoon salt; cut bacon to bits and add before serving.

Omit salt pork and cook with greens ½ to 1 cup diced leftover ham.

Mixed garden greens: Gather assorted leaves from garden, such as broccoli, outside leaves of cabbage, and young tops of carrot, radish, and kohlrabi; add a small amount of fresh herbs or horseradish leaves for seasoning. Shred and cook with salt pork or bacon.

Wild greens: Gather such wild greens as lamb's-quarters, curly and sour dock, tender poke sprouts, dandelions, deer's-tongue, peppergrass, and wild turnip, lettuce, and mustard greens; cook with salt pork as in basic recipe.

NEW ZEALAND SPINACH SAUTÉED IN BATTER

Beat to a smooth batter:

1 egg	**¾ teaspoon salt**
½ cup fresh milk	**¼ teaspoon crushed peppercorns**
¼ to ½ cup powdered milk	**1 grated onion**
¼ to ½ cup wheat germ	**1 teaspoon Worcestershire**

Cut into ¼-inch shreds enough chilled New Zealand spinach leaves and stems to make **1½ tightly packed cups**; stir shredded spinach into batter and set in refrigerator for 10 minutes.

Drop batter with spinach from tablespoon onto a hot grill brushed with:

partially hardened margarine or vegetable oil

Sauté slowly until brown on both sides; garnish with **paprika.**

VARIATIONS:

Shred spinach with other greens, using ¾ cup each.

Add finely chopped celery, fresh pimento or red bell pepper, or a few leaves of fresh tarragon, basil, or marjoram, or a pinch of dried herbs.

Instead of spinach use any greens listed on page 357.

French-fried New Zealand spinach: Drop the batter with spinach from a teaspoon into deep fat at 300° F.; drain on absorbent paper; serve garnished with **paprika.**

When shredded parsley is cooked, so many of its aromatic oils escape that it has a mild pleasant taste; it can therefore be used in large quantities with other greens without its flavor predominating. The following recipe is one of my favorites. It is particularly delicious with raw grated onion added just before serving.

PARSLEY AND SPINACH WITH BACON AND GARLIC

Pan-broil in a large utensil:

1 or 2 slices bacon

Remove bacon when crisp; keep heat moderate; shred and cook in 2 tablespoons bacon drippings:

| 2 bunches spinach | 1 bunch parsley |

Stir until wilted; cover utensil, reduce heat to simmering, and cook 4 to 6 minutes; cut into ¼-inch shreds; add:

| 1 minced clove garlic | freshly ground black peppercorns |
| ½ teaspoon salt | bacon broken to bits |

Stir well and serve.

VARIATIONS:

Sauté with bacon or add raw to cooked greens 1 chopped onion and/or ½ chilled bell pepper or pimento or stalk celery.

Instead of parsley and spinach use any greens or any combination of greens listed on page 357.

When radish tops are cooked, the prickles on the leaves soften quickly and cannot be noticed. The taste is mildly peppery and somewhat similar to that of the roots. The greens are usually enjoyed the first time they are eaten.

RADISH TOPS AND KALE WITH SOUR CREAM

Cut into ¼-inch shreds:

| 1 bunch chilled kale | tops from 1 bunch radishes |

Put shredded greens into hot flat-bottomed utensil over moderate

heat; stir or turn leaves with a pancake turner frequently until wilted; reduce heat to simmering, cover utensil, and cook 8 to 10 minutes.
Add:

½ teaspoon salt

Put greens into hot serving dish; heat slightly in the same utensil:

½ to 1 cup sour cream or yogurt   ⅛ teaspoon salt

Pour heated cream or yogurt over greens and serve.

VARIATIONS:

Cook with greens a few leaves of fresh horseradish, parsley, or other herbs, or ½ teaspoon caraway, dill, celery, or mustard seeds.

Instead of radish tops and kale use any greens listed on page 357 or any combination of greens. Radish tops are especially good with spinach.

Chilled greens: For hot-weather dinner or buffet, chill cooked greens quickly and marinate in **French dressing.**

Greens with cheese: Omit sour cream; add ½ cup diced American cheese after greens have been taken from the heat; cover utensil until cheese is melted.

Both mustard-spinach and tampala should be grown in every garden. Mustard-spinach has the delightful flavor of mustard greens, yet the tenderness of immature spinach. Tampala leaves are as tender as spinach and taste much the same except that they are sweeter and usually better liked. Both vegetables have a lower content of oxalic acid than spinach has. Since tampala grows some two feet high, it is much easier to wash than is spinach; hence fewer nutrients are lost.

The recipe which follows is my favorite for cooking all green leafy vegetables as well as shredded cabbage.

SAUTÉED MUSTARD-SPINACH

Use mustard-spinach alone or equal amounts of mustard-spinach and tampala or other less familiar greens. Wash thoroughly but quickly; whirl free from moisture. Put into salad bowl and toss with:

1 tablespoon vegetable oil

Put tossed leaves into hot utensil over moderate heat; turn frequently until heated through; cover utensil, lower heat, and steam 10 minutes without added moisture, or until tender.

Do not salt until immediately before serving.

VARIATIONS:

Rub salad bowl well with crushed garlic or cook minced garlic or chopped green onions with greens.

Instead of mustard-spinach use shredded cabbage or any greens or any combination of greens listed on page 357.

STEAMED BEET TOPS WITH ROOTS

Wash, whirl dry, and steam without added moisture:

chilled beet tops

When wilted, cut leaves and stems into ¾-inch lengths. Simmer 8 to 10 minutes. Shred and add 5 minutes before serving:

3 or 4 chilled, unpeeled beet roots

Season with:

crushed black peppercorns   2 to 4 tablespoons vinegar or
1 teaspoon salt   lemon juice

VARIATIONS:

Cook beet tops without shredded roots; to prevent discoloration of green leaves, add vinegar at the table.

Omit vinegar; dice unpeeled roots and cook in ½ cup milk; when almost tender, add tops. Shred tops in cooking utensil before serving.

If roots are no more than ½ inch in diameter, clean well and cook roots and tops together without shredding either.

Use same procedure in cooking turnip roots with tops. Use or omit vinegar.

Watercress may be served as cooked greens. It has outstanding nutritive value and, after being heated, small bulk. Because it grows wild in abundance in many parts of the country, it should be used far more frequently than it is. Care must be taken that the stems are cut into small pieces; otherwise they become tough and stringy. When watercress is cooked only a few minutes, its peppery flavor is well retained. Since it does not thrive unless the water in which it grows is pure and the soil uncontaminated, this vegetable is always "organically grown."

WATERCRESS WITH MUSHROOM SAUCE

Wash, whirl dry, and shred into ½-inch pieces:

2 bunches chilled watercress

Stir and heat to simmering:

1 can condensed mushroom soup

Drop watercress into hot sauce and mix thoroughly; simmer 5 minutes, or until tender. Taste for **salt.** Garnish with **paprika.**

VARIATIONS:

Add diced canned pimento or cook ripe bell pepper with watercress.

Instead of mushroom soup use 1 cup leftover cream gravy; add a dash of nutmeg or mace.

Instead of watercress use any greens listed on page 357.

TURNIP TOPS

Wash, whirl dry, and shred across the veins:

chilled tops of 6 to 10 turnip roots

Put into hot utensil without added moisture.

Cover utensil, keep heat moderate, and stir **frequently until leaves** wilt; reduce heat to simmering and cook 5 to 10 minutes, or until tender; add just before serving:

½ teaspoon salt	1 tablespoon chopped chives, leeks,
2 tablespoons French dressing,	or raw, sweet onion (optional)
mayonnaise, or oil	freshly ground black peppercorns

Stir well and serve.

VARIATIONS:

Omit dressing or oil and serve with partially hardened margarine or butter.

Instead of turnip tops use any greens listed on page 357.

With vinegar sauce: Turn greens into hot serving dish; put into utensil 1 tablespoon water, 1 teaspoon sugar, 3 tablespoons vinegar, 2 or 3 sliced green onions and tops; pour boiling sauce over greens and serve immediately.

"Strong-flavored" Vegetables

Although vegetables such as onions, cabbage, cauliflower, rutabagas, turnips, and Brussels sprouts are spoken of as being strong-flavored, the flavors referred to do not exist in the raw fresh vegetables, nor do they develop when the vegetables are properly cooked. Such flavors are produced only when sulfur compounds found in these vegetables are broken down. The breakdown may be brought about by enzymes during long storage or slow initial heating; by plant acids allowed to soak out of the vegetable during cooking; or by heat when the vegetable is overcooked, especially at a high temperature. Since some of the sulfur compounds are volatile, odors escaping during cooking indicate that the vegetables are being overcooked or cooked at too high a temperature. When the sulfur compounds are broken down, gases are formed from them during digestion; the person who eats such improperly cooked vegetables may suffer from discomfort and digestive disturbances.

Housewives are often advised to cook these vegetables in large amounts of water and to leave the utensil uncovered so that the volatile compounds can escape. After the cooking liquid is discarded, the vegetables—odorless, tasteless, vitaminless, and mineralless—are ready to be served. When these vegetables are put into water, the plant acids soak out and bring about the rapid breakdown of the sulfur compounds. More than any other type of vegetables, the sulfur-containing vegetables should be washed with the utmost speed and dried thoroughly and quickly. They should not be touched unnecessarily with water. Since enzymes can bring about the breakdown of the sulfur compounds, thorough chilling and quick initial heating are particularly important.

Experiments have shown that almost no sulfur compounds break down when these vegetables are cooked 8 to 10 minutes at a temperature not above boiling. If the chilled vegetable is shredded or diced, it can be thoroughly cooked in this time. When longer cooking is desired, as when cauliflower is to be cooked whole, the vegetable should be cooked in milk, which can neutralize the plant acids and thus prevent the breakdown of the sulfur compounds. Cooking in milk has the added advantages of preserving color and of ensuring that the temperature will be kept low.

If vegetables which contain sulfur are cooked in a pressure cooker, the cooking time should be checked with a stop watch; if sautéed or fried, the heat should be kept low and the vegetable cooked only a short time. When acids are neutralized or are not soaked out, when the cooking temperature is kept low and the cooking time held to the minimum, these vegetables are surprisingly sweet and mild-flavored. No fresh vegetable which is properly prepared can be called strong-flavored.

BROCCOLI WITH CREAM SAUCE

Use 1 pound chilled broccoli; cut bud ends into ¾-inch pieces; shred leaves and chop smaller stalks; peel any large stalks and cut into fingers ¼-inch thick or keep for salad.

Meanwhile heat to boiling:

1 or 2 cups cream sauce

Stir in broccoli, being careful to cover all surfaces with sauce; keep heat high until boiling, then reduce heat, cover utensil, and simmer, stirring occasionally until broccoli is barely tender, or about 10 minutes.

Add and stir:

½ teaspoon salt   ¼ teaspoon celery salt (optional)

Garnish with paprika and Parmesan cheese.

VARIATIONS:

Omit cream sauce and heat 1 cup fresh milk shaken with ¼ cup powdered milk; stir well to cover all surfaces with protein; control temperature carefully or cook in top of double boiler.

Prepare recipe in casserole; cook over direct heat; when tender, sprinkle with whole-wheat-bread crumbs, 1 cup cubed cheese, paprika; cover utensil until cheese melts; or bake in a preheated oven at 350° F. for 15 minutes.

Omit celery salt. Just before serving add any of the following: 3 tablespoons diced canned pimento; ½ cup cubed nippy or pimento cheese; a dash of nutmeg or mace; 2 tablespoons lemon juice, ½ teaspoon grated lemon rind; 1 teaspoon Worcestershire. Or before cooking add 1 grated onion, 1 teaspoon fresh or ⅛ teaspoon dried basil, marjoram, or savory or ½ teaspoon caraway, dill, mustard, or celery seeds.

Broccoli simmered in deep milk: Cook uncut broccoli in enough milk to cover, or 2 to 3 cups; simmer until tender; drain milk and save; season.

Broccoli soufflé: Add to plain or cheese soufflé (p. 194) **2 cups finely chopped broccoli;** season with **cayenne pepper, ¼ teaspoon celery salt, 1 grated onion, 1 minced clove garlic.**

Quick-cooked broccoli: Cut **1 clove garlic** in half and sauté lightly in **vegetable oil or bacon drippings;** discard garlic; cut broccoli into small pieces, add to fat, stir well, and add **2 tablespoons water;** heat quickly, cover utensil, and cook 8 to 10 minutes.

Steamed broccoli: Leave broccoli stalks uncut; stand upright in utensil containing ½ cup boiling water; steam until tender, or about 15 minutes. **Salt** and serve with oil, French dressing, mayonnaise, Hollandaise (p. 138) or cheese sauce (p. 136).

With herb butter: Heat **2 tablespoons partially hardened margarine or oil, 1 minced clove garlic, salt, pepper, ¼ teaspoon basil or orégano, ¼ cup lemon juice;** pour over steamed broccoli.

Brussels sprouts may be prepared by the recipes given for broccoli, cabbage, or cauliflower.

BRUSSELS SPROUTS WITH MUSHROOM SAUCE

Mix thoroughly and heat to simmering:

1 can condensed mushroom soup   ½ cup milk

Add:

1 pound chilled whole Brussels sprouts

Stir well to coat all surfaces with sauce; cover utensil and simmer until just tender, or 10 to 12 minutes.

Taste for **salt** and garnish with **paprika or parsley.**

VARIATIONS:

If especially soft texture is desired, cut each sprout into halves or fourths.

Cook in a small amount of water or top of double boiler or simmer in deep or shallow milk.

Creamed Brussels sprouts with celery: Cream like broccoli (p. 365); add with raw sprouts ½ cup chopped celery.

Sautéed Brussels sprouts: Cut Brussels sprouts in half; cook in frying pan brushed with **vegetable oil;** add 1 tablespoon hot water; cover utensil and cook 5 to 6 minutes over low heat. Season with ½ teaspoon salt and garnish with paprika. Or toss whole sprouts with oil before steaming.

With sour cream: Steam until tender; sauté 1 **chopped onion,** add and heat 1 **cup sour cream;** pour over sprouts.

Savoy and Chinese cabbage and collards may be prepared by any recipe used in cooking ordinary cabbage. Since they are nutritionally superior to the lighter-colored variety, they should be served more frequently when available.

STEAMED CABBAGE

Dry well after washing and shred fine on kraut cutter:

½ head chilled cabbage

Add to:

2 tablespoons boiling water

Cover utensil, heat rapidly, and reduce temperature; simmer 8 minutes.

Season with:

½ teaspoon each salt and sugar

VARIATIONS:

At the beginning of cooking add 1 or 2 teaspoons caraway seeds.

Cook shredded cabbage in ½ cup milk; or cut head into sixths without removing stalk and cook in deep milk.

Creamed cabbage: Prepare 1 cup medium cream sauce and add ½ teaspoon salt, dash each of cayenne and celery salt; add chilled shredded cabbage; stir thoroughly and simmer 8 minutes. Cubed American cheese and/or 2 tablespoons diced canned pimento may be added before serving.

Scalloped cabbage: Prepare creamed cabbage in heat-resistant casserole, cooking over direct heat; when cabbage is tender, stir in ¼ cup toasted whole-wheat-bread crumbs and ¾ cup cubed American cheese; sprinkle surface with wheat germ, cheese, and paprika; cover utensil until cheese melts; or add all ingredients to hot cream sauce and bake 15 minutes in moderate oven.

Cabbage chop suey: Chop together ½ head chilled cabbage, 4 stalks celery, 1 chilled green pepper, 1 large onion; sauté with low heat in vegetable oil for 10 minutes; add and stir in 2 or 3 tablespoons soy sauce and dash of paprika. Serve with steamed or fried brown rice.

Sautéed cabbage: Cook shredded cabbage with 1 tablespoon each hot water and oil; cover utensil and cook over low heat 8 minutes.

With bacon: Pan-broil 2 slices bacon, remove when crisp, drain fat, and sauté shredded cabbage until tender; salt, and sprinkle chopped bacon over top.

With purple cabbage: Cook equal parts shredded green and purple cabbage as in the basic recipe or any variation. Purple cabbage should be shredded finer than green cabbage so that both will be tender at the same time; if carefully prepared, this combination is both beautiful and delicious.

With sauerkraut: Combine and cook together 8 minutes without added moisture approximately 2 cups each sauerkraut and chilled shredded cabbage; if sour taste is not enjoyed, add ½ teaspoon sugar. Vary by seasoning with 1 or 2 teaspoons caraway seeds.

Unless some acid is used in cooking, purple cabbage changes color more quickly than does any other vegetable. Cook it preferably in stainless steel, glass, or enamel rather than in aluminum; and shred it paper-thin for quick cooking.

The following recipe is one of my favorites for guest dinners.

SWEET-SOUR PURPLE CABBAGE

Use large utensil; pan-broil until crisp:

1 slice bacon

Remove bacon and add:

¼ cup each vinegar and brown   ½ teaspoon salt
   sugar   ½ head finely shredded purple
2 tablespoons water   cabbage

To prevent discoloration, stir or toss cabbage until well moistened with vinegar. Cover utensil and simmer 20 minutes, or until tender. Increase heat to evaporate off moisture.

VARIATIONS:

Omit vinegar and decrease sugar to 1 tablespoon; add 2 tablespoons lemon juice, 2 diced tart apples, dash of nutmeg.

Purple cabbage with onion: Sauté until transparent 1 or 2 chopped onions with bacon; add ¼ tablespoon French dressing or lemon juice, omitting vinegar.

Purple cabbage with sour cream: Cook shredded purple cabbage in ½ cup heated sour cream; season with ½ teaspoon salt and 1 teaspoon crushed caraway or cardamon seeds; simmer until tender.

If whole cauliflower is cooked in enough milk to cover, the vegetable can be snowy white when tender and completely without odor during the cooking.

WHOLE CAULIFLOWER WITH CHEESE SAUCE

Heat to simmering in utensil just large enough to hold cauliflower:

1½ to 2 cups fresh or reconstituted milk

Trim, wash, and put into the hot milk:

1 entire head cauliflower

Add more milk if needed to cover head. Simmer about 20 minutes, or until barely tender. Put cauliflower on serving platter. Meanwhile make thickening by mixing to a paste:

2 or 3 tablespoons whole-wheat-   ½ cup milk used to cook cauli-
   pastry flour   flower

Add thickening to remaining hot milk; stir well, simmer 8 minutes and add:

1 cup diced Cheddar-type cheese

As soon as cheese melts, serve sauce over salted cauliflower. Garnish with paprika.

VARIATIONS:

Omit thickening. Remove from heat and stir 2 beaten eggs, ½ teaspoon salt, and cheese into milk. Let stand 5 minutes.

Break cauliflower into 1½-inch pieces. Cook in ½ cup milk or 1 cup medium cream sauce. Stir well to coat surfaces with milk protein. Simmer 10 minutes, or until barely tender. Season with salt, paprika, butter or partially hardened margarine.

Omit cream sauce, saving milk for cream soup; mix together 2 tablespoons each partially hardened margarine or butter and ½ cup slivered almonds. Heat and sprinkle over top.

Cauliflower with tomatoes: Sauté **1 clove garlic and 1 chopped onion in 1 tablespoon vegetable oil**; discard garlic and add **¼ teaspoon crushed black peppercorns, 1 teaspoon salt, ¾ cup canned or raw diced tomatoes or tomato purée**; bring to boiling and add raw cauliflower broken into pieces; stir well and add **1 teaspoon fresh or pinch of dry basil, orégano, or thyme**; cover utensil and cook 10 minutes; serve sprinkled with **Parmesan cheese. Bell pepper, pimento, or celery** may be sautéed with garlic, or **chopped parsley** may be added before serving.

Steamed cauliflower: Break cauliflower into 2-inch pieces and rinse with 1 cup water containing 1 tablespoon vinegar; steam about 10 minutes, or until just tender, using the least water necessary to prevent burning; serve with salt, paprika, and partially hardened margarine or butter, or with French dressing, mayonnaise, or Hollandaise sauce (p. 138).

Leeks might be described as overgrown green onions. Their flavor is similar to that of green onions or sweet dry onions, except that they are more mild, sweet, juicy, and, to most people, more delicious. Any person who enjoys the flavor of onions in small amounts will probably be enthusiastic about leeks.

Leeks may be prepared by recipes given for onions. As much as 2 to 3 inches of the green leaves should be used. Leeks are especially delightful when cooked in milk and served with Hollandaise or cheese sauce.

Onions are almost invariably overcooked, and as a result their delightful fresh flavor is sacrificed. They should be served while still slightly crisp, or cooked only until translucent. Dry onions contain about 15 per cent sugar. If they are peeled after they are cooked, no sugar is lost and they are far sweeter and more delicious than when prepared by the usual methods.

BROILED ONIONS

Select flat white or purple onions no more than 1 inch thick but as large as available; do not skin or cut.

Set on the broiler rack 2 inches from heat; keep heat as high as possible without burning skin; broil 8 to 10 minutes; turn, lower heat, and continue broiling until tender, or about 10 minutes longer; remove from heat; peel off skin and outside layer.

Cut petal-fashion toward root; sprinkle with salt, paprika, and dots of butter or partially hardened margarine.

VARIATIONS:

If flat onions are not available, bake large round ones 20 to 30 minutes, or until tender; remove skin just before serving.

Broiled onion slices: Cut large onions into ½-inch slices; set on oiled baking sheet, brush both sides with **oil** and sprinkle with **paprika**; place 2 inches from broiler under moderate heat; when they start to brown, or in about 6 minutes, turn with pancake turner; brown the other side slightly and lower heat to finish cooking; **salt.** Garnish with **paprika.**

Creamed onions: Select small white onions, peel, and simmer in ½ cup hot milk until almost tender; add ¾ teaspoon salt, thickening for cream sauce, ¼ teaspoon paprika; or add ¼ cup diced green pepper or pimentos before cooking, or 2 tablespoons parsley or ½ cup cubed cheese before serving. If it is more convenient, steam unpeeled onions on rack above water until tender; peel and drop into hot cream sauce.

Creamed green onions: Cut off tops of 2 bunches green onions, retaining 2 inches or more of green; keep parallel and drop into **1 cup simmering milk**; add ¼ teaspoon crushed white peppercorns; simmer until barely tender, or 10 to 12 minutes; put onions on serving plate and sprinkle with **salt**; thicken milk, season with ½ teaspoon salt, ¼ teaspoon paprika; pour sauce on onions without covering green tops and white base; garnish with **parsley sprigs or pimento strips.**

Scalloped onions: Prepare creamed whole or sliced onions in heat-resistant casserole over direct heat; when onions are tender, sprinkle with ½ cup each toasted wheat germ or whole-wheat-bread crumbs and cubed American cheese; garnish generously with paprika. Cover utensil until cheese melts, or brown under broiler.

French-fried onion rings: Cut onions into ½-inch slices, separate into rings, and dip in **batter** (p. 158); set on oiled paper to dry 10 minutes or longer; fry a few rings at a time in hot fat at 300° F. for 2 to 4 minutes; drain on brown paper. Vary by mixing **shredded cheese** with batter. With onions fry rings of **chilled bell pepper or fresh chili pepper.**

Onion casserole: Slice 4 large onions and put into hot casserole containing 2 tablespoons each water and vegetable oil; cover casserole and bake in preheated moderate oven until transparent, or about 15 minutes; sprinkle with salt, chopped parsley, and ½ cup cubed or grated cheese; turn off heat and leave in oven until cheese melts. If mild flavor is desired, omit water and add ½ cup top milk.

Onions cooked in sour cream: Add small white onions or ⅓-inch rings of red and white onions to 1 cup heated sour cream; simmer until tender, or about 10 to 12 minutes; add ½ teaspoon salt and dash of cayenne.

Sautéed onions: Cut large onions into ¾-inch slices; sauté gently in oil; turn once, cooking 10 to 12 minutes. Garnish with paprika and Parmesan cheese or chopped parsley.

Spiced red onions: Slice large red onions ⅓ inch thick and put into hot casserole; or alternate slices of white and red onions; add 1 tablespoon each vinegar, brown sugar or dark molasses, water, bacon drippings; season with 3 whole cloves and small piece of cinnamon bark; heat quickly, then simmer or bake until tender. Serve while rings are slightly crisp.

Steamed onions: Set dry unpeeled onions on rack above boiling water; steam until tender, or 15 to 20 minutes; peel, sprinkle with salt and paprika. Vary by putting cooked peeled onions in flat baking dish; sprinkle with wheat germ or toasted crumbs, grated cheese, paprika; heat slowly under broiler until cheese melts.

Stuffed onions: Remove centers from large onions, leaving 4 to 6 meaty outside layers; fill with heated stuffing of leftover diced carrots or other vegetables, diced leftover meat, chopped pepper or pimento, and celery; add salt and pepper; or prepare half the meat-loaf recipe (p. 108) and use for stuffing; cover with tomato sauce or concentrated canned tomato soup; bake in hot oven 15 to 18 minutes.

RUTABAGAS

Peel 1 to 3 chilled rutabagas and cut into wedges or fingers ½-inch thick; dice old and fibrous rutabagas into small cubes; drop into:

½ cup hot milk

Stir to coat surfaces with milk protein; cover utensil; heat rapidly, and simmer for 15 minutes, or until tender, stirring occasionally; season with:

½ teaspoon salt
dash of cayenne

partially hardened margarine or butter

VARIATIONS:

Cook rutabagas by any recipe suggested for turnips (p. 374).

Mash rutabagas by pressing through a hot colander or ricer; season as in basic recipe or add a dash of nutmeg.

Before serving, add to rutabagas 1 tablespoon chopped chives, green onions and tops, or 3 to 4 tablespoons parsley.

Cut rutabagas into quarters and steam until tender; season as in basic recipe.

Baked rutabagas: Leave young and tender rutabagas whole; otherwise cut into halves or quarters; do not peel; brush all surfaces with oil and bake in preheated oven at 350° F. for 40 to 50 minutes, or until tender; or steam until rutabagas start to be tender; finish cooking in oven. Serve like baked potatoes.

Leftover rutabagas: Beat 1 egg slightly and add ½ teaspoon salt, 1 or 2 cups mashed rutabagas; shape into patties, roll in **whole-wheat flour,** and sauté at low temperature.

SAUERKRAUT WITH CARAWAY SEEDS

Put into utensil for waterless cooking:

1 pound sauerkraut   **1 to 2 teaspoons crushed caraway seeds**

Stir well, cover utensil, and simmer 15 minutes. If time permits, allow seasoned kraut to stand ½ hour or longer.

Reheat, and add:

1 or 2 tablespoons vegetable oil, bacon drippings, or fat from ham or spareribs

Taste for **salt.**

VARIATIONS:

Omit caraway seeds and cook ½ cup crushed pineapple with sauerkraut. Use or omit fat.

Pan-broil ham; heat sauerkraut quickly in same utensil without added moisture.

Cook sauerkraut with an equal amount of shredded green or purple cabbage.

Sauerkraut with apples: Omit or use caraway seeds; add 2 diced unpeeled red apples, 1 tablespoon ham or bacon drippings, 1 teaspoon dark molasses.

Sauerkraut with tomatoes: Sauté in vegetable oil 1 each chopped onion and celery stalk; add ½ cup canned or diced fresh tomato; heat to boiling, and stir in sauerkraut. Cut 2 or 3 wieners into ½-inch pieces and add 2 minutes before serving.

Sauerkraut with wieners: Prepare sauerkraut as in basic recipe, laying wieners on top; serve as soon as heated through.

Use yellow, or golden ball, turnips in preference to white turnips. After they are washed and wiped dry, try not to touch them with water.

CRISP SHREDDED TURNIPS

Shred **4 to 6 chilled unpeeled turnips** and put immediately into:

2 tablespoons hot top milk

Stir well, cover utensil, and cook 5 minutes; season with:

½ teaspoon salt   **dash of cayenne**
freshly ground black peppercorns

Serve while slightly crisp.

VARIATIONS:

Salt shredded turnips and cook in oiled hot casserole in preheated oven 6 to 8 minutes; or sauté with ½ clove garlic; discard garlic; salt.

Baked turnips: Select whole baby turnips or flat ones no more than 1½ inches thick; toss or brush with oil and heat rapidly by steaming 5 minutes or by putting under broiler for 10 minutes; bake until tender, or about 10 to 15 minutes. Serve like baked potatoes.

Creamed turnips: Cut unpeeled turnips into quarters; simmer in ¾ cup top milk seasoned with crushed white peppercorns until almost tender, or about 15 minutes; add thickening for cream sauce, dash of nutmeg.

Mashed turnips: Cut unpeeled turnips into 4 to 6 wedges each and steam in ½ cup top milk until tender; pass through hot ricer or food mill; season with **partially hardened margarine or butter, salt, pepper, and milk** left from cooking them.

Sautéed turnips: Slice **4 to 6 chilled unpeeled turnips;** sauté in vege· table oil over low heat; cover utensil, turn frequently, and cook 8 to 10 minutes; season with ½ **teaspoon salt and dash of paprika;** or sauté sliced turnips with carrots, kohlrabi, onions, green peppers, pimentos, rutabagas, or potatoes. In combining vegetables, those which require a longer cooking time should be cut into thinner slices than others.

Scalloped turnips: Use slicer and cut chilled unpeeled turnips paper thin; cook in casserole in ½ **cup hot milk** seasoned with ½ **teaspoon salt and** ¼ **teaspoon crushed black peppercorns;** sprinkle with **crumbs, shredded cheese, paprika;** cover casserole and bake in preheated oven at 400° F. for 10 to 15 minutes, or until just tender.

Steamed turnips: Steam whole unpeeled turnips 10 to 18 minutes, or until tender; cut petal-fashion and season with **salt, paprika, oil or** French dressing, mayonnaise, or ⅓ **cup grated cheese.**

Respect the Potato

Since millions of people eat potatoes daily, it is especially important to form habits of cooking them so that their nutrients are retained. Aside from calories, the contribution white potatoes can make to health, if allowed to do so, is the cumulative amount of vitamin C and iron they offer, although they contain other vitamins and minerals as well. A medium-size potato supplies an average of 33 milligrams of vitamin C, or approximately the amount in a glass of tomato juice, and 1.5 milligrams of iron, the amount in an egg. During the winter months, potatoes may be the chief source of these nutrients for many families. Yet both iron and vitamin C are often extracted or thrown away before the potatoes reach the table.

View critically, for example, the atrocious but common method of preparing mashed potatoes for Sunday dinner. The potatoes are often peeled in the early morning and left swimming in water at room temperature while the family goes to church. This water is usually poured off and more water is added before the potatoes are put on to boil; this water is also thrown away. Yet even unpeeled potatoes have been found to lose 83 per cent of their iron and 100 per cent of their vitamin C if boiled 20 minutes.

If you wish to retain the nutritive value, prepare potatoes like any other fresh vegetable which contains iron and vitamin C. Scrub them thoroughly with a brush and dry them immediately. If they are to be peeled, sliced, diced, or grated, chill them in advance to inhibit enzyme action when the cut surface is exposed to the air; thus discoloration and loss of vitamin C are prevented. If old potatoes need to be freshened, put them into the refrigerator pan for 24 hours; keep enough crisped potatoes ahead for one or two meals. When potatoes must be cut in advance of cooking, put them in a plastic bag in the refrigerator without added moisture. Avoid peeling them for most uses. Heat them as quickly as possible, and use all the liquid in which they have been cooked.

Mashed potatoes prepared by steaming them unpeeled and then passing them through a hot ricer or food mill have far more flavor than those which have been peeled and boiled. When equipment for waterless cooking is available, potatoes can be baked on top of the range more easily and economically and with less loss of nutrients than in an oven.

To avoid needless destruction of food value, do not cook potatoes twice except to use leftovers. Potatoes to be French-fried or pan-fried, for example, should be uncooked.

Although sweet potatoes and yams are not rich in vitamin C or iron, they supply from 3500 to 5000 units of vitamin A per serving. When they are available, use them interchangeably with white potatoes.

BAKED POTATOES

There are three methods of baking potatoes, of which the slow but customary oven method is the least desirable.

Select 4 to 6 medium-size potatoes, preferably long slender ones; scrub and dry them; brush surfaces with oil.

Method I: Put potatoes into a preheated utensil designed for waterless cooking; cover utensil, keep heat moderate for 6 minutes, then set over simmer burner until potatoes are tender, or 20 to 30 minutes; set lid of utensil to one side during the last 5 minutes of baking.

Method II: Set oiled potatoes under the broiler near moderate heat for 10 to 15 minutes, turning to heat all sides; finish baking in moderate oven at 350° F. for 15 to 20 minutes.

Method III: Place in hot oven at 425° F. and bake until tender, or 40 to 45 minutes.

Remove from utensil or oven and make two crosswise gashes on top of each potato; pinch to open gashes, insert a piece of **partially hardened margarine or butter** in each potato, sprinkle with **salt, freshly ground peppercorns, and paprika.** Serve at once.

VARIATIONS:

Bake large potatoes until nearly tender; split lengthwise and spread each half with 1 teaspoon prepared mustard; sprinkle with salt, Worcestershire, 1 teaspoon grated onion, whole-wheat-bread crumbs, chopped leftover bacon or grated cheese; finish baking until tender.

Baked new potatoes: Place small new unpeeled potatoes in waterless-cooking utensil or flat baking dish; bake over direct heat or in oven until tender, or from 15 to 25 minutes; shake utensil twice during baking to rotate potatoes.

Baked sweet potatoes or yams: Prepare and bake by any method suggested in basic recipe; yams cook in about half the time required for white or sweet potatoes.

Glazed sweet potatoes or yams: Bake or steam unpeeled sweet potatoes or yams until nearly tender; cut in half lengthwise, place in flat baking dish; brush with **dark molasses,** dot with **partially hardened margarine or butter;** bake until tender in moderate oven.

Stuffed sweet potatoes or yams: Cut 4 hot baked sweet potatoes or yams in half lengthwise; salt, fluff pulp with a fork, mix in 2 tablespoons **top milk or drained crushed pineapple;** garnish with **paprika,** dot with **partially hardened margarine or butter,** reheat under broiler.

When white potatoes are stuffed immediately after being baked, oxygen is whipped into them; the baking time is needlessly prolonged, and vitamin C has little chance of escaping destruction. Use stuffed potatoes largely as a means of making leftover baked potatoes interesting. If the pulp is chilled before being mashed, little loss of vitamin C occurs except that destroyed during reheating.

STUFFED WHITE POTATOES

Cut in half lengthwise:

2 or more baked potatoes

Scoop out pulp, mash, and mix with:

½ cup shredded yellow cheese ½ teaspoon salt
4 tablespoons top milk freshly ground peppercorns
2 tablespoons chopped parsley

Pack mixture into skins; sprinkle with paprika and put in hot oven at 400° F. for 10 minutes.

VARIATIONS:

Stuff leftover baked potatoes; freeze and serve later.

Mix with potato pulp any one or more of the following: 1 minced clove garlic; 1 or 2 teaspoons caraway seeds; 1 teaspoon Worcestershire; 1 grated onion or finely chopped green-onion tops; chopped and lightly sautéed celery, mushrooms, or green peppers; sliced stuffed olives; anchovies; diced canned pimento; 2 teaspoons minced fresh dill or dill seeds; diced leftover vegetables or meat; or ¼ cup chopped almonds.

Omit milk and cheese and add 2 tablespoons mayonnaise; combine with potato pulp any leftover creamed ham, chicken, dried beef, fish, or vegetables.

Hash-browned potatoes: Dice leftover white or sweet potatoes, preferably unpeeled; season with salt and pepper; sauté quickly in vegetable oil or bacon drippings; add chives, minced green-onion tops, or diced leftover meat or other vegetables.

Leftover baked sweet potatoes or yams: Cut leftover sweet potatoes or yams lengthwise into slices and brush with dark molasses; place in alternate layers in shallow oiled baking dish with pineapple slices or thick applesauce; sprinkle applesauce lightly with grated lemon rind, nutmeg, or cinnamon; bake in moderate oven until heated through.

The following recipe is a substitute for French-fried potatoes. It requires little fat and is easier than French frying, although the end result is much the same.

OVEN "FRENCH FRIES"

Cut into ⅓-inch sticks:

3 or 4 chilled unpeeled potatoes

Toss in salad bowl with:

1 or 2 tablespoons vegetable oil

If a rich brown color is desired, sprinkle generously with paprika before tossing.

Place on oiled baking sheet and put in hot oven at 450° F. until brown, or about 8 minutes; lower heat and cook until potatoes are tender; sprinkle with:

½ teaspoon salt

VARIATIONS:

Instead of baking, cook under broiler; turn once.

Baked or broiled sweet potatoes or yams: Cut chilled unpeeled sweet potatoes or yams lengthwise into ⅓-inch slices; brush top surface with oil and bake or broil as in basic recipe; season with **salt and grated orange rind.** Or after cooking a few minutes, sprinkle with **brown sugar** or brush with **dark molasses.**

With bananas: When slices of sweet potatoes or yams are almost tender, cut **bananas** in two lengthwise, then in half, and put one section of banana on each slice of potato; brush with **molasses** and cook until well browned.

Broiled yams on skewers: Cut partly cooked yams into ¾-inch cubes; arrange on metal skewers with cubes of raw apple; brush with oil and broil on oiled baking sheet until almost tender; on ends of skewers put **cubes of baked ham, fresh or leftover lamb, or pineapple;** continue broiling with low heat until potatoes are tender.

CREAMED WHITE POTATOES

Leave small new potatoes whole; cut chilled large ones into 1-inch sections or cubes.

Heat to simmering:

¾ cup top milk

Add and stir:

8 or 10 new potatoes or 3 or 4 large ones, preferably unpeeled

Cover utensil and simmer until potatoes are almost tender, or about 12 minutes; add:

2 tablespoons whole-wheat flour   ½ teaspoon salt
  beaten with ½ cup milk   freshly ground peppercorns

Simmer 10 minutes longer.
Serve sprinkled with **paprika**.

VARIATIONS:

Add to milk any one or more of the following: ½ to 2 teaspoons caraway, dill, or celery seeds; grated onion; a pinch of thyme or basil; or season with ½ teaspoon paprika, 1 teaspoon Worcestershire, 5 drops Tabasco, or minced fresh dill or chives.

Omit cream sauce and simmer potatoes in ½ cup milk; garnish with chopped parsley and paprika; or cook potatoes in chicken stock instead of milk; add pinch of sage.

Instead of plain cream sauce, use dill, caraway, pimento, egg, cheese, piquant, mock Hollandaise, or other cream sauce (pp. 135–138).

With peas: Add 1 or 2 cups fresh peas after thickening has been added.

AMERICAN FRIED POTATOES

Slice thin:

4 to 6 chilled unpeeled white potatoes

Heat:

3 or 4 tablespoons vegetable oil or partially hardened margarine

Drop potatoes into fat; fry over moderate heat, turning frequently; add:

½ to ¾ teaspoon salt   **freshly ground black peppercorns**

Cook until tender and well browned, or about 15 minutes.

VARIATIONS:

Brown 1 clove garlic in fat and discard before adding potatoes; fry with potatoes 1 or 2 sliced dry onions or green onions with tops; or season with ¼ teaspoon celery salt or 1 or 2 teaspoons caraway seeds.

Instead of white potatoes slice chilled unpeeled sweet potatoes and fry as in basic recipe; keep heat moderate to prevent shrinking. Fry in fat left from ham or pork chops when available. Vary by frying diced apples with sweet potatoes; or cut sweet potatoes lengthwise into ½-inch slices and fry with pineapple slices or rings of cored unpeeled red apple.

Fried leftover potatoes: Slice potatoes; keep heat high and cook the shortest time necessary for browning; sprinkle with **parsley.**

Fried whole potatoes: Use small new white potatoes; leave unpeeled; shake utensil during frying to keep potatoes well greased; cook 8 to 15 minutes; when tender, **salt,** and add **1 tablespoon each chopped chives, parsley, or mixed fresh herbs,** such as tarragon, basil, marjoram, sage.

Potato patty shells: Fry shredded white or sweet potatoes without browning until almost tender; arrange against sides and on bottom of deep greased muffin pans, pressing firmly; bake in hot oven at 450° F. for 10 minutes; serve filled with creamed peas, spinach, or other vegetables or with creamed shrimps, chicken, or ham.

Potatoes to be served with a roast: When a roast is cooked at low temperature, potatoes, carrots, and onions baked around it require almost 2 hours to become tender; as a substitute, cut **unpeeled potatoes and carrots** in half lengthwise and fry with **whole peeled onions** in ¼ **cup or more of fat** dipped from the dripping pan; keep heat moderate and turn as surface browns; cook with utensil covered 20 to 25 minutes; sprinkle with **salt,** pepper, paprika; serve around roast.

Spanish-fried potatoes: Fry with white potatoes **1 minced clove garlic, 1 each chopped bell pepper and onion;** ½ **cup cooked diced ham** may be added.

FRENCH-FRIED POTATOES

Chill **3 or 4 large potatoes** thoroughly; do not peel.
Heat to 360° F., using cooking thermometer:

2 to 3 cups vegetable oil, bacon drippings, lard, or cooking fat

If oil is used, add contents of a 100-unit capsule of vitamin E to prevent oxidation (p. 157). Put wire basket in oil to heat; when thermometer reading is about 340° F., cut unpeeled potatoes into sticks ⅓ inch thick; lay on heated basket and put in hot fat; watch thermometer carefully and do not allow temperature to exceed 325° F. after the potatoes are added; if fat becomes too hot, potatoes shrivel.

Fry until golden brown, or 8 to 10 minutes; drain on absorbent paper, sprinkle with salt, and serve immediately.

VARIATIONS:

Cut potatoes into shoestrings, slices, or lattice slices; fry until brown.

Use whole unpeeled new potatoes the size of large marbles; fry until tender, or about 7 minutes; drain, salt, and sprinkle with parsley.

Potato chips: Using slicer, cut chilled unpeeled white or sweet potatoes into extremely thin slices; fry at 360° F. until brown, or 3 to 5 minutes; drain on paper, salt. Chips of sweet potatoes are delicious, especially if served hot.

MASHED POTATOES

Scrub, chill, and cut into pieces 1 inch thick:

3 to 5 unpeeled potatoes

Drop into:

½ cup hot top milk seasoned with   ¼ teaspoon crushed peppercorns

Cover utensil and simmer 10 to 15 minutes, or until tender.

Meanwhile heat ricer, colander, or food mill by setting it on utensil holding potatoes; press potatoes through ricer or food mill as soon as they are tender.

Add:

½ to ¾ teaspoon salt	top milk left from steaming
2 tablespoons partially hardened margarine or butter	¼ cup cream

Beat vigorously, taste for seasonings, and serve at once.

VARIATIONS:

Instead of white potatoes use sweet potatoes, yams, or peeled banana squash or rutabagas.

Dice potatoes into ¼-inch cubes without peeling them. Cook and season as in basic recipe. Mash. The peeling adds to the flavor and does not detract too much from the appearance.

Cook and mash together equal quantities of potatoes and rutabagas or winter squash; cut squash or rutabagas into smaller pieces than potatoes; season as in basic recipe.

Steam whole unpeeled potatoes on rack above boiling water or cook without added moisture in waterless-cooking utensil; proceed as in basic recipe.

If equipment with a tight-fitting lid is not available, simmer potatoes until tender in enough hot milk to cover; drain milk into a wide-mouthed jar and save.

MASHED POTATO PATTIES

Stir into 1 or 2 cups leftover mashed potatoes:

2 tablespoons chopped parsley

Make into patties and roll in:

wheat germ, whole-wheat-bread crumbs, or whole-wheat flour

Heat grill and brush with vegetable oil or partially hardened margarine. Brown patties quickly on both sides, cooking only 6 to 8 minutes.

VARIATIONS:

See **Shepherd's pie**, p. 214.

Add leftover flaked fish or canned salmon or clams with 1 teaspoon dill seeds, or diced leftover ham, chicken, or other meat with a pinch each of savory and basil.

Add to mashed potatoes ½ cup shredded cheese and mix well; while patties are browning, sauté 1 chopped onion; put browned patties on serving platter, heat with onion 1 cup tomato purée; salt and serve over patties.

Potato puffs: Beat 1½ cups leftover mashed potatoes with 1 egg, ¼ cup powdered milk, ½ teaspoon salt, 3 diced pimentos; drop onto flat oiled baking dish, sprinkle with cheese and paprika, and bake at 350° F. for 15 minutes. Vary by adding flaked salmon or other fish or diced leftover meat, 1 to 3 teaspoons each chopped onion and fresh dill or 1 teaspoon dill seeds.

Fried potato puffs: Combine ingredients, drop onto hot oiled grill, and brown on both sides.

In most potato casserole dishes, the sliced or diced potatoes are placed in a cold casserole, cold liquid is added, and the potatoes are baked uncovered for an hour or more; so much surface is exposed to oxygen and the dry heat penetrates so slowly that vitamin C is largely destroyed. If you do not have a heat-resistant casserole which can be used on top of the range, have the liquid hot before adding the potatoes and keep the casserole covered throughout most of the baking time.

SCALLOPED POTATOES

Combine in casserole and heat to simmering over direct heat or in moderate oven:

1 cup top milk	¼ teaspoon crushed white pepper-
¾ teaspoon salt	corns

Slice thin and dust with 2 tablespoons whole-wheat flour:

3 cups chilled unpeeled potatoes

Add potatoes to hot milk; cover casserole and simmer over direct heat 10 to 15 minutes; or bake in moderate oven at 350° F. for 20 minutes; remove cover, sprinkle with wheat germ or whole-wheat-bread crumbs and paprika; brown.

VARIATIONS:

If oven is to be used, omit flour and stir potatoes into 1 cup hot cream sauce.

Before browning potatoes, sprinkle top with ½ cup shredded cheese; add or omit crumbs.

Instead of milk, cook potatoes in ¾ cup chicken stock seasoned with a pinch of sage, or ¾ cup ham stock seasoned with 1 teaspoon dill or caraway seeds; thicken sauce.

Omit 1 cup of potatoes and use 1 cup thinly sliced carrots, turnips, kohlrabi, onions, celery root, or salsify.

Add 2 tablespoons chopped parsley or bell pepper.

Cook potatoes in 1 cup tomatoes instead of milk; add 1 chopped onion, bell pepper, or celery stalk, 1 minced clove garlic, 2 tablespoons vegetable oil, a pinch of basil. Vary by adding diced leftover meat, flaked fish, or crisp bacon cut to bits before putting casserole under broiler.

Omit flour and salt; cook white or sweet potatoes in 1 can condensed mushroom soup diluted with ¼ cup milk; add peppercorns, ¼ teaspoon paprika.

Sweet potato or yam casserole: Heat in casserole ¾ **cup pineapple juice, 2 tablespoons dark molasses;** add **unpeeled sweet potatoes or yams** cut lengthwise into ⅓-inch slices; cover casserole; simmer over direct heat or bake in moderate oven 15 to 20 minutes until almost tender; cover with **pineapple slices,** dot with **partially hardened margarine or ham or bacon drippings,** and brown under broiler. Vary by broiling thin slices of ham over sliced pineapple.

Sweet potatoes or yams with apples: Alternate **sliced sweet potatoes and thinly sliced apples** in an oiled heat-resistant casserole; sprinkle layers with **salt, cinnamon, grated lemon rind;** add 2 tablespoons each **hot water and bacon drippings, margarine, or butter;** simmer over direct heat until tender, or about 15 minutes. Brown top under broiler.

Potato salad should be served, not as a substitute for a salad, but as a cooked vegetable. The nutrients it supplies are entirely different from those furnished by green leaves and uncooked fruits and vegetables. The same is true of other so-called salads made of cooked vegetables.

AMERICAN POTATO SALAD

Quarter and steam until tender in or above a small amount of water:

4 to 6 unpeeled potatoes

Chill quickly, peel, and slice; combine and add:

⅓ cup vinegar   1 chopped onion
⅓ cup water left from steaming   ½ teaspoon freshly ground black
¾ teaspoon salt   peppercorns

Let stand until moisture is absorbed, stirring 2 or 3 times; add:

½ cup chopped celery   ¼ cup oil or ½ cup mayonnaise
2 to 4 tablespoons chopped parsley   or cooked dressing

Mix well, let stand in refrigerator until ready to serve, and turn onto nest of **lettuce or watercress.**

VARIATIONS:
Add any one or more of the following: 1 diced red unpeeled apple; 1 or 2 chopped bell peppers or pimentos; 2 or 3 sliced hard-cooked eggs; 2 or 3 tablespoons sliced stuffed olives; 1 diced cucumber; 1 minced clove garlic; 1 tablespoon chives or minced fresh dill **or** 1 or 2 teaspoons dill or caraway seeds.

GERMAN POTATO SALAD

Quarter and steam in jackets:

4 or 5 medium-sized potatoes

Meanwhile, sauté until crisp:

6 strips bacon

Remove bacon, drain off all except 3 or 4 tablespoons drippings; add and bring to simmering:

½ cup cider vinegar   ¼ cup finely shredded onion
½ cup or more water left from   2 tablespoons sugar
   steaming potatoes   1 teaspoon salt

Peel and slice potatoes; put hot potatoes into vinegar mixture and stir until they appear to be glazed; they should not be dry.

Crumble bacon and stir part into salad; sprinkle remainder over top. Let stand several hours or overnight. Reheat or serve chilled.

VARIATIONS:

Add to salad or put over top 2 or 3 sliced hard-cooked eggs or 2 tablespoons finely chopped parsley.

One of the most delightful ways of preparing potatoes is to shred and quick-cook them. So much surface is exposed that if high heat is used, a large proportion of the sugar caramelizes, making the taste delicious. Potatoes prepared in this way should take the place of the customarily overcooked hash-browned potatoes.

QUICK HASH-BROWNED POTATOES

Heat:

4 to 6 tablespoons vegetable oil or partially hardened margarine

Quickly shred directly into hot fat:

4 thoroughly chilled unpeeled potatoes

Keep heat high and turn frequently; cook until golden brown, or about 5 to 8 minutes. Add:

½ teaspoon salt   **dash of paprika or cayenne**

VARIATIONS:

Cook 1 or 2 shredded onions with potatoes.

Stir in any one of the following a few minutes before serving: chopped chives, parsley, fresh dill, green-onion tops, a few minced leaves of fresh marjoram, orégano, or sage; celery or onion salt.

Baked shredded potatoes: When oven is being used, put shredded potatoes into an oiled preheated casserole; add **½ teaspoon salt and freshly ground black peppercorns;** cover and bake 7 to 10 minutes. Vary by combining potatoes with an equal amount of **shredded turnips,**

carrots, parsnips, or rutabagas, or add 1 grated onion or finely chopped bell pepper, pimento, or celery; potatoes may be sprinkled with ½ cup shredded cheese.

Creamed shredded potatoes: Heat to simmering 1 cup cream sauce, ¾ teaspoon salt; 6 minutes before time to serve, stir in 2 cups shredded raw potatoes; cover utensil and simmer; garnish with chopped parsley or chives and paprika. Vary by using any of the following sauces: caraway, celery, mustard, cheese, curry, dill, mushroom, olive, onion, or pimento (pp. 136–137).

Potato pancakes: Grate or shred fine 4 unpeeled chilled potatoes and 1 onion; add 1 tablespoon whole-wheat flour, 1 teaspoon salt; drop from spoon into 1 tablespoon hot oil or partially hardened margarine; brown quickly on both sides. Serve with applesauce.

With vegetables: Make pancakes of equal amounts of potatoes and turnips, carrots, parsnips, or rutabagas. Serve with chopped parsley.

STEAMED POTATOES

Leave small unpeeled potatoes whole and cut large ones into halves lengthwise; drop into:

¼ cup boiling water

Cover utensil and cook 12 to 18 minutes, or until tender.

Serve with skins on or remove skins; if peeled before serving, sprinkle with ½ teaspoon salt, parsley, and freshly ground black peppercorns.

VARIATIONS:

If utensil does not distribute heat, steam potatoes on a rack above water.

Peel steamed potatoes; combine and heat 2 tablespoons each oil, chopped chives and chopped parsley, 3 tablespoons lemon juice, ½ teaspoon salt, freshly ground black peppercorns; pour sauce over steamed potatoes.

Peel and sprinkle over hot potatoes 1 teaspoon chopped fresh orégano, thyme, and/or basil or dill.

Peel steamed potatoes and sprinkle with ½ cup grated cheese; add seasonings as in basic recipe.

Leftover steamed potatoes: Peel and slice cold steamed potatoes; sauté quickly in bacon drippings with 1 grated onion; add salt, freshly

ground peppercorns, 1 tablespoon each chopped bell pepper and parsley. Vary by heating in ½ cup top milk or well-seasoned leftover gravy.

Potato Substitutes Lend Variety

There are a number of foods which may be substituted for potatoes in that they supply approximately the same number of
calories per serving: dry beans, dry peas, lentils, rice, corn, whole
buckwheat, unground wheat, bananas, and the more solid varieties of squash. None of these foods should be served with potatoes, not because the combination is harmful but because they
are similar to potatoes in composition. They do not supply the
same vitamins and minerals which could be obtained from the
less starchy vegetables. The higher protein furnished by beans,
lentils, peas, and grains than that supplied by potatoes is healthful.

Several vegetables not listed with the following recipes, such as
parsnips, rutabagas, and almost any fried vegetable, have approximately the same calorie content as potatoes and may be substituted for them. Foods prepared as meat extenders, such as dry
beans, buckwheat, macaroni, spaghetti, rice, and unground wheat,
can serve as a substitute for both meat and potatoes. When these
foods are to be served in addition to meat, or purely as a substitute for potatoes, prepare them by the recipes given on pages
172 to 196, omitting the meats suggested.

SAUTÉED BANANAS

Whenever possible, sauté bananas on a grill which has been used for
pan-broiling ham, pork chops, or pork sausage; otherwise use 1 tablespoon bacon drippings or oil seasoned with a small amount of smoke-
flavoring.

Remove skins from:

4 large firm bananas

Put on hot grill; keep heat high and turn as each side is browned;
when golden on all sides, or in about 6 minutes, sprinkle with salt.
Serve with meat.

VARIATIONS:

Choose red bananas or plantains when available; cut plantains in half lengthwise and crosswise; after browning, cook 10 to 12 minutes with the utensil covered.

Baked bananas: Wrap each banana in a **strip of partially cooked bacon** or a thin **slice of boiled ham;** put in shallow baking dish and bake in hot oven at 425° F. about 8 minutes, or until bacon or ham is light brown. If bacon is used, pan-broil it first with extremely low heat without browning.

Bananas fried in batter: Cut bananas in ¾-inch pieces and drop into **batter** (p. 158); fry in 4 tablespoons hot fat or French-fry at 350° F. until golden brown. Serve with lemon slices.

Bananas with cheese: Bake, sauté, or broil bananas and sprinkle with **Parmesan cheese or grated American or pimento cheese;** vary by rolling in **wheat germ or crumbs and grated cheese** before broiling or baking.

Broiled bananas: Put bananas on oiled baking sheet; sprinkle with **paprika;** set 2 inches from broiler under high heat until lightly browned, or for about 2 minutes; turn and brown on all sides; **salt.**

Glazed bananas: Brush bananas with **dark molasses;** broil or bake; sprinkle lightly with **salt and cinnamon or nutmeg** and serve with lemon slices.

FRIED APPLES

Use tart, slightly green apples, preferably "Early Transparents"; core and slice or dice the pulp from:

6 to 8 chilled unpeeled apples

Put into frying pan with:

2 tablespoons partially hardened margarine or butter

Keep heat high, turn apples frequently, and brown well; if they are not tender by the time they are browned, cover utensil and steam until tender. Add 5 minutes before taking up:

¼ cup brown sugar (optional)   ⅛ teaspoon salt

Serve with meat.

VARIATIONS:

Core and cut large apples into rings ⅓ inch thick; brown on both sides; sprinkle lightly with sugar and nutmeg. Serve with ham or pork.

Hulled barley is not refined and has a delicious flavor in comparison with pearl barley, which is mostly starch. Either barley or millet may be used in soups and casseroles or as a substitute for rice or potatoes.

HULLED BARLEY OR MILLET

Bring to boiling:

2 cups beef bouillon

Add so slowly that boiling does not stop:

1 cup hulled barley or millet   **1 teaspoon salt**

Reheat to boiling, lower temperature, and simmer 15 minutes; add:

½ cup shredded onion
¼ cup finely chopped parsley
freshly ground black peppercorns

2 tablespoons partially hardened margarine or butter

Simmer 5 minutes longer. Serve instead of rice or potatoes.

VARIATIONS:

Omit salt; use 2 cups water and 2 to 4 beef or chicken bouillon cubes.

Stir in ½ cup slivered almonds or pine nuts. Sprinkle more nuts over top before serving.

Use heat-resistant casserole; simmer over direct heat 15 minutes, add other ingredients and bake 20 minutes at 350° F.

Add ¼ to ½ teaspoon thyme, sage, basil, or rosemary.

Instead of barley or millet use buckwheat groats or cracked wheat; cook buckwheat 15 minutes, cracked wheat 45 minutes.

RED BEANS MEXICAN STYLE

Wash quickly without soaking:

1½ cups dry red beans

Heat to boiling:

2½ to 3 cups vegetable-cooking water, soup stock, or diluted canned consommé

Add beans slowly to rapidly boiling liquid; reduce heat and simmer until beans are tender, or about 2 to 2½ hours, when they should be almost dry.

Add 15 minutes before serving:

1 finely chopped dry onion or 2 green onions and tops	½ teaspoon cumin seeds
1 minced clove garlic	2 or 3 tablespoons vegetable oil
	1 teaspoon salt

Immediately before serving add:

¼ cup chopped parsley

VARIATIONS:

Add chopped raw onion and 1 chopped bell pepper or fresh chili pepper just before serving.

If fresh red beans are used, follow same procedure but shorten cooking time to 30 or 40 minutes.

Omit cumin seeds and add ½ teaspoon rosemary, orégano, or marjoram.

Omit oil and add 1 or 2 slices of diced bacon or salt pork when beans are almost tender; or use bacon drippings instead of oil.

Before serving add 2 tablespoons cider vinegar or lemon juice or ½ cup dry wine.

Instead of kidney beans use dry or fresh lima beans, black or pink beans, pinto beans, or chick peas, known in the West as garbanzo beans.

Buckwheat, often sold as buckwheat groats, has a delightful flavor and is well liked by almost everyone who tastes it. It is a good source of the B vitamins. The more highly seasoned recipes are perhaps best for introducing it, but the simple ones soon become favorites. If any is left over, it may be served as a cereal.

STEAMED BUCKWHEAT GROATS

Heat to boiling:

2 cups soup stock, vegetable-cooking water, or consommé

Add so slowly that boiling does not stop:

1 cup unwashed whole buckwheat   1 teaspoon salt

Boil rapidly 1 minute; cover utensil, lower heat, and simmer 15 minutes; remove lid of utensil and let steam escape, so that each grain is fluffy and separate.

Serve with partially hardened margarine or butter.

VARIATIONS:

If water is used, add 2 chicken or beef bouillon cubes; salt to taste.

Sauté in 2 tablespoons oil 1 each chopped onion and bell pepper, 1 minced clove garlic; add liquid and buckwheat; proceed as in basic recipe. Or add 1 cup slivered almonds just before serving.

Instead of buckwheat use 1 cup lentils, hulled barley, whole millet, or cracked wheat; simmer 30 minutes, or until tender; season as basic recipe or any variations.

Just before serving add 2 diced canned pimentos and 1 can mushrooms, or add diced leftover vegetables in time to heat through.

Corn on the cob is a delightful but long mistreated vegetable. Ideally it should be brought from the garden immediately before time to cook it. If bought at the market, it should be kept in the coldest part of the refrigerator and not husked until just before cooking. When the husks are removed, enzymes quickly change much sugar to starch, causing loss of flavor. It should be washed quickly in running water and dried immediately to prevent the sugars from being dissolved out. Corn is almost invariably overcooked. It becomes tough if heated to boiling temperature longer than 2 or 3 minutes. Allow it only to heat through; the less it is cooked after it is hot, the more delightful its flavor

Although the popular method of cooking corn on the cob seems to be to wrap it in aluminum foil, it is difficult to tell whether such corn is still raw or overcooked.

CORN ON THE COB

Take off outer husks, leaving 1 or 2 layers to prevent corn from drying out during cooking. Fold these husks back, remove silks, bad spots, and wash quickly.

Dry immediately, spread with **butter or partially hardened margarine**, and sprinkle with **salt and pepper**.

Replace husks and put ears into hot oven at 400° F.; roast 10 to 12 minutes, or until just heated through.

Remove husks before serving if corn is to be eaten immediately; leave husks on second servings.

VARIATIONS:

Roast no longer than 8 minutes if all husks are removed.

If frozen corn on the cob is used, thaw completely at room temperature before putting it on to cook; steam on rack above water.

Put bed of husks in bottom of waterless-cooking utensil; husk corn, put into preheated utensil, and cook without added moisture 6 to 8 minutes.

Broiled corn: Prepare corn as in basic recipe, leaving 1 or 2 layers of husks on cob; set on broiling rack or baking sheet under moderate heat; broil 4 to 5 minutes on each side if corn is chilled, or less if warm.

Leftover corn: Hold cob upright and cut downward, being careful not to cut too near cob; scrape cob with blunt edge of knife; use corn in salad, reheat to simmering in a little top milk, or add to string beans, carrots, peas, or other vegetables just before serving.

Steamed corn: Leave on 1 or 2 layers of husks so that condensed steam cannot touch corn during cooking; set on a rack above rapidly boiling water; cover utensil and steam 4 to 6 minutes; if corn is husked, steam only 3 to 5 minutes; serve immediately.

If corn must be cut from the cob before time to cook it, put it into the refrigerator immediately and keep near freezing unit. Since the corn germ, containing the greatest nutritive value, is at the base of each kernel, the cob should be scraped thoroughly after the corn is cut.

Canned or dried corn may be prepared by any of the following recipes. Dried corn should be soaked overnight in milk, 1 cup milk being used for each cup corn; it should be heated in the same milk.

CORN COOKED IN MILK

Quickly cut from cob, scraping cob with knife to get fluid and corn germ from base of kernels:

2 cups corn

Keep chilled until 3 minutes before serving; then add to:

⅓ cup simmering top milk

Stir, heat rapidly to simmering; cover utensil, lower heat, simmer 2 minutes; add:

½ teaspoon salt   **freshly ground white peppercorns**

VARIATIONS:

If frozen corn is used, put into hot milk while still frozen; add ½ teaspoon sugar. Serve as soon as heated through.

Corn baked in milk: When oven is being used, preheat casserole with 2 tablespoons top milk; add 2 cups corn and ½ teaspoon each salt and sugar; cover casserole and heat in moderate oven 5 to 8 minutes.

With cheese: Put corn, top milk, and seasonings into flat preheated baking dish and cover with **grated cheese;** heat in oven until cheese is melted, or about 8 to 10 minutes.

Corn fritters: Stir 1 cup canned corn and liquid or fresh or thawed frozen corn with 2 egg yolks; combine in sifter ½ cup whole-wheat flour, ¼ cup powdered milk, 1 teaspoon salt, ⅛ teaspoon paprika; sift into eggs and corn; fold in 2 stiffly beaten egg whites; drop from teaspoon into deep fat at 350° F. and fry until delicately brown, or about 5 minutes; drain on paper towels. Or fry in shallow fat as patties.

Corn and pepper fritters: Add to fritter batter 1 **finely diced** stalk celery, 1 chopped chilled bell pepper or 3 tablespoons canned or fresh pimento; or add **any leftover vegetables,** such as peas or carrots. Vary by frying in shallow fat.

Corn patties: Beat well 1 egg, ½ cup each powdered milk and fresh milk, ⅛ teaspoon each paprika and dry mustard; add ½ cup wheat germ, 1 cup corn, ½ teaspoon salt; drop from teaspoon onto hot grill and sauté until brown on both sides.

Corn pudding: Heat to simmering in heat-resistant casserole 1½ cups fresh milk; meanwhile beat together 3 eggs, ½ cup each fresh milk and powdered milk, 1¼ teaspoons salt, ¼ teaspoon crushed black peppercorns; stir into milk and add 2 cups fresh, frozen, or canned corn; drain liquid from canned corn and use instead of part of the milk. Bake uncovered in slow oven at 325° F. for 35 minutes, or until firm.

Corn soufflé: Add 2 cups fresh, canned, or frozen corn to plain soufflé (p. 194).

Creamed corn: Prepare 1 cup medium cream sauce and add ½ teaspoon salt, ¼ teaspoon crushed white peppercorns, 2 cups fresh or frozen and thawed corn; stir, cover utensil, and simmer 3 minutes, or until heated through. Drain juice from canned corn, and use in making sauce.

Scalloped corn: Prepare creamed corn in casserole; cover with ⅓ cup wheat germ and ¾ cup grated American cheese; garnish with paprika, and let cheese melt in oven or under broiler.

Smothered corn: In utensil which retains heat, melt 1 tablespoon partially hardened margarine or butter; add 2 cups fresh corn, stir, cover utensil, and let stand until corn is heated through, or 5 to 7 minutes.

Lentils contain 25 per cent protein, cook quickly, are inexpensive, and are so similar in flavor and texture to cooked dry beans that they are usually enjoyed the first time they are eaten. They deserve greater popularity than they have thus far received in America.

SWEET-SOUR LENTILS

Heat to boiling:

2 cups vegetable-cooking water,   1 crushed bay leaf
    soup stock, or water with 2 to   ½ to 1 teaspoon salt
    4 chicken or beef bouillon cubes

Add so slowly that boiling does not stop:

1 cup washed lentils

Lower heat and simmer 25 minutes; add:

1 minced clove garlic   **2 tablespoons each oil, vinegar,**
dash of nutmeg or cloves   **and brown sugar**

Stir and cook 5 minutes longer, or until quite tender.

VARIATIONS:

Instead of lentils, use hulled barley or millet, buckwheat groats, or cracked wheat.

Omit sugar, oil, and vinegar; pan-broil 2 strips bacon until crisp; before serving lentils, stir in 2 tablespoons bacon drippings; sprinkle crumbled bacon over top.

When lentils are almost tender, add ½ cup chopped onions, celery, bell pepper or fresh or canned chili pepper; or season with ½ teaspoon basil, orégano, marjoram, or savory; or add 1 teaspoon chili powder or crushed dill, caraway, or coriander seeds.

"CREAMED" RICE

Heat to boiling:

2 cups water   **1 teaspoon salt**

Add so slowly that boiling does not stop:

1 cup brown or converted rice

Reduce heat; simmer brown rice 45 minutes, converted rice 15 minutes.

Evaporate off any remaining moisture; combine and stir into hot rice:

1 cup fresh top milk   **½ cup instant powdered milk**

Heat to simmering and pour into serving dish. Garnish with paprika and sprigs of parsley.

VARIATIONS:

Cook in rice 1 cup peas, diced raw carrots, celery, or mushrooms; add only in time to become tender; or 5 minutes before serving stir in diced leftover meat or vegetables.

Cook rice in soup stock, using chicken or ham stock when available; season with ¼ teaspoon crushed white peppercorns and ½ cup shredded onion or sliced mushrooms; add or omit milk.

Just before serving stir in 2 tablespoons finely chopped chives, green onions, or parsley.

Rice cooked with tomatoes: Add rice to **2 cups boiling tomato juice;** season with ¼ teaspoon crushed black peppercorns, 2 tablespoons vegetable oil, 1 minced clove garlic, 1 finely chopped onion, ¼ crumbled bay leaf, 2 teaspoons molasses or sugar. Omit milk.

Wild rice: Omit milk; otherwise cook as in basic recipe.

Whole unground wheat is an excellent food which should be served more often than it is, especially to growing children or to any person whose calorie requirements are high. Families who are accustomed to eating it are usually enthusiastic to the extreme. Its chewiness, which may seem objectionable at first, becomes its charm.

STEAMED UNGROUND WHEAT

Put **1 cup unground wheat** in a wire strainer and wash quickly under running water; add to:

3 cups boiling water, soup stock, or tomato juice

Cover utensil, reduce heat to simmering, and cook until tender, or 3 to 4 hours; uncover utensil during last of cooking and evaporate any remaining moisture; add:

**1 tablespoon partially hardened   1 teaspoon salt
margarine or butter**

Serve with chicken or other meat.

VARIATIONS:

Cook in pressure cooker 25 to 30 minutes, using 2 cups liquid to 1 cup wheat.

When wheat is almost tender, add 1 or 2 tablespoons bacon drippings, 1 minced clove garlic, 1 chopped onion or ½ cup sliced mushrooms.

A few minutes before serving add ½ cup or more cream sauce, salt, ground white peppercorns, diced canned pimento; or add leftover gravy, 2 tablespoons minced onion, a pinch of sage. Vary by cooking in chicken stock with crushed white peppercorns until wheat is almost tender; add salt, ½ cup diced celery, 1 cup raw or frozen peas, 1 chopped pimento, a pinch each of thyme and basil.

Cook in tomato juice; when wheat is almost tender, add ¼ teaspoon cumin seeds, a pinch of orégano, 1 each chopped bell pepper and onion, 1 minced clove garlic.

Cracked wheat has the advantages of being inexpensive, of cooking in a much shorter time than the unground grain, yet having sufficiently large particles to give a chewy quality. It serves as an interesting occasional substitute for potatoes and can also be eaten as a cereal or used in stuffing for fowl or fish.

CRACKED WHEAT

Heat to boiling:

2 cups vegetable-cooking water

Add so slowly that boiling does not stop:

1 cup cracked wheat	2 teaspoons instant chicken bouil-
½ teaspoon salt	lon

Simmer 20 minutes and stir in:

½ cup chopped onion	freshly ground black peppercorns
½ cup sliced celery or mushrooms (optional)	1 or 2 tablespoons partially hard-ened margarine, butter, or oil

Simmer 10 minutes longer and serve.

VARIATIONS:

Instead of seasonings suggested above, add ½ teaspoon basil, marjoram, orégano, or cumin seeds.

Omit seasonings and stir in 1 cup sour cream just before serving.

Although fresh soybeans contain no starch, they are rich in sugar. Some varieties are so sweet that they taste like new peas. To prevent the protein from becoming tough, do not submit them to temperatures higher than simmering. Fresh lima beans may be cooked by the same recipe.

FRESH SOYBEANS OR LIMA BEANS

Add **2 to 3 cups fresh chilled soybeans or lima beans** to:

½ cup hot milk

Stir to cover beans with milk protein; cover utensil, heat quickly, then simmer 15 to 20 minutes.

Add:

½ teaspoon salt

Garnish with **paprika.**

VARIATIONS:

Steam soybeans or lima beans in vegetable-cooking water or soup stock.

Until a taste for soybeans is acquired, steam a few of them with fresh lima beans.

After removing soybeans from heat, add chopped canned pimento and ½ cup melted cheese.

Season steamed soybeans with one or more of the following: chopped chives, onions, celery, pimento, green-onion tops, crisp bacon or bacon drippings, smoke-flavoring, minced garlic or parsley, or sliced stuffed olives.

Chilled soybeans: Quickly chill cooked soybeans and marinate in **French dressing.** Serve cold or add to salads.

Creamed soybeans or lima beans: Prepare beans as in basic recipe, using top milk; a few minutes before serving add **thickening for cream sauce.**

Winter squashes include all the solid squashes: banana, Danish, acorn, Hubbard squashes, crookneck and straightneck squashes, green warted squashes, and Boston marrow, or basket pumpkin. All these squashes and pumpkin can be prepared by the following recipes. Since squashes are difficult to peel, it is usually easier to cook them unpeeled and cut off the peel before they are served or to serve them unpeeled. The cooking time varies somewhat with the type of squash.

BROWNED WINTER SQUASH

Wash the peel, remove seeds and stringy parts, and cut into serving sizes:

1½ to 2 pounds winter squash

Set peel side down on rack above a small amount of boiling water; cover utensil and steam 10 to 15 minutes, or until squash is tender; set on baking sheet and brush with **dark molasses and vegetable oil, butter, or partially hardened margarine;** sprinkle with:

salt	celery salt or nutmeg
freshly ground black peppercorns	paprika

Broil under moderate heat until squash is brown, or about 10 minutes.

VARIATIONS:

Instead of cooking under broiler, bake in moderate oven at 400° F. for 20 minutes. Or omit steaming, brush with oil and molasses, salt, and bake for 50 minutes.

Acorn squash: Cut in half and prepare as in basic recipe; before placing under broiler or in oven, put into each half 1 tablespoon molasses, 2 tablespoons top milk or evaporated milk, 1 teaspoon butter or partially hardened margarine. Vary by putting into each half 1 tablespoon each sherry, brown sugar, partially hardened margarine, and sprinkling of nutmeg.

Stuffed acorn squash: Steam squash until slightly tender; salt, stuff with **crumb dressing** (p. 129), and bake 20 minutes at 350° F., or until tender. Vary by serving baked squash filled with **creamed chicken, ham, peas, or other leftover creamed meat or vegetables.**

Mashed squash: Steam squash until tender; scrape out pulp with a spoon, mash, season with **partially hardened margarine or butter, salt, paprika.** Vary by adding any one of the following: **1 teaspoon minced fresh basil or mint leaves; 2 tablespoons chopped parsley; ½ cup crushed pineapple with 1 tablespoon molasses; or ½ cup steamed raisins, dash of nutmeg, cinnamon, 1 tablespoon brown sugar.**

Leftover mashed squash: Put into flat oiled baking dish, cover with thick **applesauce** or with **2 strips bacon;** bake in moderate oven until heated through and bacon is crisp. Vary by folding into squash **1 or 2 beaten eggs, ½ cup each fresh and powdered milk.**

Steamed squash: Cut squash into strips, peel, and dice into 1-inch cubes; put into preheated utensil with 1 or 2 tablespoons boiling water; cook over simmer burner or in top of double boiler until tender, or about 15 to 20 minutes; season with **salt, margarine or butter, and cayenne or dark molasses.** Set lid of utensil to one side to let moisture escape during last 5 minutes of cooking.

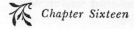

Chapter Sixteen

If You Want to Bake Bread

For those of us who live in areas where excellent breads made of stone-ground, whole-grain flour are available, baking bread at home seems scarcely worth while. In many localities, however, almost all commercial bread is made of highly refined flour loaded with chemical softeners, whiteners, agers, fresheners, preservers, and mold- and fungus-growth preventers. Even breads labeled "whole-wheat," unless purchased from a health-food store, often contain most of these same chemicals. In addition, sprays poisonous to insects and human beings alike have been dropped from planes onto the growing grains and onto soils already badly contaminated by many previous years' spraying. The recipes in this section, therefore, are for the health-conscious housewife who cannot buy wholesome bread for her family and therefore wishes to bake it. Fortunately, delicious stone-ground flours made from a wide variety of carefully selected grains and without the addition of chemicals of any kind are available throughout America (see page 542).

The public has been misled into believing that fortified breads and flour are equally as nutritious as the unrefined products. Vitamin E, some 16 B vitamins, many minerals, and the most valuable protein—that in the germ—are removed during refining. Only three substances are added to "enriched" breads and flour: two-thirds as much vitamin B_1 and one-third as much iron and the B vitamin niacin as the grain originally contained. Many millers, I am told, have found that stirring the iron and vitamins into their white flour is an expensive, time-consuming, and, to their way of thinking, unnecessary nuisance; hence they do not do it, yet still label their products "enriched." Even if fortification were always carried out honestly, it is as logical to say that you are enriched by a burglar who robs you of twenty-five or more articles but drops three small ones during his get-away as to claim that flour is enriched by being robbed of twenty-two or more nutrients. It is the cumulative contribution from using unrefined breadstuffs retaining all the original nutrients instead of white-flour products which pays nutritional dividends.

Not only do breadstuffs of unrefined flours contribute iron, vitamin E, many B vitamins, and valuable protein, but they can be made still more health-producing by the addition of such valuable foods as powdered milk, wheat germ, and soy flour. For example, almost every recipe for quick breads in this section calls for milk solids in addition to liquid milk; hence they furnish more calcium, excellent protein, and vitamin B_2 than do the usual recipes for such foods. Fresh wheat germ is by far the most nutritious part of the grain and should be used as much as palatability permits. Because the oil and vitamin E has been extracted from most of the toasted wheat germ on the market, it cannot be recommended. At a fraction of the cost, soy flour supplies two or three times more adequate protein than meat does.

But alas! Breads also contribute calories. Persons leading sedentary lives should probably eat no more than one slice of bread or one roll, muffin, or biscuit a day. When overweight is a problem, all breadstuffs should be foregone. It is only when calories will be utilized that home baking can be heartily recommended. Nevertheless every kitchen should know the fragrant odor of home-baked bread occasionally, and every housewife has the right to discover that bread baking can be a rewarding hobby even if she must give most of her delicious creations to her slender friends.

Women who think it impossible to make delicious breads of whole-grain flours should remember that our great-grandmothers, who took much pride in their baking, used only whole-grain flour because no other was available. They also used only stone-ground products. Since the heat of friction during fast commercial milling precooks the flour and brings about a marked loss in flavor, stone-ground flour is demanded by epicures. The taste difference is comparable to that between last night's warmed-over steak and a fresh one sizzling from the grill. One of my neighbors, accustomed to the texture and full nutty flavor of whole-grain breads, declares that the white varieties now taste to him "like fluffed-up plaster of Paris."

Freshness of all ingredients, of course, is absolutely essential to good bread making. The oil in wheat germ can quickly become rancid. Whole-grain flour can support growth; therefore weevils may infest it. Wheat germ should be refrigerated as carefully as milk or butter. Except for small amounts kept out for immediate use, whole-grain flour should be kept in a cool place or, if held longer than a week, in the refrigerator; all flour keeps well when frozen.

Never shall I forget a dinner to which a friend invited me, saying, "I'm going to prepare everything from your cookbook." It was her first attempt to use whole-wheat flour and powdered milk. She had tried to make yeast bread of rancid pastry flour and still more rancid wheat germ, purchased from a market where the turnover was slow. She had added to the bread powdered milk which should have been sweet-smelling and as fine as face powder but which had an offensive odor and looked like crushed rock; such changes occur when powdered milk has been left exposed to the air. It was impossible to say who was the more embarrassed, my hostess or myself. We ate cold cereal, however, and remained friends. But I shudder when I think of how many other housewives may have unknowingly obtained products of inferior quality.

Pointers on Making Yeast Breads

Success in making yeast breads depends upon the gluten, or wheat protein, content of the flour and upon how well the dough is beaten, stirred, or kneaded. A good yeast-bread flour must be rich in gluten. If you attempt to make yeast bread of a pastry or "all purpose" flour, you will produce only heavy, flat loaves.

When dough is stirred, beaten, and kneaded, the bits of gluten in each tiny particle of flour are brought into contact with each other; they stick together and form rubbery, elastic sheets throughout the dough. As the live yeast liberates bubbles of carbon dioxide, the elastic gluten stretches like thin rubber sheets and holds the gas in the loaf, thus making it large in volume and light in texture. The entire point of stirring, beating, and kneading dough is to bring these particles of gluten together and thus make it possible for such rubber-like sheets to be formed. If the flour is low in gluten, if the dough is beaten insufficiently, or if substances are added which mechanically separate the gluten particles, the bubbles of carbon dioxide escape in the same way they do from a glass of beer; the resulting loaf will be flat and the bread heavy.

Rye flour contains only a trace of gluten; all other flours and ingredients added to breads not only lack gluten but "dilute" the gluten content of the wheat flour. If you are a beginner at bread making, temporarily avoid adding rye, soy, or buckwheat flour, corn meal, powdered milk, and other gluten-lacking products even though their nutritive value and flavor are desirable. When you can make beautiful high loaves of bread, then add other ingredients as you wish, but only after the gluten has been developed by thorough beating and the dough is smooth and elastic.

There is available delicious stone-ground, whole-wheat-bread mix* to which only water and yeast need be added. Any woman can probably make perfect bread the first time she tries merely by following the simple directions on the package; such a mix is a good starting point for an amateur.

Yeast itself is a rich source of B vitamins. In addition to the familiar cakes of fresh compressed yeast, quick-acting granular bakers' yeast is also available. It is sold in packages containing one tablespoon, or enough for a single baking, or in quarter- and

---

* Sold nationally through health food stores and supplied by El Molino Mills, 3060 W. Valley Blvd., Alhambra, California.

half-pound packages, enough for 16 or 32 bakings. Purchasing yeast in the bulk is not only less expensive but enables one to make bread on the spur of the moment.

The more yeast added to breadstuffs, the greater its nutritive value and the more quickly the dough rises. Pancakes, waffles, and quick breads can be ready to bake in almost as short a time when made with yeast as with baking powder if sufficient active yeast is used. If three cakes of yeast or the equivalent are added to waffles, for example, they will be ready to bake soon after they are prepared. If only one cake is used, time must be allowed for the yeast to grow into the equivalent of several cakes. The longer yeast is allowed to grow, the more the yeast plants multiply, the more tiny bubbles of carbon dioxide are liberated, and the finer is the texture of the baked product. When convenient, therefore, allow the dough to rise twice before it is cooked.

Bakers' yeast is a live plant; it must be treated much like a potted geranium. It grows best at 80 to 85° F., or the temperature of a warm summer day. Just as a geranium does not grow in cold weather or is killed if put into a hot oven, so does yeast stop growing when chilled and is killed when overheated. If yeast dough is allowed to rise too much or if it is not kept sufficiently warm while the yeast is growing, the dough becomes sour. Unless you desire sour bread, stir or knead down the dough each time it has doubled in bulk; keep it near 85° F. or else chill it so completely that the yeast cannot grow. Since eggs and fat inhibit the growth of yeast, they are added to refrigerator rolls to prevent the dough from souring.

Yeast bread will keep moist for many days if a cooked cereal, such as wheat germ cooked in milk, is added to the dough. The cooked starch holds moisture in the bread, somewhat as applesauce does when added to a cake. If you use only a little bread, keep the loaves fresh by wrapping and freezing them.

Wheat germ contains enzymes which, if not destroyed by heat, can digest both starch and gluten in a slow-rising dough, causing it to become runny. Except when breads are to be baked within 3 hours after being made, wheat germ should first be slightly toasted or simmered in milk before being added.

Flour for yeast bread need not be sifted except when it is necessary to mix it with powdered milk. Flours differ considerably in their moisture content; each bread recipe can therefore be only approximate.

Despite the difficulties, bread making can easily become a successful hobby which your family may not let you give up.

WHOLE-WHEAT BREAD

If flour, honey, or other ingredients have been refrigerated, allow them to warm to room temperature.

Combine in a large mixing bowl:

3 cups warm water   **2 or 3 tablespoons, packages, or**
¾ cup honey   **cakes bakers' yeast**

Allow yeast to soften 5 minutes or longer. Add:

¼ cup oil, butter, or partially hardened margarine (optional)
5 cups unsifted high-protein, stone-ground whole-wheat flour
1 scant tablespoon salt

Beat by hand 100 or more strokes or 7 minutes with electric mixer at low speed. If dough is not beaten sufficiently, the bread will be heavy. Add and stir well:

2 to 3 cups more whole-wheat flour, or enough to make a stiff dough

Sprinkle approximately 1 cup flour over a bread board or pastry cloth, and turn dough onto it.

Knead until dough is smooth and elastic; use more flour if required to prevent sticking.

Put into oiled bowl smooth side down, then turn greased side up; cover, and let rise in a warm place (85° F.) until double in bulk, or about 1 hour. If oven with pilot light or other warm place is not available, set bowl in a sink of very warm water.

When double in bulk, knead or punch to original size. Cover and let rise again until double in bulk.

Knead to original size. If 1-pound loaf pans are to be used, divide dough into 3 equal parts; divide into 2 parts for 1½-pound loaf pans; shape into loaves. Place in loaf pans greased with lard, butter, or margarine; bread sticks to pans greased with vegetable oil.

Let rise until dough reaches to top of pan; the dough will continue to rise in the oven.

Bake in a preheated oven at 350° F. for 50 minutes for 1-pound loaves, 70 minutes for 1½-pound loaves, or until well browned. Turn out onto wire rack to cool. If crispness is desired, brush crust with cream, butter, or margarine while bread is still hot.

VARIATIONS:

Decrease honey to ¼ or ½ cup or use ¼ to ½ cup dark molasses instead of honey.

If chewy bread is enjoyed, omit fat.

Use graham flour instead of whole-wheat if desired.

Before putting loaves into pans, brush with beaten egg white and roll in sesame or poppy seeds.

Make rolls, coffee cake, or pizza from a third of the dough, following directions on p. 188.

Use 3 cups warm milk instead of water. If fresh milk is not pasteurized, heat to simmering to destroy molds and wild yeasts which affect flavor of bread.

If a crunchy bread is desired, knead into dough ¾ cup steamed cracked wheat or soy grits before forming into loaves.

After beating dough, add ½ cup powdered milk, sifting it with 1 cup flour; stir well before adding enough more flour to make a stiff dough; ½ to 1 cup leftover mashed potatoes or any cooked cereal may also be added.

Omit kneading; beat dough 70 or more strokes and let rise; stir to original size and let rise again before forming into loaves.

Instead of baking bread in loaf pans, bake in large juice cans if tall loaves are desired; or use several small cans. Fill cans half full of dough. Vary baking time with size of can.

Instead of 1 cup whole-wheat flour, stir into dough after beating 1 cup of any one of the following: soy, buckwheat, or rye flour; bran; rice polish; or stone-ground yellow corn meal; or add 2 to 4 tablespoons brewers' yeast. These ingredients cause the bread to be somewhat heavy unless ½ cup gluten flour is used with them.

Adjust your bread making to your work schedule. Use 1 tablespoon, package, or cake of yeast, and allow 2 hours for dough to rise if you must be away for that length of time. Or make dough in evening, let rise once, knead down, keep in refrigerator overnight, remove and let rise, and bake the following morning. Or make sponge by adding 2 cups whole-wheat flour to water, yeast, and honey; keep warm, stir sponge down whenever double in bulk, and proceed when convenient.

Directions for Making Bread

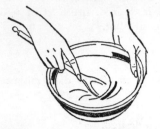

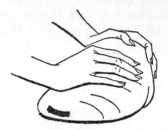

1. Measure warm liquid (110° F.) into large bowl. Add yeast and stir until dissolved. Add other ingredients. Beat by hand 100 or more strokes or 7 minutes with electric mixer at low speed. Add 2 to 3 cups more whole-wheat flour, or enough to make a stiff dough.

2. Turn dough onto floured canvas or board. Grease or flour hands and knead dough by folding it toward you, then pushing it away with heels of your palms; use more flour if required to prevent sticking. Give dough a quarter turn, and continue to fold, push, and turn until dough is smooth and elastic.

3. Place dough, smooth side down, in greased bowl, then turn so greased side is up. Cover with cloth or lid and set in warm place (about 85° F.) until double in bulk, or about 1 hour.

4. Knead or punch dough down thoroughly, pressing out all air bubbles. Turn dough smooth side up and let rise 20 to 30 minutes, or until double in bulk.

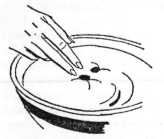

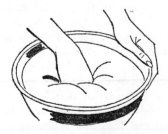

Drawings based on illustrations from El Molino Mills, Alhambra, California

5. Turn dough onto lightly floured canvas or board and knead out air. If making more than one loaf, divide into desired portions. Shape each portion into loaf by pressing into oval shape.

6. Fold dough into half lengthwise, and flatten again. Lift dough by ends and stretch into rectangle.

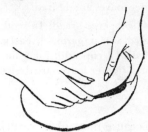

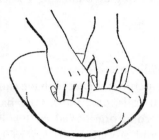

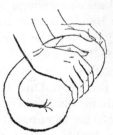

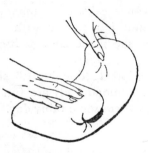

8. Roll dough toward you, sealing well with heels of your palms. Place, with smooth side down, in well-greased 8½- by 4½-inch loaf pan; then turn greased side up. Dough should fill pans about ⅔ full. Cover and let rise approximately 30 minutes, or until dough reaches to top of pan.

7. Bring ends of dough to center and overlap, pressing down firmly to seal.

9. When dough is slightly rounded above pans, preheat oven to 350° F. Bake 50 minutes for 1-pound loaves, 70 minutes for 1½-pound loaves, or until well browned. Remove from pans, place on rack, and cool.

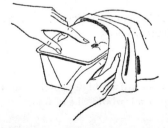

Rye bread: Add **2 cups rye flour** after beating dough. Proceed as in basic recipe; or omit honey and let dough rise in a cool place overnight if sour rye bread is desired. Bake in ordinary loaf pans. This is a heavy bread but extremely delicious. Sift **½ cup gluten flour** with rye flour if lighter loaves are desired.

Wheat-germ bread: Instead of 1 cup flour stir in after beating **1 cup toasted wheat germ, wheat germ and middlings, or wheat germ simmered in 1 cup milk** for 5 minutes. Sift **½ cup gluten flour** with wheat flour if lighter loaves are desired.

Because most of us rarely prepare rolls, it seems scarcely worth the effort to make only one pan at a time; hence I have suggested making enough for forty 2-inch rolls, or 2 pans. One pan might be served immediately and a second one baked only sufficiently to stop the growth of yeast and stored or frozen to be browned and served later. Or the dough may be divided into halves, thirds, or fourths, and rolls, coffee cake, and cinnamon buns prepared. One friend, snowbound last winter with 100 pounds of whole-wheat flour, told me she made enough bread and rolls for an entire year.

The braids, twists, and oversized clipped "doughnuts" suggested for coffee cake and orange and almond rolls are fun to make and have a professional look. Try them some rainy day.

WHEAT-GERM ROLLS

Combine in large mixing bowl:

2 cups warm water
¾ cup honey or dark molasses

2 tablespoons, packages, or cakes
bakers' yeast

Let stand 5 minutes or longer. Add:

⅔ cup vegetable oil, butter, or
partially hardened margarine
2 eggs

3 cups unsifted high-protein, stone-
ground whole-wheat flour

Stir until ingredients are combined, then beat by hand 100 strokes or with an electric mixer 10 minutes at low speed.

Add and stir thoroughly:

1 cup wheat germ	1 tablespoon salt and
1 cup whole-wheat flour	⅔ cup powdered milk
sifted with	

Stir in ½ cup more flour if needed to make a stiff dough. Cover bowl, set in a warm place at 85° F. or in very warm water until double in bulk, or about 1 hour. Stir down and let rise again. Turn onto floured bread board or pastry cloth, knead to original size, and make into 2 pans of rolls; or make half the dough into rolls, a fourth into coffee cake, and the remaining fourth into cinnamon rolls.

Bake in preheated oven at 350° F. for 20 to 25 minutes for rolls to be served immediately. Bake 15 to 20 minutes for rolls to be frozen and browned later.

This recipe makes forty 2-inch rolls.

VARIATIONS:

To make Parker House rolls, cut with biscuit cutter, brush top with oil, crease center with knife and fold in half. For dinner rolls, cut with small biscuit cutter, make circle of thumb and forefinger of left hand, push dough through circle, squeezing cut edges together; set close together in baking pan. For 3-leaf-clover rolls, place 3 small balls of dough in greased muffin tin. Make scones by rolling dough into a 9-inch circle; cut into 10 pie-shaped wedges and roll each wedge from outside toward center. For butterhorns, bend scones into semicircles and set far apart on baking sheet.

Instead of water, use 2 cups fresh warm milk. If milk is not pasteurized, heat to simmering and cool before adding yeast.

If time permits, use 1 tablespoon, package, or cake of yeast; if in a hurry, increase yeast to 3 tablespoons, packages, or cakes.

Instead of 1 cup whole-wheat flour, sift with salt and powdered milk and stir in after beating 1 cup rice polish or rye, buckwheat, or soy flour; or add 2 tablespoons brewers' yeast.

Almond roll: Use a fourth of the dough; roll into a thin rectangle and sprinkle with 1 cup slivered almonds and ½ cup sugar into which has been stirred 1 teaspoon almond extract; add ¼ cup finely diced citron if desired. Press almonds into dough. Roll like a jelly roll and transfer to a greased baking sheet, forming into a circle like a huge doughnut; with wet scissors cut from outside margin almost to center at 1-inch intervals and turn each slice diagonally, overlapping the next. Sprinkle top with sugar and almonds. Bake when double in bulk.

Cinnamon buns: Prepare half the basic recipe; after beating, sift in with other ingredients 2 tablespoons cinnamon, ½ cup sugar; add 1 cup seedless raisins which have been soaked 5 minutes in ¾ cup boiling water. After dough rises, make in shape of buns; bake 10 minutes and brush top with glaze of ½ cup sugar boiled 2 minutes with ¼ cup water; brush again 5 minutes before removing from oven. If hot-cross buns are desired, make crosses with icing (p. 506).

Cinnamon rolls: Use a fourth of the dough; roll into a rectangle ¼ inch thick; brush with butter or partially hardened margarine, and sprinkle generously with sugar and cinnamon. Roll like jelly roll, cut into 1-inch pieces, and set close together on greased 8- by 8-inch pan. Vary by adding steamed raisins or broken walnuts or pecans with cinnamon. Bake when double in bulk.

Coffee cake: Use a fourth of the dough and roll into a rectangle no more than ¼ inch thick; sprinkle with ⅓ cup brown sugar, ½ cup each chopped walnuts or pecans and seedless raisins soaked 5 minutes in ¼ cup boiling water; add cinnamon or nutmeg if desired. Or spread with steamed currants, nuts, and sweetened raw apples cut paper-thin. Roll as jelly roll, then twist 4 times or more before placing on greased baking sheet; or cut 3 or 4 deep diagonal gashes across top after setting on baking sheet. Bake when double in bulk.

Orange roll: Use a fourth of the dough and roll into a rectangle ¼ inch thick; sprinkle with ½ cup sugar and finely shredded rind of 2 oranges; cut dough lengthwise into 3 strips and fold each over, also lengthwise, to prevent sugar and rind from falling out; braid and transfer to greased baking sheet. Bake when double in bulk.

Pizza: See page 188.

BUTTER ROLLS

Combine in mixing bowl:

1 cup warm water	1 or 2 tablespoons, packages, or
⅔ cup honey	cakes bakers' yeast

Let stand 5 minutes or longer; add:

½ cup vegetable oil	2½ cups high-protein, stone-
3 eggs	ground, whole-wheat flour

Stir until ingredients are combined, then beat by hand 100 strokes or 10 minutes with an electric beater at low speed.

Sift in:

¾ cup whole-wheat flour   2 teaspoons salt
⅓ cup powdered milk

Stir well, set in a warm place or in very warm water; stir down when double in bulk, and let rise again. Beat dough to original size before turning onto floured bread board or pastry cloth. Try not to work any more flour into dough while making rolls than is absolutely necessary; the charm of these rolls lies in their lightness.

Press or roll dough ¼ inch thick and spread with **butter or partially hardened margarine;** roll like a jelly roll, cut into 1-inch pieces, and set close together on 2 greased 8- by 8-inch pans. Let rise until double in bulk.

Bake in moderate oven at 350° F. for 20 to 25 minutes if for immediate use. Bake 15 to 20 minutes if to be browned and served later. Makes thirty small rolls.

VARIATIONS:

Shape dough into dinner rolls (p. 413).

Divide dough into 2 parts; make half into rolls and keep other half in plastic bag in refrigerator overnight; when double in bulk, knead without removing from bag. Make into rolls the following day.

Make half the dough into rolls and use the remainder for any variation suggested for wheat-germ rolls.

Butterhorns: Roll dough in the form of scones (p. 413); dip top of each into **beaten egg white** and then into **sesame or poppy seeds** or into **sugar and shaved almonds;** curve scones in semicircles; arrange 2 inches apart on greased baking sheet. Bake when double in bulk.

Tips on Quick Breads

When soda is used in baking, many of the B vitamins in whole-wheat flour and wheat germ are quickly destroyed. As long as powdered milk, soy flour, wheat germ, or other ingredients rich in protein are included, 2 teaspoons of baking powder can be substituted for each ½ to 1 teaspoon of soda called for in any recipe. Such proteins neutralize the lactic acid in sour milk, buttermilk, and yogurt so completely that they can be used with baking powder to give a pleasant but not sour flavor. Although the valuable bacteria in yogurt are destroyed in cooking, I have suggested using it because you may have it when sour milk or buttermilk is unavailable.

Pancakes, waffles, muffins, and cornbread, however, are more nutritious and delicious when made with yeast rather than baking powder; and they can be made almost as quickly. The delightful aroma which fills the house when these foods are cooking is justification enough for using yeast.

In baking quick breads, flour should be sifted before being measured. If you do not wish to bother with sifting, stir the flour thoroughly with a spoon and then use approximately 7/8 cup flour for each cup called for.

The flour used for quick breads should be low in gluten and the dough stirred as little as possible. If a dough is stirred vigorously or kneaded, the particles of gluten stick together and the texture becomes tough. Slight stirring or kneading, however, is necessary to make the dough hold together. In quick breads, both the gluten and the crust, formed rapidly by the high oven temperature, hold in the bubbles of carbon dioxide liberated by baking powder or yeast and make a light texture possible. Since soy flour contains no gluten whatsoever, it cannot hold in the carbon dioxide bubbles, and stiffly beaten egg whites must be relied upon as the leavening agent in making pancakes or waffles largely of soy flour.

Both soy flour and powdered milk burn easily; pancakes containing these ingredients should be baked slowly on a moderately hot griddle. If crisp bacon, diced ham, nuts, crushed pineapple, or mashed banana is added to pancakes or waffles, there is less temptation to accompany them with concentrated sweets. Whenever possible, serve creamed chicken or tuna, thick applesauce, or crushed fresh or frozen strawberries, peaches, or raspberries with waffles or pancakes.

PANCAKES MADE WITH BAKING POWDER

Sift into a mixing bowl:

1 cup stone-ground whole-wheat-pastry flour	1 teaspoon salt
½ cup powdered milk	2 teaspoons double-acting baking powder

Add:

1½ cups sweet or sour milk, buttermilk, or yogurt	2 tablespoons vegetable oil
2 eggs	½ cup fresh wheat germ

Stir with no more than 50 strokes. Drop from tablespoon onto moderately hot griddle; bake slowly; turn and brown the other side. Makes 10 to 12 pancakes 5 inches in diameter.

Serve with bacon, eggs, and crushed fresh fruit.

VARIATIONS:

Instead of flour and wheat germ, use 1½ cups wheat germ and middlings; add ¼ cup extra liquid.

Substitute for ½ cup whole-wheat flour any one of the following: rice polish, yellow corn meal, or rye, buckwheat, or soy flour. Add 1 teaspoon caraway seeds with rye flour if desired.

Add any of the following: ½ cup well-drained crushed pineapple, fresh or canned blueberries, or mashed banana; or ¼ cup peanut butter or crushed walnuts or pecans; or diced ham or 3 or more slices crisp bacon crumbled to bits.

Buckwheat pancakes: Instead of wheat flour use 1 cup buckwheat flour; add 1 tablespoon dark molasses.

Corn-meal pancakes: Omit both wheat germ and whole-wheat flour; use 1½ cups coarse yellow stone-ground corn meal; fold in stiffly beaten egg whites just before baking. If you enjoy the taste of coarse corn meal, these pancakes are delicious. They somehow have an honest, early-pioneer flavor. If a daintier texture is preferred, use 1 cup finely ground corn meal and ½ cup whole-wheat flour.

Soy pancakes: Omit wheat germ and use 1 cup soy flour with ½ cup whole-wheat flour. Add other ingredients of basic recipe. Fold in stiffly beaten egg whites just before baking.

PANCAKES MADE WITH YEAST

Stir in mixing bowl:

½ cup warm water
1 to 3 tablespoons, packages, or
cakes bakers' yeast

1 tablespoon honey, molasses, or
sugar

Let stand 5 minutes or longer; add:

1 cup sweet or sour milk, buttermilk, or yogurt
2 eggs

2 tablespoons vegetable oil
½ cup wheat germ

Sift into liquid:

1 cup whole-wheat-pastry flour
½ cup powdered milk

1 teaspoon salt

Stir and bake immediately if 3 tablespoons of yeast or equivalent
are used; let rise in a warm place 30 minutes or longer if 2 tablespoons
of yeast are used, or overnight if 1 tablespoon is used.

Bake slowly on a moderately hot griddle. Serve with applesauce or
crushed fresh fruit.

VARIATIONS:

Use any variations suggested for baking-powder pancakes; buckwheat
pancakes made with yeast are especially delicious.

THIN PANCAKES

Combine and stir:

1½ cups milk

3 egg yolks

Sift in and stir well:

⅔ cup whole-wheat-pastry flour
½ cup powdered milk

1 teaspoon salt

Beat stiff and fold in:

3 egg whites

Bake on a moderately hot griddle; use 3 tablespoons batter for each pancake, making it about 5 inches in diameter. Stack and serve immediately or use for blintzes (p. 199) or crêpes suzette (p. 504).

Since waffles are so frequently served for late breakfasts or Sunday guest suppers, I have given a recipe which makes 8 waffles.

BAKING-POWDER WAFFLES

Sift into a mixing bowl:

1¼ cups stone-ground whole-wheat-pastry flour
½ cup powdered milk

1 teaspoon salt
3 teaspoons double-acting baking powder

Add and stir well:

2 cups sweet or sour milk, buttermilk, or yogurt
2 tablespoons honey, dark molasses, or sugar

⅔ cup vegetable oil
1 cup wheat germ
3 egg yolks

Beat stiff and fold in:

3 egg whites

Bake on a preheated waffle iron. Serve with creamed chicken or tuna, crushed sweetened berries, or maple syrup.

VARIATIONS:

If any batter is left over, keep in refrigerator; thin slightly with milk and bake as pancakes.

Omit flour and wheat germ and use 2¼ cups wheat germ and middlings; or instead of ½ cup flour use ½ cup yellow corn meal, rice polish, or soy flour. Add 1 or 2 tablespoons brewers' yeast if desired.

Use ¼ cup oil and add 6 tablespoons peanut butter.

Add ½ to 1 cup of any of the following: ground or crushed walnuts or pecans; finely diced ham; drained crushed pineapple or chopped and well-drained cooked apricots or prunes; diced banana; fresh or drained canned blueberries; or combine pineapple or banana with nuts, ham, or bits of crisp bacon.

Buckwheat waffles or pancakes: Omit whole-wheat flour and use 1¼ cups buckwheat flour; bake as waffles or add ½ cup fresh milk and bake as hotcakes.

Corn-meal waffles: Use sour milk, buttermilk, or yogurt; omit flour and add 1¼ cups coarsely ground yellow corn meal.

Gingerbread waffles: Use 1½ cups sour milk, yogurt, or buttermilk and ⅔ cup dark molasses; sift with dry ingredients 2 tablespoons sugar, 1 teaspoon cinnamon, 2 teaspoons ginger. Serve with whipped cream or ice cream. If you can borrow a few extra waffle irons, gingerbread waffles, which are delicious, are wonderful for guest suppers.

Rye waffles: Use buttermilk; instead of whole-wheat-pastry flour use 1¼ cups unrefined rye flour; add grated rind of 2 oranges or 1 teaspoon caraway seeds as desired.

A friend, who has three big waffle-loving sons, tells me that formerly she hated to make waffles because it occupied her entire Sunday mornings, but that the waffles made by the following recipe are so satisfying that each of her sons can eat only two and she now has time to attend church.

YEAST WAFFLES

Combine in a mixing bowl and stir:

½ cup water
2 tablespoons honey or sugar

1 or more tablespoons, packages, or cakes bakers' yeast

Allow yeast to stand 5 minutes or longer. Add and stir well:

1½ cups sweet or sour milk, buttermilk, or yogurt
3 egg yolks

⅔ cup vegetable oil
1 cup fresh wheat germ

Sift in:

1¼ cups whole-wheat-pastry flour
½ cup powdered milk

1 teaspoon salt

Stir enough to blend; let rise in a warm place for 2 hours or longer, stirring down each time batter has doubled in bulk; just before baking, beat stiff and fold in:

3 egg whites

Bake on preheated waffle iron. Serve with applesauce or crushed strawberries or raspberries.

VARIATIONS:

To bake immediately, use 3 tablespoons, packages, or cakes yeast; if made 1½ hours before serving, use 2 tablespoons yeast or the equivalent.

If more convenient, prepare batter, let rise once or twice, stir down and set in refrigerator overnight; remove from refrigerator 30 minutes before baking; stir egg yolks into batter just before folding in whites.

Add more liquid to any leftover batter and bake as pancakes.

Use any variations suggested under baking-powder waffles (p. 419).

If you have not used coarse yellow stone-ground corn meal, I urge you to do so. In addition to supplying vitamin A, or carotene, which the white meal lacks, it has a far more delicious flavor than the corn meal held for months on a grocer's shelf. Keep your corn meal frozen or refrigerated.

QUICK CORNBREAD

Sift together into a mixing bowl:

2 cups coarse yellow stone-ground corn meal
1 teaspoon salt

½ cup powdered milk
2 teaspoons double-acting baking powder

Add and stir well:

1 cup sweet or sour milk, buttermilk, or yogurt
½ cup wheat germ
2 tablespoons vegetable oil

2 tablespoons honey or sugar (optional)
1 egg

Pour into a well-greased 8- by 8-inch pan. Bake in preheated oven at 425° F. for 20 to 25 minutes.

VARIATIONS:

Double the recipe and divide into 2 pans; bake one pan 15 to 18 minutes, cool on wire rack, freeze, and brown and serve later.

If light texture is desired, use 2 eggs; fold in stiffly beaten whites just before baking.

Instead of wheat germ, use rich polish or soy flour.

Bake 15 minutes in muffin tins or paper baking cups; fill half full.

Add ¼ to ½ cup soy grits.

RAISED CORNBREAD

Combine in mixing bowl:

1 to 3 tablespoons honey or sugar	1 or more tablespoons, packages,
⅓ cup warm water	or cakes bakers' yeast

Let sit 5 minutes or longer and add:

⅔ cup sweet or sour milk, butter-milk, or yogurt	3 tablespoons vegetable oil or bacon drippings
1 egg	½ cup wheat germ

Sift in and stir well:

1¼ cups coarse yellow stone-ground corn meal	1 teaspoon salt
¼ cup whole-wheat-pastry flour	½ cup powdered milk

Let rise in a warm place 30 minutes or longer. Pour into a greased 8- by 8-inch pan, and let rise 10 minutes. Bake in a preheated oven at 350° F. for 30 to 35 minutes or until brown.

VARIATIONS:

To bake cornbread immediately, use 3 tablespoons yeast or the equivalent; use 2 tablespoons if bread is prepared 1 hour before time to bake, 1 tablespoon if mixed 2 hours or longer before baking time.

Fill paper baking cups or well-greased muffin tins half full; let rise 10 minutes or longer; bake 15 to 20 minutes.

Add ¼ to ½ cup soy grits or use soy flour instead of wheat germ.

If light texture is desired, use 2 eggs and fold in stiffly beaten whites just before baking.

Add ½ cup grated or shredded carrots or finely chopped celery; or add 1 teaspoon crushed dill seeds.

WHEAT-GERM MUFFINS

Sift into mixing bowl:

1 cup sifted whole-wheat-pastry
flour
1 teaspoon salt

3 teaspoons double-acting baking
powder
¼ cup powdered milk

Add and stir only enough to moisten:

1 cup wheat germ
1 cup sweet or sour milk, buttermilk, or yogurt
2 eggs

¼ cup honey or dark molasses
2 tablespoons vegetable oil
½ cup raisins (optional)

Fill paper baking cups or well-greased muffin tins two-thirds full. Bake at 400° F. for 15 to 20 minutes, or until brown. Makes a dozen large muffins.

VARIATIONS:

If light texture is enjoyed, separate eggs and fold in stiffly beaten whites immediately before baking.

Omit ½ cup of wheat flour and add ½ cup rice polish or soy, buckwheat, or rye flour; or add 1 tablespoon brewers' yeast or ¼ cup soy grits.

Add ½ cup or more of any of the following: walnuts, pecans, chopped dates, ground dried apricots, shredded carrots, finely diced raw apple, chopped drained cooked prunes, or thick applesauce; or add 1 tablespoon grated onion or a pinch of marjoram, basil, or thyme.

Blueberry muffins: Use ⅓ cup sugar, omitting honey or molasses; before stirring add 1 cup fresh or well-drained canned blueberries.

Bran muffins: Increase salt to 1¼ teaspoons; add 1 cup bran or bran flakes, ½ cup each raisins and nuts.

Cheese muffins: Omit molasses or honey and fat; blend 1 cup grated cheese with dry ingredients. Vary by adding chopped parsley and/or 1 teaspoon dill or caraway seeds.

Corn-meal muffins: Omit whole-wheat flour and use 1 cup each yellow corn meal and wheat germ; use honey rather than molasses if flavor of corn meal is particularly enjoyed. These are delicious muffins.

Oatmeal muffins: Add ½ cup raw rolled oats or leftover cooked oatmeal; fold in stiffly beaten egg whites.

Orange muffins: Use sugar; add grated rind of 2 oranges.

Rice muffins: Add ½ to 1 cup cooked brown or converted rice and ½ cup raisins or chopped dates.

Rye muffins: Omit wheat germ; use 1 cup each wheat and rye flour; add 1 or 2 tablespoons caraway seeds or grated orange rind.

Yeast muffins: Omit baking powder; soak 1 tablespoon or more bakers' yeast in moisture ingredients; sift in dry ingredients and proceed as in basic recipe.

BAKING-POWDER BISCUITS

Sift into a mixing bowl:

1½ cups whole-wheat-pastry flour	4 teaspoons double-acting baking powder
1¼ teaspoons salt	
¼ cup powdered milk	

Add:

½ cup wheat germ	4 tablespoons vegetable oil

Add and stir with 25 strokes:

¾ cup sweet or sour milk, buttermilk, or yogurt

Turn onto floured canvas; knead 10 times; pat 1 inch thick and cut with biscuit cutter.

Place close together on greased baking sheet; bake in hot oven at 450° F. for 12 to 15 minutes.

VARIATIONS:

Instead of ½ cup whole-wheat flour use ½ cup rice polish or soy, rye, or buckwheat flour; knead 20 times.

Cut dough with doughnut cutter; serve covered with creamed ham, tuna, or chicken.

Add any of the following: ¼ cup finely shredded parsley; ¼ teaspoon thyme, basil, or marjoram; 3 tablespoons finely diced pimentos, celery, or grated onion; 2 teaspoons or more poppy, sesame, or caraway seeds. Don't miss herb biscuits; they are delicious.

Cheese biscuits: Use 2 tablespoons oil; blend with dry ingredients ¾ cup grated nippy cheese.

Cobblers: Sift 4 tablespoons sugar with dry ingredients; mix 3 cups sweetened sliced fresh or canned fruit or berries with 2 or 3 tablespoons whole-wheat-pastry flour; put in bottom of shallow baking dish, cover with dough rolled ¼ inch thick, and bake as in basic recipe; if fruit, such as apples, will not cook in 15 minutes, steam first until almost tender.

Drop biscuits: Use 1¼ cups milk; drop from spoon onto greased baking sheet.

Fruit or nut biscuits: Before adding oil mix with dry ingredients ½ cup chopped dates, seedless raisins, ground dried apricots or peaches, or broken walnuts, pecans, or other nuts; if desired, sift with flour 2 tablespoons sugar and ¼ teaspoon each cinnamon and nutmeg.

Peanut-butter biscuits: Use 2 tablespoons oil and ¼ cup peanut butter; add 1 tablespoon honey with milk.

Sour-cream biscuits: Use 2 tablespoons oil; add 1 cup sour cream instead of milk.

Many women tell me that they do not make steamed bread because they have nothing to steam it in. All you need is any covered utensil large enough to hold two pint cans. The cans may be those in which fruits or fruit juices have been purchased. If you haven't a rack, jar lids or crumpled foil may be used to keep the bread away from the direct heat.

STEAMED BROWN BREAD

Sift into mixing bowl:

½ cup whole-wheat-pastry flour
½ cup yellow stone-ground corn meal
⅓ cup powdered milk

½ teaspoon salt
2 teaspoons double-acting baking powder

Drop into dry ingredients and stir until each piece is coated:

1 cup raisins or chopped dates (optional)

Add and stir well:

1 cup sweet or sour milk, buttermilk, or yogurt

½ cup dark molasses
½ cup wheat germ

Pour into 2 well-greased pint cans; cover with lids or heavy paper tied on with string.

Use a large cooking utensil and set cans on a rack, jar lids, or crumpled foil; add boiling water until it comes halfway up around cans; cover utensil and keep water boiling slowly for 1½ to 2 hours.

VARIATIONS:

Instead of corn meal use ½ cup rice polish or rye, buckwheat, or soy flour.

Add ½ cup soy grits, bran flakes, broken walnuts, or pecans; or add 2 to 4 tablespoons brewers' yeast.

Raised brown bread: Omit baking powder and soak **1 or more tablespoons, packages, or cakes bakers' yeast in ¼ cup water;** use ¾ cup milk, buttermilk, or yogurt. Proceed as in basic recipe, sifting dry ingredients into moist ones. Let rise until almost double in bulk before starting to steam.

NUT BREAD

Sift into mixing bowl:

1½ cups whole-wheat-pastry flour
⅓ cup powdered milk
1 teaspoon salt

2 teaspoons double-acting baking powder

Add and mix until covered with flour:

1 cup broken walnuts, pecans, or other nuts

Add:

1¼ cups sweet or sour milk, buttermilk, or yogurt
3 tablespoons vegetable oil

⅓ cup honey or dark molasses
½ cup wheat germ

Stir with no more than 40 strokes. Line bottom of loaf pan with heavy paper and grease well; pour batter into pan, forcing it into corners; make indentation lengthwise through center. Bake at 350° F. for 45 minutes.

VARIATIONS:

Instead of nuts add ½ cup soy grits soaked in ¼ cup milk and 1 teaspoon black-walnut flavoring or ¼ teaspoon almond extract.

Add 2 tablespoons brewers' yeast to basic recipe or any variation calling for molasses; omit 2 tablespoons of flour.

Instead of ½ cup wheat flour use ½ cup rice polish, yellow corn meal, or rye, buckwheat, or soy flour.

Almond bread: Use sugar or honey instead of molasses; add 1 cup chopped almonds and 1 teaspoon almond extract.

Apricot-nut bread: Sweeten with honey; mix with dry ingredients ½ to 1 cup ground dried apricots; use 1½ cups milk; or omit milk and add 1¼ cups cooked dried apricots or canned apricots beaten or blended in liquefier.

Banana-nut bread: Use honey; instead of liquid add 1¼ cups mashed bananas; add grated rind of ½ lemon.

Date-nut bread: Add 1 cup finely chopped dates; or add dates to banana-nut bread or other variations.

Orange-nut bread: Add finely shredded or grated rind of 2 oranges.

Peanut-butter bread: Omit fat and nuts; blend ¾ cup non-hydro-genated peanut butter with dry ingredients, using pastry cutter; add other ingredients.

Pineapple-nut bread: Instead of other liquid use 1¼ cups crushed pineapple and juice; add grated rind of ½ lemon.

Spiced honey-nut bread: Use honey; sift 1 teaspoon each nutmeg and cinnamon with dry ingredients.

Prune-nut bread: Instead of other liquid use 1½ cups pitted cooked prunes and juice; chop prunes or leave whole.

Cheese puffs, a delightful accompaniment to any soup or salad, are surprisingly easy to make and add a festive touch when guests drop in unexpectedly. They may be prepared in advance and stored or frozen.

CHEESE PUFFS

Heat to simmering:

¼ cup butter or partially hard-   ½ cup milk
ened margarine

Sift flour before measuring, then sift directly into milk:

½ cup whole-wheat-pastry flour   ⅛ teaspoon salt

Cook the batter, stirring constantly, until it leaves the sides of the pan and forms a large ball, or about 2 minutes. Remove from heat and beat in one at a time with rotary beater:

2 eggs

If convenient, chill 30 minutes or longer; otherwise bake immediately;

chilling causes the puffs to be larger. Heap teaspoons of the batter on a greased baking sheet 1½ inches apart, making high 1- or 2-inch mounds.

Put into a hot oven at 425° F. and bake until the peaks are a delicate brown, or about 6 minutes; lower temperature to 300° F., open oven door 1 minute, then bake slowly 12 minutes for 1-inch puffs, 20 minutes for 2-inch ones.

Cut a gash in side of each puff and fill with **cream cheese or grated American, pimento, or Jack cheese;** season cheese with **dill or caraway seeds, chopped ripe or stuffed olives** as desired. Return to oven for 5 minutes, or until cheese has heated. Serve at once.

This recipe makes twenty 1-inch puffs or eight to ten 2-inch puffs. Chill, store or freeze any not needed for immediate use.

VARIATIONS:

Instead of cheese, fill puffs with creamed or curried shrimps, chicken, lamb, ham, or other meats.

Cream puffs: Chill puffs; fill with **sweetened whipped cream or chilled pie filling (p. 491).** Serve as dessert.

Many busy housewives quite understandably prefer to prepare quick breads from a mix rather than to measure the ingredients separately for each baking. An all-purpose mix, nutritionally superior to commercial ones, can be made in a few minutes.

My system of mix preparation is to put a plastic bag into a large bowl and turn the top of the bag down over the sides. After the major ingredients have been sifted directly into the bag, the wheat germ can be added, the top of the bag held together, and the final mixing done by a squeeze-and-punch method which seems more efficient to me than stirring. The mix for immediate use can then be poured into a cannister and the remainder stored in the freezer in the same bag in which it is made.

NUTRITIOUS QUICK-BREAD MIX

Measure without sifting; combine and then sift into a large bowl, cannister, or plastic bag:

6 cups stone-ground whole-wheat-
pastry flour

2 cups soy flour

2 scant tablespoons salt

⅓ cup double-acting baking powder

1 cup powdered milk (not instant)

Add and mix thoroughly:

2½ cups wheat germ

Keep part of the mix in a cannister for immediate use. Store the remainder in a cool place, preferably in refrigerator or freezer.

Instant powdered milk should not be used in the mix. It is so bulky that measurements will be inaccurate when you adapt the mix to your own recipes.

To use this mix for your favorite recipes, merely substitute it for the amount of flour called for and omit salt and baking powder or soda. Even if a recipe specifies sour milk or buttermilk, no soda is needed; the protein in the mix will neutralize acid. Spices may be stirred into the dry mix before liquid ingredients are added. From then on you proceed as directed in the original recipe.

The following recipes show how the mix may be used, but are by no means the only ones. Since flours vary considerably in moisture content, at times you may find a batter too thin and will need to add slightly more mix; on other occasions, somewhat more liquid may be required. Friends who have used the mix, however, have been enthusiastic about it. One of them remarked, "The recipes which the mix can be used for are limited only by a woman's imagination and by how much she enjoys baking."

PANCAKES

Combine in mixing bowl:

1 egg
1 cup sweet or sour milk, buttermilk, or yogurt

2 or 3 tablespoons vegetable oil
1½ cups nutritious mix

Stir until smooth; bake on moderately hot grill. This recipe make ten 5-inch pancakes.

If very light pancakes are desired, use 2 eggs and fold in stiffly beaten whites just before baking.

See page 417 for pancake variations.

WAFFLES

Combine in mixing bowl:

2 egg yolks	½ cup vegetable oil
1 cup sweet or sour milk, butter-milk, or yogurt	1½ cups nutritious mix

Mix until smooth and fold in:

2 stiffly beaten egg whites

Serve with creamed chicken or tuna.
See pages 419–420 for waffle variations.

BISCUITS

Combine in mixing bowl and stir:

⅓ cup vegetable oil or melted par-tially hardened margarine	⅔ cup sweet or sour milk, but-termilk, or yogurt

Add and stir no more than 25 strokes:

2¼ cups nutritious mix

Turn onto floured canvas or bread board. Knead lightly and pat 1 inch thick; cut with biscuit cutter and place close together on greased baking sheet.
Bake in a hot oven at 450° F. for 12 to 15 minutes.
Use same dough for cobblers, quick pizza, or drop biscuits (p. 425).

MUFFINS

Combine in mixing bowl:

2 eggs	2 tablespoons honey or dark mo-lasses
1 cup sweet or sour milk, butter-milk, or yogurt	2½ cups nutritious mix
2 tablespoons vegetable oil	

Mix until ingredients are well moistened. Fill paper baking cups or greased muffin pans two-thirds full. Bake at 400° F. for 15 minutes if to be served immediately; or bake half the muffins 12 minutes, cool, wrap, and freeze to be browned and served later. Makes 16 muffins. If light texture is desired, fold in stiffly beaten egg whites just before baking.

For muffin variations, see pages 423–424.

SPICE COOKIES

Combine and sift into mixing bowl or stir until blended:

2¼ cups nutritious mix   ½ teaspoon nutmeg
1 teaspoon cinnamon

Add:

1 cup tightly packed brown sugar   ⅔ cup vegetable oil
2 eggs

Stir until creamy. Drop from teaspoon onto greased brown paper or baking sheet or on aluminum foil; bake at 400° F. about 8 minutes, or until brown. If baked on foil, do not remove until cold. Keep in refrigerator if crispness is desired.

For cookie variations, see pages 519–520.

NUT LOAF

Stir until nuts are coated with flour:

3 cups nutritious mix   1 cup coarsely chopped walnuts

Add and mix until well moistened:

1 egg   ¾ cup sugar
1 cup sweet or sour milk, butter-   ½ cup vegetable oil
milk, or yogurt

Pour into a well-greased 1-pound loaf pan and bake at 350° F. for one hour. Turn on rack to cool.

For variations see nut bread, page 426.

COFFEE CAKE

Combine and mix until ingredients are well moistened:

1 egg	½ cup sugar
¼ cup vegetable oil	1½ cups nutritious mix
¾ cup milk	

Pour into a well-greased 8- by 8-inch pan.
Prepare topping by stirring together:

1½ teaspoons cinnamon	1 tablespoon vegetable oil
¼ cup tightly packed brown sugar	½ cup chopped nuts

Sprinkle crumbly mixture over top; bake at 375° F. for 30 minutes.
Serve hot or cold.

SPICE CAKE

Combine and allow to soak:

1 cup seedless raisins	¾ cup boiling water

Meanwhile cream together:

1 cup tightly packed brown sugar	½ cup partially hardened margarine

Add and beat well:

1 cup sweet or sour milk, buttermilk, or yogurt	2 egg yolks

Sift into moist ingredients:

1¾ cups nutritious mix	½ teaspoon cloves
1 teaspoon cinnamon	

Before stirring, drain raisins on a paper towel and add, being careful
to coat each with flour; then stir all ingredients until well blended.
Fold in:

2 stiffly beaten egg whites

Pour into a well-greased 8- by 8-inch pan and bake at 350° F. for 30 minutes.

When cool dust with **confectioners' sugar** or spread with **uncooked icing** (p. 506).

To make applesauce cake use **1 cup applesauce** instead of milk.

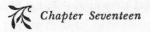

Chapter Seventeen

Fortify Your Cereals

Research has shown that anyone wishing to experience maximum well-being and minimum fatigue must eat breakfasts supplying 20 grams or more of protein. Yet a cereal, which may constitute the entire meal for children and parents alike, supplies an average of 6 to 8 grams of protein if it is one of the usual cooked varieties, and about half as much if it is a cold one. Even whole-grain cereals, which do furnish vitamin E, iron, the B vitamins, and protein, are 60 per cent or more starch. Such cereals are nevertheless excellent for children and for any family whose budget is limited provided they are eaten with other protein foods or fortified with such high-protein foods as wheat germ, soy grits, or powdered milk.

"Enriched" cereals, like "enriched" flour, have been robbed of some twenty nutrients; little worth mentioning is put back. Most packaged cereals have been far more successful as money makers than as health builders. Their nutritive value can be greatly increased by mixing ½ to 1 cup or more of toasted wheat germ into a 10-ounce package as soon as it is opened. Most of the quick-cooking and precooked cereals have also lost many of their original nutrients. If the achievement of health is to be the goal, such cereals as wheat germ and middlings, old-fashioned oatmeal, steel-cut oats, and stone-ground whole-grain cereals should be served almost exclusively. These cereals have the added advantage of being much more flavorful than the quick-cooking varieties.

Cooking a cereal a long time or at a high temperature decreases the health-building quality of the protein and causes partial destruction of several of the B vitamins. The practice of cooking cereal in the evening and reheating it for breakfast is unwise for the same reason. With the exception of unground wheat, cereals should not be cooked under pressure. Although the shorter cooking time is better, little loss of vitamin B_1 occurs when cereals such as steel-cut oats are cooked as long as 30 minutes.

Since few foods contribute so much to health as does wheat germ, it should be added to as many cereals as palatability permits. Wheat germ and middlings cooked alone as a cereal are usually enjoyed the first time they are eaten. A taste for pure wheat germ has to be developed. If it is new to your family, start by adding only 1/2 teaspoon to a serving of any cooked cereal and increase the amount gradually as the taste becomes familiar. When once the taste is enjoyed, pure wheat germ can be used alone as an uncooked cereal, toasted and eaten with uncooked cereal, or cooked 5 minutes, preferably in milk.

A number of cereals not generally used are excellent and usually enjoyed. For example, steel-cut oats have not been submitted to the high temperature necessary before oats can be rolled; they are therefore nutritionally superior to rolled oats and deserve wider use. Soy grits, or cracked soybeans, can be mixed with any cereal to be cooked. Whole buckwheat is especially appreciated by anyone who enjoys buckwheat pancakes. Triple-cleaned, unground wheat, purchased at stock-feed stores, makes an excellent cereal. Because of its large percentage of starch, however, any whole-wheat cereal has a considerably lower vitamin and protein content than wheat germ.

The protein, calcium, and vitamin B_2 can be increased, and refined sugar, when used, decreased if powdered milk is added to cooked cereals. Several brands of instant milk can be stirred into the cereal just before it is served, thus eliminating the use of a double boiler, although a few brands will lump. The instant milk is twice as bulky as the old-fashioned variety, and far more nutrients can be obtained if non-instant powdered milk is mixed with the dry cereal before it is cooked. Many mothers have told me that the addition of powdered milk has caused their children to enjoy cereals much more than ever before.

Except for pure wheat germ, the most valuable cereal is wheat germ and middlings; hence it should be served more often than any other.

WHEAT GERM AND MIDDLINGS

Heat to boiling:

2 cups water   1 teaspoon salt

Stir constantly while sprinkling into water:

1 cup wheat germ and middlings

Lower heat and simmer 12 to 15 minutes; add more water if needed to keep cereal moist; remove from heat and add while stirring rapidly:

1 cup instant powdered milk

Let set 2 or 3 minutes before serving.

VARIATIONS:

Mix 1 cup each dry cereal and non-instant powdered milk; prepare cereal in top of double boiler; cook over direct heat 3 to 5 minutes and finish cooking over boiling water.

Instead of using water, cook cereal in fresh milk.

Use 2½ cups water and add ½ cup soy grits.

Instead of wheat germ and middlings, use yellow corn meal, whole buckwheat, converted rice, or any finely ground whole-grain cereal. These cereals cook in 15 minutes. Stir 1 cup instant milk into each before serving; or mix an equal amount of non-instant powdered milk and any ground cereal before cooking, and prepare in a double boiler.

Cook 1 cup of the following cereals in 2½ cups of water and ½ cup soy grits for 30 minutes: steel-cut oats, oatmeal, brown rice, millet, hulled barley, or any coarsely ground whole grain; add more water if needed; 3 minutes before serving stir in instant milk. Use the same method in cooking cracked wheat but simmer for 1 hour.

Simmer unground wheat in water 2 or 3 hours or cook under pressure 30 minutes.

Although some of the vitamin B_1 and folic acid in wheat germ are harmed by being heated, most persons find wheat germ considerably more palatable if it is toasted sufficiently to lose its raw flavor. Toasting it at home is far more economical than purchasing the pre-toasted varieties, many of which have the fat and vitamin E removed. Since ½ cup of natural wheat germ supplies 19 grams of complete protein (more than 3 eggs) in addition to vitamin E, many B vitamins, unsaturated fatty acids, and iron, wheat germ makes an ideal cold cereal for breakfast. Toasting it with honey makes it somewhat crisp and crunchy as well as sweeter.

TOASTED WHEAT GERM

Mix thoroughly:

4 cups fresh wheat germ   ½ cup warmed honey

Spread wheat germ on a low baking pan. Roast in a moderate oven at 300° F. for 10 minutes. Cool, pour into a plastic bag, and keep refrigerated. Serve with milk as a cold cereal or mix with any cold whole-grain cereal before serving.

VARIATIONS:

Omit honey if natural flavor is enjoyed.
Use instead of crumb-topping for desserts.

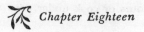 *Chapter Eighteen*

Milk Cannot Be Overemphasized

Milk is such a valuable food that a quart daily should be drunk by each person, regardless of age. Almost every individual who does not drink milk shows signs of deficiencies of protein, calcium, and riboflavin, or vitamin B_2. People who do not use milk as a beverage have been found to have an average intake of only 0.3 gram of calcium daily; yet they wonder why they suffer from insomnia and are often highstrung and nervous. One should learn to enjoy the taste of milk and drink it with meals and between meals, as a substitute for water. People often remark, "I don't drink milk but I take calcium tablets," implying that calcium is a substitute for milk. Such a remark is like saying, "I do not have a car but I do have a fender."

The best milk available is medically certified raw milk, the production of which is carefully supervised by the American Medical Milk Commission. Unfortunately, only a few certified herds exist in the United States. Most persons in our country over fifty were brought up on raw milk, and such milk is still preferable provided it comes from disease-free cows and is carefully handled. Pasteurization causes a loss of calcium and the destruction of enzymes, antibodies, and hormones. When the sources and methods of handling milk are unknown and medically certified milk is not available, however, pasteurized milk should be used.

If milk is exposed to light, vitamin B_2 is gradually destroyed. For example, when milk in a clear bottle is left in the sunshine, 33 per cent of the vitamin is lost in 1 hour, 69 per cent in 2 hours. As much as 48 per cent of the vitamin is destroyed in 10 minutes when milk is heated in a glass utensil compared to 22 per cent when heated in an uncovered metal utensil; when heated in a covered metal utensil, no loss occurs. If you cannot be at home when milk is delivered, arrange for the milkman to cover it with a box or a dark cloth. Cartons which do not admit light are preferable to bottles for delivering milk which cannot be taken in immediately. Be particularly careful to use opaque utensils rather than glass ones for preparing milk soups, custards, puddings, and milk drinks unless the pudding or custard is to be baked in a dark oven. Keep these foods covered as much as possible not only during cooking but also while they are cooling.

Although persons who rely entirely on milk drinks for their supply of milk rarely obtain sufficient amounts to produce a high degree of health, milk drinks are particularly valuable during illnesses and infections, and in the summer when parents must compete with the soft-drink industry if health is to be maintained. Ingredients can be kept on hand so that malted milks and milkshakes may be prepared at home. Since raw egg white prevents the absorption of the B vitamin, biotin, and therefore should not be served, especially to children or ill persons, eggnogs should be cooked or made only of egg yolks.

Skim milk contains the nutrients in which people are so often deficient: protein, calcium, and riboflavin; it also supplies a variety of other minerals and small amounts of many B vitamins. Calcium, however, must react with fat to form a soap in the intestines; only after this soap dissolves can the calcium pass into the blood. Because most meals supply some fat, skim milk can be drunk at meals with reasonable assurance that the calcium will be absorbed. If skim milk is drunk between meals, some food such as a cracker with peanut butter or a tablespoon of nuts should be taken with it to supply fat.

In addition to milk served as a beverage, the more milk you can work into your cooking, the better health your family will probably enjoy. Whenever you can, use evaporated milk without diluting it. It may be added to custards and ice creams and used in gelatin desserts instead of whipped cream. Half the water having been evaporated, the milk supplies (if not diluted) twice the amount of nutrients found in fresh milk. Its taste, if disliked, can be disguised with lemon juice and flavorings.

Few foods can offer so much to your family's health as can powdered skim milk, provided it is used not as a substitute for fresh milk but to fortify foods, thus adding to their content of protein, calcium, and vitamin B_2. Only when persons live in localities where it is impossible to obtain clean, fresh milk, such as in parts of India and Japan, should they use heat-treated powdered milk instead of fresh milk as a beverage. Dr. Frances M. Pottinger and others have shown that the less milk is heated, the greater is its nutritional value. The present popularity of instant milk instead of fresh milk as a beverage is one more factor in bringing about physical deterioration.

All recipes in this book have been tested with non-instant, or spray-process, powdered milk. This milk is as fine as face powder, beautifully white, and has a mild, delicate taste and odor. One-half to ⅔ cup of non-instant powdered milk is equivalent to a quart of fresh milk, whereas 1⅓ cups of instant milk is equal to a quart of liquid milk. Companies which produce instant powdered milk and maintain large test kitchens have informed me that instant milk cannot be used in concentrated form in cooking. It does not dissolve readily after being mixed with dry ingredients; it causes bakery products to become gummy and other foods to be chalky. Yogurt prepared with instant milk is stringy, and uncooked foods, such as cake icings and candies, are gritty. My experience has been that some brands of instant powdered milk are wonderful for fortifying cooked cereals and fresh milk to be used as a beverage. Reconstituted milk made of the instant powder can be used economically in cooking instead of fresh milk. My feeling is that any housewife truly interested in building health should keep both instant and non-instant powdered milk on hand at all times.

The spray-process powdered milk, preferable for most cooking, can be purchased directly from milk companies, bakers, and health-food stores. If your health-food store does not carry non-instant powdered milk, ask that it be ordered for you. This non-instant powdered milk must be kept in a tightly closed container; if left uncovered or in a paper bag, it can absorb almost 10 per cent water in a single foggy or rainy day. Moist powdered milk becomes lumpy and is difficult to mix. The moisture causes decomposition of protein to set in; eventually a disagreeable odor and flavor develop. I have seen and certainly smelled powdered milk which could not possibly be used because it had been left open a few days, yet if not exposed to air, it will keep almost indefinitely. Store it in a cannister or a 2-pound coffee can.

Yogurt is another form of milk which is nutritionally excellent. It can be prepared inexpensively at home by adding either yogurt culture or already prepared yogurt to liquid milk. As long as the milk is kept warm, the yogurt bacteria grow; they thrive on milk sugar and change some of it to lactic acid, which causes the milk to thicken. As soon as the yogurt becomes thick, it should be immediately chilled to stop bacterial growth; otherwise so much acid may be liberated that the milk curds separate from the whey and the yogurt becomes too sour to be palatable.

Yogurt is nutritionally superior to sweet milk in many ways. The milk protein in yogurt is partially predigested by the bacteria; some of the calcium dissolves in the lactic acid. If digestion is below par, the protein and calcium from yogurt are more available to the body than are these substances in sweet milk. The bacteria in yogurt thrive in the intestines, whereas bacteria found in ordinary sour milk and buttermilk are killed at 90° F., or below body temperature. The yogurt bacteria living in the intestines break down milk sugar into lactic acid; since the bacteria which cause gas and putrefaction cannot live in lactic acid, they are largely destroyed. It is for these reasons that persons suffering from digestive disturbances or milk allergies can usually tolerate yogurt without difficulty; and that yogurt is especially valuable to use as a formula for sick infants. Furthermore yogurt bacteria synthesize, or make, the entire group of B vitamins in amounts sufficient for both themselves and their host; thus the person who uses yogurt liberally has a "B-vitamin factory" in his intestines.

When antibiotics are given by mouth, valuable intestinal bacteria are destroyed; in their absence, fungus, molds, and wild yeast grow rapidly and often infect the intestine itself and the area around the anus, resulting in severe itching which may last for years. The infestation is sometimes carried to the mouth, especially by small children, where it causes thrush. Such conditions usually clear up quickly if 1 to 3 cups of yogurt are eaten daily. They can be largely prevented if yogurt is eaten at each meal during the time an antibiotic must be taken by mouth or during convalescence from the illness.

If yogurt is new to you, do not expect to enjoy it immediately. Cultivate a taste for it gradually, then serve it frequently. Yogurt is particularly delicious if made into a sundae with frozen undiluted orange juice. When health is below par, it is often advisable to use as much as a quart of yogurt daily, substituting it entirely for fresh milk. Bacteria are killed by heat, therefore to use yogurt in cooking has no nutritional advantage.

A form of milk which cannot be recommended is chocolate milk; yet surveys have shown that about 90 per cent of the milk purchased in school cafeterias is in this form. Experiments have shown that animals fed chocolate milk absorbed less calcium and phosphorus than did animals given plain milk; their growth was retarded, and their bones were much smaller and more fragile. Calcium deficiencies are already widespread, and mothers are unwise to entice their children to drink milk by making it into cocoa. If chocolate and cocoa are used, powdered milk may be added to supply extra calcium.

In preparing meals for your family, use a combination of all types of milk: fresh milk, evaporated milk, "tiger's milk," buttermilk, yogurt, and both instant and non-instant powdered milk; use them all liberally.

Regardless of the form it takes, milk can rarely be overemphasized.

VANILLA MILKSHAKE

Shake, beat, or blend in liquefier until smooth:

1 cup chilled fresh milk	⅛ teaspoon vanilla flavoring
¼ cup powdered milk	½ to 1 cup vanilla ice cream
2 or 3 teaspoons sugar	

Pour into chilled glass and serve.

VARIATIONS:

Add any one of the following: crushed fresh strawberries; mashed banana; crushed pineapple; apricot purée; date pulp; orange juice and grated rind or orange extract; crushed and sweetened loganberries or raspberries.

Instead of vanilla flavoring use almond or a drop each of almond and lemon; lemon and banana; black walnut, maple, peach, or pineapple flavorings.

Use any fruit ice cream or sherbet.

Omit ice cream and add 3 tablespoons sweetened whipped evaporated milk.

PINEAPPLE FLOAT

Beat, shake, or blend in liquefier until smooth:

1 cup pineapple juice	¼ cup powdered milk

Pour into a glass and add:

¼ cup vanilla ice cream or whipped cream

VARIATIONS:

Omit pineapple juice and use any of the following juices: apricot, pear, loganberry, strawberry, raspberry, boysenberry, black cherry, grape, peach, or orange; use juices from canned fruits when available.

Omit ice cream and add evaported milk whipped with lemon juice and sweetened to taste.

MALTED MILK

Shake, beat, or blend in liquefier until smooth:

1 cup fresh milk	⅓ cup powdered milk
1¼ tablespoons malted milk	½ to 1 cup ice cream
½ to 1 teaspoon brewers' yeast	¼ teaspoon vanilla
1 or 2 teaspoons sugar	

Pour into chilled glass and serve.

VARIATIONS:

Add ¼ cup crushed pineapple, strawberries, or other fruit, purée, or juice.

Omit sugar and add 1 teaspoon or more dark molasses; add vanilla, maple, or rum flavoring.

Omit ice cream, heat to simmering, and sprinkle generously with nutmeg.

EGGNOG

Shake, beat, or blend in liquefier until smooth:

1 cup fresh milk	¼ cup powdered milk
2 egg yolks	pinch of salt
3 teaspoons sugar	½ teaspoon vanilla

Serve chilled or hot sprinkled with nutmeg.

VARIATIONS:

Use 2 teaspoons sugar and add 1 teaspoon or more dark molasses; or add maple, rum, or brandy flavoring.

Omit vanilla and add 1 tablespoon brandy or rum.

RASPBERRY YOGURT

Shake, beat, or blend in liquefier until smooth:

1 cup chilled juice from canned raspberries	⅓ cup powdered milk

Add and beat slightly:

1 cup yogurt

Pour into chilled glasses and serve.

VARIATIONS:

Instead of raspberry juice use 1 cup of any of the following juices: apricot, orange, Concord grape, pineapple, prune, pear, peach, strawberry, or other berry juice; sweeten to taste.

Use fresh milk instead of yogurt in basic recipe or any variation.

ORANGE SHAKE

Combine in liquefier:

2 cups chilled fresh or diluted frozen orange juice	1 tablespoon sugar
½ cup powdered milk	few drops vanilla

Blend until smooth; add 3 tablespoons crushed ice to each serving.

VARIATIONS:

Instead of orange juice use the following fruits and/or juices: apricot, pear, strawberry, raspberry, boysenberry, loganberry, black cherry, peach, grape, pineapple; omit vanilla except for apricot and peach shake; add 1 tablespoon lemon juice to berry and pineapple shake; omit sugar when juices from canned fruits are used. Don't miss Concord grape shake; it is delicious.

COCOA

Heat to simmering:

3 cups fresh or reconstituted milk

Meanwhile shake or blend in liquefier and add to hot milk:

1 cup liquid milk	pinch of salt
3 tablespoons sugar	1 teaspoon vanilla
3 tablespoons cocoa	½ cup non-instant powdered milk

Do not boil. Serve as soon as hot.

VARIATIONS:

Use 3 cups boiling water; beat cocoa, sugar, salt, and 1 cup non-instant or 1½ cups instant powdered milk with 1 cup water. Stir in 5 minutes before serving.

For foamy cocoa, use 3½ cups liquid milk; whip ½ cup chilled evaporated milk and stir in just before serving. The evaporated milk adds to both texture and flavor.

Omit cocoa; drop into warm milk and stir until melted 1 square bitter chocolate; or omit sugar and use sweet chocolate.

Chill cocoa; pour into glasses and add ½ cup vanilla ice cream to each serving.

POSTUM

Beat, shake, or blend in liquefier until smooth:

¾ cup fresh milk   3 tablespoons powdered milk

Heat to simmering; pour over:

1 teaspoon Postum

Stir well and sweeten to taste.

VARIATIONS:

Omit fresh milk; blend ¼ cup powdered milk with ¾ cup water and heat to simmering.

Instead of Postum use any other powdered coffee substitute.

Tiger's milk is amazingly high in protein and the B vitamin and can be made to supply the daily need for unsaturated fatty acids. Anyone who wishes to enjoy the greatest well-being with the least effort would do well to drink 1 or more glasses of it daily. It is also excellent for persons who like to drink breakfast rather than eat it; and for individuals whose health is below par.

Brewers' yeast, which tiger's milk contains, is extremely rich in phosphorus. To maintain an ideal calcium and phosphorus ratio, ¼ cup of powdered calcium lactate should be stirred into each pound of yeast, especially if yeast is to be used daily.

TIGER'S MILK*

Blend in liquefier:

½ cup frozen, undiluted orange juice	1 or 2 teaspoons vanilla
	1 to 3 teaspoons safflower or soy
1 cup fresh skim milk	oil

Blend at low speed 1 minute; without stopping motor add:

½ cup non-instant powdered skim milk	¼ to ½ cup brewers' yeast

Pour into plastic refrigerator pitcher; add and stir:

2 or 3 cups fresh skim milk

Serve no more than ½ cup (4 ounces) at first. Drink with meals and/or for midmeals.

VARIATIONS:

Instead of non-instant powdered milk, add ¾ cup instant milk; 1⅓ cups of instant milk give the nutritional equivalent of the above recipe but cause the drink to be extremely thick.

If no liquefier is available, beat with egg beater or electric mixer or shake in quart jar.

When flavor of yeast becomes familiar, increase to ¾ cup.

If more calories are desired, increase oil to 3 tablespoons.

Instead of orange juice, use fresh, canned, or frozen berries, chunk or grated canned pineapple, banana, or a combination of fruits.

Add 1 or 2 egg yolks and dash of salt.

Although yogurt has been made for hundreds of years by persons who never heard of thermometers, it is much easier to make with a thermometer. Yogurt bacteria grow rapidly between the

---

* Instant tiger's milk, convenient for traveling or for mixing in juice or milk at restaurants (a fourth cup or more can also be added to almost any highly seasoned food) is available from Plus Products, 2302 East 38th Street, Los Angeles 58, California. Balanced B yeast, Red Star yeast, and calcium lactate are also available from the same source.

temperatures of 90 and 120° F. They are killed by high temperatures; below 90° F. they grow slowly if at all. The bacteria which produce ordinary sour milk multiply rapidly at warm room temperatures, or between 65 and 85° F., but are killed at 90° F. If you attempt to make yogurt and fail to keep the milk warm enough, you will have ordinary sour milk instead of yogurt. The trick of making yogurt is in keeping the milk quite warm until it thickens.

An electric yogurt maker,* which maintains a constant ideal temperature, holds 6 pints or more of yogurt, and takes the guesswork out of yogurt making, is a worth-while investment for persons who eat yogurt frequently.

Cows are given penicillin frequently these days, and the penicillin in the fresh milk destroys the bacteria and prevents the yogurt from thickening. For this reason I recommend that yogurt be made with powdered milk, although fresh milk may be used if it is known to be penicillin-free.

Should whey separate from the milk curds in your yogurt, the incubation time has been too long, or the yogurt has not been chilled quickly enough. Beat, sweeten to taste with honey or dark molasses, and serve as "buttermilk."

When yogurt does not thicken, the temperature during incubation may have been so high that the bacteria were killed or so low that the bacteria could not grow; incubation time may have been too short; you may have forgotten to add the starter or culture; or the starter or culture may have been old. Add more starter, check temperature carefully, and incubate longer.

If yogurt has an unpleasant taste, molds and foreign bacteria are probably responsible. Get a new starter and be sure to heat fresh milk, if used, to simmering and then cool it before adding the bacteria.

"Old-country" yogurt was usually made from milk which had been allowed to evaporate on the back of the stove for two or three days. The following recipes, to which evaporated milk is added, has a particularly delicious old-country flavor.

---

* Yogurt makers and pure yogurt culture are available from the International Yogurt Company, 628 North Doheny Drive, Los Angeles 69, California.

YOGURT

Beat or blend in liquefier:

2 cups tepid water   yogurt culture or 3 tablespoons
1½ cups non-instant powdered   commercial or previously made
    skim milk   yogurt

Pour mixture into a pitcher containing:

1 quart tepid water   1 large can evaporated milk

Stir well and pour into drinking glasses or pint jars. Set glasses or jars in dry yogurt maker. If yogurt maker is not used, put into large pan of warm water; bring water level to rim of glasses or jars. Cover pan, and set over pilot light or in warming oven where a temperature of 100 to 120° F. can be maintained.

Check consistency at end of 3 hours. Chill immediately after milk thickens. Yogurt will keep in refrigerator 5 days or longer.

Serve as a sundae with frozen undiluted orange juice or lemonade.

VARIATIONS:

Serve with brown sugar and cinnamon, honey and finely shredded orange or lemon rind, or sweetened berries, peaches, or other fresh fruit.

Omit evaporated milk and use 1½ quarts of fresh whole or skim milk to which ½ to 1 cup of powdered milk is added. After culturing, beat slightly and serve instead of buttermilk. This yogurt can be used for an infant's formula.

Make yogurt of goat's milk; omit or use powdered and evaporated milks.

Yogurt popsicles: Stir together 1 pint yogurt, 1 small can frozen orange juice, 2 teaspoons vanilla. Pour into paper cups, put tongue compressor in center, and freeze. Add ¼ cup instant tiger's milk if desired.

Because it is exposed to high temperatures during the drying process, powdered milk is nutritionally inferior to fresh milk as a beverage. If milk is to be cooked, however, as it is in custards, cream soups, hot milk drinks, and many other foods, money can be saved by using reconstituted rather than fresh milk.

RECONSTITUTED MILK

Stir or shake in a quart jar until smooth:

2 cups cold water   1⅓ cups instant powdered milk

Fill jar with cold water. Refrigerate.
Or put into a liquefier:

1 to 2 cups cold water

Start motor at low speed and pour into vortex:

⅔ cup non-instant powdered milk

Turn off motor as soon as water and milk are blended. Pour into a quart jar or milk bottle and fill with cold water. Refrigerate.

VARIATION:

To save refrigerator space, stir or blend powdered milk with 2 cups water; before using, dilute milk with an equal amount of water.

When the budget is limited, mix 2 cups of instant or 1 cup of non-instant powdered milk into 1 quart of water; fill drinking glass with half fresh milk, half reconstituted milk.

To add nutritional value to your own favorite recipes as well as to save storage space, beat 2 cups each water and non-instant powdered milk until smooth; store in refrigerator without diluting; when making cream soups, soft custards, milk drinks, cream sauces, puddings, and other foods containing fresh milk, for each cup of fresh milk called for in the recipe, use ¾ cup fresh milk and ¼ cup undiluted powdered-milk mixture. Stir in the powdered-milk mixture 2 or 3 minutes before removing food from heat.

Most of the buttermilk on the market, known as cultured buttermilk, is made from skim milk to which lactic-acid bacteria and bits of butterfat are added. Cultured buttermilk contains more protein, calcium, and vitamin B_2 than does churned buttermilk and is, therefore, nutritionally superior to the churned variety. Since whole milk usually contains 4 to 5 per cent butterfat, buttermilk 2 per cent, and skim milk none, the person who wishes to drink buttermilk yet remain on a low-animal-fat diet can prepare it himself. Home-cultured buttermilk is also considerably cheaper than the commercial varieties, especially if made from reconstituted milk.

CULTURED BUTTERMILK

Shake in quart jar or milk bottle:

3½ cups fresh or reconstituted   ½ cup commercial buttermilk
  skim milk

Cover jar or bottle and set in a warm place overnight (perhaps on a hot-water heater), or for 10 to 12 hours. The temperature should be about 80 to 85° F.

When milk has coagulated, shake or stir well and refrigerate.

VARIATIONS:

Use half fresh skim milk and half reconstituted milk; or combine and shake together ½ cup buttermilk, 2 cups water, 1⅔ cups instant powdered milk; after shaking, fill jar or bottle with water and culture as in basic recipe.

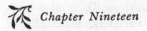 *Chapter Nineteen*

Freezing, Canning, and Pickling

Persons who are so fortunate as to be able to grow their own fruits and vegetables on naturally mineralized, composted, and mulched soil not only experience rare flavor treats but can achieve a higher degree of health than can millions of other people in our country. Furthermore they can grow foods almost impossible to buy in city markets: fresh vitamin-C-rich pimentos and paprikas, tampala, Chinese celery and cabbage, crisp kohlrabi, and many other delicious foods. Any surplus of this bounty can be frozen or canned for the winter months.

Even if you must buy your fruits and vegetables at a market, home-frozen and -canned foods are less expensive and usually more nutritious and delicious than commercially prepared ones. If you do purchase foods for freezing or canning, get acquainted with the wholesale produce markets. Late on Saturday morning foods which will not keep well over the week end can be obtained at bargain prices. When gallons of vegetables, fruits, and juices are stored away, larger quantities are eaten, fewer pastries and sweets are desired, and a higher degree of health is assured.

The same rules for preserving nutrients in cooking should be applied in freezing and canning fruits and vegetables. The foods should be washed without a moment's unnecessary soaking. Loosen the skins of peaches and tomatoes by steaming them a few minutes rather than by soaking them in hot water. Do not use lye to remove the skins of peaches; it not only destroys vita-

min C but may cause the fruit to become so alkaline that botulism, or fatal food poisoning, may develop. Whenever possible,
chill the food before cutting it. So that enzymes will be quickly
destroyed, syrup which is to be poured over fruit should be boiling and the initial heating should be as rapid as possible.

Space permits only a short discussion of freezing, canning, and
pickling here. More detailed instructions may be obtained from
your State Department of Agriculture.

Freezing Fruits and Vegetables

Fruits and vegetables to be frozen should be prepared and frozen
with all possible speed to prevent loss of vitamin C. Fruits which
discolor easily, such as apricots, and all vegetables retain greater
nutritive value and better color and flavor if they are precooked,
or blanched, to destroy enzymes before being frozen. Uncooked
fruit should be cut sufficiently so that it can be solidly packed
without air spaces between the pieces of fruit. Crushed or puréed
raw fruit, for example, has been found to retain more vitamin C
than whole or halved fruit because it packs more solidly.

If you must purchase your fruits and vegetables for freezing,
buy them in the early morning and prepare them immediately.
If you have your own garden and freezing unit, spend a lazy day,
taking a long nap in the afternoon; then gather the various foods
at dusk after a sunny day, when the vitamin content has been
found to be at its highest, and pack and freeze them in the cool
of the evening.

PREPARATION OF FRUITS FOR FREEZING

Wash fruit quickly without soaking; peel or stem; cut as for table use,
preparing only 3 to 5 cups at one time; when facilities permit, chill
before washing.

Loosen skins of peaches by steaming 5 minutes over boiling water.

Sweeten fruit to taste, using approximately ¼ cup sugar to each 3
cups sliced California persimmons, guavas, very ripe apricots; ½ cup

sugar for 3 cups sliced peaches, nectarines, seeded black cherries, firm apricots, or sweet berries; ¾ cup sugar for sour cherries, gooseberries, or other sour berries. Mix fruit well with sugar, let stand in refrigerator until sugar is melted.

Pack fruit in containers; put on lids; label and date containers; if fruit cannot be frozen immediately, keep in very cold refrigerator. Molds and bacteria may cause fruits, particularly soft berries, to spoil before they are frozen.

Place in quick-freezing unit and freeze at —20° F. or at a lower temperature; store at 0° F. or below.

Before serving let fruit thaw slowly in refrigerator; serve immediately after thawing.

VARIATIONS:

Instead of mixing dry sugar with fruit, prepare a heavy syrup of 3 cups each sugar and water; heat until sugar is dissolved; store in refrigerator until thoroughly chilled. Place fruit in container and fill with cold syrup to within 1 inch of the top; if any fruit floats, push down into syrup before sealing package.

Frozen cooked fruits: For any fruit which would be more palatable cooked than raw, such as cranberries, rhubarb, gooseberries, underripe peaches or apricots, steam in 2 or 3 tablespoons water until just soft, or 4 to 8 minutes; chill thoroughly, sweeten to taste, pack, freeze, and store.

Frozen fruit purées: Use overripe fruits or small unattractive berries, apricots, or other fruits. Chill thoroughly and mash, crush, or blend in liquefier. Sweeten to taste; pack, freeze, and store. Use for making ice cream, gelatin salads or desserts, sherbets, or serve as a sauce alone or over rice, ice cream, or baked custard. Prepare applesauce or apricot purée as for canning (pp. 457–458); chill, pack, and freeze.

Frozen fruit juices: Prepare tomato, berry, grape, or any fruit juice as for canning (pp. 457–458); chill thoroughly, pack into suitable containers, freeze, and store.

Frozen vegetables: Prepare vegetables as if for table use; wash quickly, cut, sort for sizes; break broccoli and cauliflower into sizes suitable for serving; slice string beans. Prepare no more than 2 pounds of vegetables at one time. Place vegetables in a cloth bag; set on a rack *above* rapidly boiling water in utensil with tight-fitting lid; shake bag so that vegetables are loose and steam can easily surround them. Steam asparagus, string beans, lima beans, broccoli, Brussels sprouts, cauliflower, and diced zucchini or summer squash 5 minutes; steam peas and corn cut from cob 2 minutes, spinach and other greens 3 minutes, artichokes 8 minutes. Lift bag of vegetables and immerse immediately in ice water to which are added several teaspoons of salt; do not soak longer than 1 minute, or only long enough to chill. Drain. Pack in cellophane bags, seal with a hot iron, package, label, freeze, and store.

Frozen vegetable purées: Blanch vegetables as directed above; chill in ice water, drain, and blend in liquefier; salt to taste, pack, freeze, and store. Use for soufflés, cream soups, or gelatin salads. Prepare large amounts of these vegetables if you must cook for a person staying on a smooth diet, an elderly person, or a small baby. Put purées on to heat while still frozen.

Cold-Pack Canning

In cold-pack canning the uncooked fruit is packed into clean jars, hot syrup is poured over it, and the fruit is cooked in the jar. By far the easiest method is to cook it by steam. Set the jars on a rack above boiling water in any large utensil which can be tightly covered. If the steam is held in, it is the same temperature as that of boiling water. The jar and lid are sterilized as the fruit cooks.

Do not fasten the lids tightly until after the fruit is cooked; the steam inside the jars must be allowed to escape. When the lid is tightly fastened, the steam pressure often causes the jars to break or even explode, resulting in serious accidents from flying glass and scalding liquid.

If the top of the fruit discolors, enzyme action has occurred before the fruit was cooked. When discoloration occurs after the food is canned, it indicates that the fruit was not sufficiently cooked to destroy the enzymes. If the fruit comes to the top of the jar, the syrup used is heavier than the fruit or much juice has been cooked out of the fruit, causing it to be light. These conditions do not mean that the fruit is spoiled. If the syrup becomes cloudy or mold develops, discard the fruit without tasting it. Botulinus gives no warning odor, color change, or taste.

Vary the cooking time and the syrup used according to the

condition of the fruit. Use a somewhat longer cooking time when fruit is unusually solid or put into the jars so compactly that little or no hot syrup can be added. Use heavier syrup for very sour fruits and those tightly packed. Fruits may be canned without sugar and sweetened just before being used. Since sugar penetrates fruit slowly, it is more evenly distributed when added before the fruit is canned.

COLD-PACK APRICOTS

Wash fruit quickly, cut into halves, and remove seeds, decay, and bruised parts; pack into clean jars to within 1 inch of the top. Put 3 or 4 pits in each jar for flavor.

Fill to within ½ inch of the top with boiling water or syrup; slip a silver knife down the inside edge of jar to allow liquid to be evenly distributed.

Wipe off glass edges and adjust rubber and lid; fasten lid with thumb and little finger; it must be loose enough to turn easily.

Set jars on a rack above boiling water in a large utensil such as a turkey roaster or electric cooker; cover utensil.

Bring water under rack to a rolling boil; start counting cooking time when water begins to boil; steam 16 minutes for pint jars, 20 minutes for quart jars, 30 minutes for half-gallon jars.

At the end of cooking period, tighten tops; leave jars upright; if ring tops are used, remove rings after 24 hours; store in a cool dark place.

VARIATIONS:

For sweet loosely packed fruits, make light syrup of 1 cup sugar to 3 cups water; make medium syrup of 1 cup sugar to 2 cups water, or heavy syrup of 1 cup each sugar and water; use heavy syrup for soft, tightly packed fruits or sour fruits.

Steam pint and quart jars of berries, precooked apples, precooked rhubarb, and small plums 15 minutes, half-gallon jars 24 minutes. Steam pints or quarts of cherries, freestone peaches, very ripe or small pears, or large plums 20 minutes, half gallons 30 minutes; steam quarts of fresh prunes, cling peaches, firm unpeeled pears, peeled grapefruit sections, and pints of tomatoes 30 minutes; half gallons of the fruits and quarts of tomatoes 40 to 45 minutes.

Follow basic recipe in canning berries, cherries, grapes, peaches, pears, and plums; loosen skins of tomatoes and peaches by steaming over boiling water. Leave high-quality pears unpeeled; put 2 or 3 pits in each jar of freestone nectarines or peaches.

Canned apples: Prepare 1 quart light syrup with 1 cup sugar to 1 quart water; bring to boiling; meanwhile wash, core, and remove bruised and wormy spots from apples; do not peel or touch with water after they are washed; dice, slice, or quarter and drop directly into boiling syrup; boil 4 minutes; pack into clean jars, fill with hot syrup, and steam 15 minutes; seal. Add ½ teaspoon each cloves and a small piece of cinnamon as desired. Repeat the process as syrup is used, preparing only 2 or 3 pounds of apples at a time.

Canned peppers: Since peppers are such a rich source of vitamin C, any excess grown in the garden should be frozen or canned; use red bell peppers, ripe pimentos, and paprikas when available; wash, remove stem ends and seeds, cut into halves or quarters; pack into jars, add ½ teaspoon salt for each pint, fill with boiling water, and steam 55 minutes for pint or quart jars, or 40 minutes at 5 pounds pressure; or add 2 tablespoons vinegar and steam without pressure 40 minutes.

Canned rhubarb: Wash, cut into 1-inch lengths, steam with 2 tablespoons water until soft, or about 15 minutes; pack boiling hot without adding water or sugar; steam 15 minutes, seal. After opening, sweeten to taste; let stand before serving.

Canned tomatoes: By far the easiest way to can tomatoes is to remove stem ends, pack solidly into jars, squeezing out enough juice to fill jar; add 1 teaspoon salt per quart and steam 45 minutes for quart jars, 60 minutes for half-gallon jars. After opening a jar of tomatoes, lift off and discard skins. If peeling before canning is desired, steam the washed tomatoes over boiling water, cool slightly, and remove skins; do not immerse in either boiling or cold water; pack solidly into jars; salt but do not add water.

Canning Juices and Sauces

The purpose of cold-pack canning, or cooking the fruit in the jars, is to prevent the fruit from mashing by being handled after it is cooked. When mashing is not a problem, the easiest method of canning fruits is the open-kettle method in which the juice or cooked fruit is brought to a boil, poured into clean jars, and sealed. The pasteurization point is 140° F.; therefore, the jar is sterilized by the hot fruit or juice.

Tart sauces and juices should be sweetened just before being used rather than before they are canned.

TOMATO JUICE AND PURÉE

Use small tomatoes or irregular sizes; wash quickly, remove decayed spots, and put into a large utensil; do not peel, quarter, or remove stem ends.

Set over high heat; use a large knife and cut through many tomatoes at one time, bringing knife from one side of utensil to the other; mash tomatoes slightly to squeeze out juice. Add:

1 teaspoon salt for each quart of tomatoes

If seasoned juice is desired, add celery leaves, green pepper stalks and seeds, onion tops, a few sliced carrots.

Cover utensil; keep heat high and cook until tomatoes are tender, stirring occasionally to ensure even heating.

Press tomatoes through a cone-shaped colander; collect thin juice in one utensil; change utensils and keep thick purée separate.

Bring juice to a rolling boil; set jar in pan of warm water to prevent breaking; pour boiling juice into jar to within ⅛ inch of top; wipe edge of glass, adjust rubber and lid, and seal.

Invert jar to sterilize lid. Let stand in a place free from draft. Do not move the jars until cool. If screw top is used, remove ring after 24 hours.

Use purée for making catsup (p. 460); or bring to a rolling boil, stirring frequently; pour into clean jars and seal. Use for sauces and soups.

VARIATIONS:

Use the same procedure in making sauces and/or juices from the following fruits: apricots, apples, plums, berries, grapes, cherries, peaches, pears, nectarines, or yellow tomatoes. Use small or especially ripe fruits not desirable for other canning. Do not remove stems from strawberries or stones from small apricots or cherries. If clear berry, plum, or grape juice is desired, strain through a cloth after passing through colander. Do not peel, core, or cut apples except to remove damaged spots. Add only enough water at the beginning of cooking to prevent sticking. Pass fruits through colander and proceed as in basic recipe.

Cider: Obtain cider as soon as possible after it is made; heat quickly to destroy enzymes, bring to a rolling boil, pour into clean jars, and seal.

Canned tomatoes: To can tomatoes by the open-kettle method, loosen skins by steaming over boiling water; peel, remove stem ends, quarter; cook until tender in a covered utensil, or about 10 to 15 minutes; pour into clean jars and seal.

Tomato Catsup and Sauces

Few recipes need revising so much as do those customarily used for making catsup, chili sauce, and barbecue sauce. Instead of laboriously peeling the tomatoes and cooking them for 3 hours or more to evaporate off gallons of delicious juice, season and can the juice and make the sauces of the remaining purée. By this procedure, no sauce need be cooked longer than a few minutes.

CHILI SAUCE

Put through the meat grinder, using large knife:

½ cup celery
½ cup onion
2 cloves garlic

½ cup green peppers, preferably green chili peppers
1 teaspoon salt

Steam vegetables in a small amount of tomato juice until onion is transparent; add:

1 quart tomato purée
½ cup vinegar
1 teaspoon crushed black peppercorns

1 tablespoon minced fresh or ½ teaspoon dried basil and/or orégano
⅓ cup brown sugar

Heat to a rolling boil; pour into clean pint jars and seal; invert jars to sterilize lids.

Serve with meat or fish.

VARIATIONS:

For spiced chili sauce add ½ teaspoon each cinnamon, allspice, nutmeg, ¼ teaspoon ground cloves.

Barbecue sauce: Prepare as in basic recipe, adding the following ground and cooked vegetables to 1 quart purée: 1 cup each celery and onions; or ½ cup each celery, onions, green or red bell pepper, chili pepper, or pimentos; or omit onions and use 1 cup celery or ½ cup each celery and sweet peppers.

Spiced barbecue sauce: Add ½ teaspoon each cinnamon, allspice, nutmeg, ¼ teaspoon cloves.

Italian sauce: Add a pinch each rosemary, marjoram, savory, basil, orégano. Serve with ravioli, fish, and meat. Vary by adding 1 cup ground unpeeled carrots with other vegetables.

Mexican sauce: Add ½ cup each chopped red bell pepper and green chili peppers, ½ teaspoon cumin seeds; season with orégano; if only bell peppers are used, add 1 tablespoon chili powder.

Tomato catsup: Omit vegetables except garlic; add ¼ teaspoon ground cayenne, 1 teaspoon each ground mace, dry mustard, crushed celery seeds.

Pickling

Tomatoes, peppers, cabbage, and most of the fruits and vegetables used in making pickles and relishes are rich sources of vitamin C. Vinegar retards the action of the enzymes which destroy this vitamin. Carefully prepared pickles, therefore, can be sufficiently rich in vitamin C to make a contribution to health, especially in localities where few fresh fruits and salads are eaten during the winter.

When vegetables are soaked, whether in brine or in ice water, many vitamins and minerals are drawn out and discarded. The purpose of such soaking is to make the ingredients crisp and to prevent shriveling when sugar is added to them. The same purpose can be accomplished without loss of nutritive value if the vegetables are soaked in the pickling liquid to which is added a small amount of a calcium salt, calcium chloride. This salt is much more effective than is table salt and is used commercially to produce the delightful crispness of small cucumber pickles and gherkins. It may be purchased inexpensively at a drugstore, or any druggist can order it for you. Fifty cents' worth will probably be all you can use. This salt adds to the nutritive value of the pickles and makes the difference between mediocrity and perfection.

GREEN TOMATO RELISH

Put through meat grinder, using largest knife:

6 green unpeeled tomatoes	3 green or red bell peppers, or
4 stalks celery	green chili peppers
2 large onions	

Mix well and bring to boiling:

1 pint cider vinegar	1 teaspoon freshly ground black
¼ cup mustard seeds	peppercorns
1 tablespoon salt	¼ teaspoon cayenne
¼ cup white or brown sugar	

Add vegetables to boiling liquid, simmer 10 minutes without covering, pack into clean jars, and seal.

VARIATIONS:

Add sugar to taste if sweet relish is desired.

Tie 2 tablespoons pickling spices in a cheesecloth bag and cook with tomatoes.

Add 2 cups finely chopped green or purple cabbage.

Omit tomatoes and use 8 medium ground cucumbers.

Cabbage relish: Omit tomatoes and mustard seeds; add 1 finely shredded head cabbage, 1 teaspoon turmeric.

Cauliflower relish: Instead of the tomatoes grind and add 1 cauliflower and 2 to 4 carrots.

Celery-horseradish relish: Use white mustard seeds; increase celery to 2 cups when ground; add ½ cup horseradish, 2 teaspoons each whole cloves, cinnamon bark, allspice berries; stir in horseradish immediately before putting into jars.

Corn relish: Add 2 cups fresh corn to relish 4 minutes before putting into jars.

Pepper relish: Omit tomatoes and celery; use 6 green and 6 red peppers.

PICKLED BELL PEPPERS, PIMENTOS, PAPRIKAS, AND OTHER SWEET PEPPERS

Bring to boiling the estimated amount of liquid needed, using the following proportion:

1 cup vinegar   1 cup water

Remove stems and seeds from:

red or green bell peppers, fresh pimentos, paprikas, or other peppers

Cut peppers into halves or thirds and drop into boiling liquid; simmer 5 minutes and pack firmly into pint or quart jars; add to each quart:

½ teaspoon salt   1 teaspoon sugar

Finish filling jars with hot liquid; seal and store.

VARIATIONS:

Add to each jar ¼ bay leaf and 1 small clove garlic.

To remove skin from fresh chili peppers, sear with high heat under broiler; wrap quickly in a towel, cool, and peel; or can as directed above and remove skin before using.

If crispness is desired, cut peppers and soak overnight in water, vinegar, sugar, salt, and 1 teaspoon of calcium chloride per quart.

Instead of canning, pack into small cardboard cartons and freeze.

CUCUMBER PICKLES

Wash cucumbers thoroughly with a cloth; combine in a pottery bowl or earthenware jar:

2 cups vinegar   3 pounds small whole cucumbers,
1 cup water   or as many as can be covered by
1 tablespoon salt   liquid
¾ teaspoon calcium chloride   ¼ to 1 cup white or brown sugar

Let soak overnight.

Drain liquid into saucepan and add:

seasonings suggested in variations, tied in cloth bag

Bring to boiling and add:

cucumbers

Simmer 10 minutes without boiling; pack into clear jars and seal.

VARIATIONS:

Add any of the following groups of seasonings: 1½ tablespoons mixed pickling spices; 1 tablespoon each white mustard seeds and crushed white peppercorns; 1 crushed bay leaf, 1 clove garlic, ¼ teaspoon cayenne; 1 teaspoon each whole cloves and allspice berries, 1 stick cinnamon bark; 1 tablespoon each mustard seeds and cloves.

Cut cucumbers in half lengthwise if they are 3 or 4 inches long; cut larger cucumbers into fourths lengthwise or into chunks 1 inch long.

If liquid is left after canning pickles, add sliced cucumbers or chopped mixed vegetables, simmer 10 minutes, and seal.

In the following variations, soak ingredients overnight in vinegar, water, calcium chloride, and salt in proportions given in basic recipe; add spices to vinegar; follow exact procedure of basic recipe except as noted.

Bread-and-butter pickles: Use 2 quarts sliced cucumbers, 2 large sliced onions; add 3 tablespoons mustard seeds, 1 tablespoon celery seeds, and ¼ teaspoon cayenne.

Cauliflower pickles: Break 1 small head cauliflower into pieces, dice stalk; add 2 tablespoons mustard seeds and 1 teaspoon ground turmeric. Vary by adding 2 sliced red or green bell peppers and/or 1 cup pickling onions or diced cucumbers.

Dill pickles: After soaking, put cucumbers directly into jars; heat with vinegar for each quart of pickles 1 tablespoon dill seeds, ½ teaspoon mustard seeds, ½ teaspoon crushed white peppercorns.

Gherkins: Use tiny cucumbers with 1 cup of sugar; after soaking, pack into pint jars; add 1 small clove garlic; heat liquid with ½ teaspoon each mustard seeds and crushed white peppercorns for each pint.

Pickled onions: Omit cucumbers and use 1 quart pickling onions; add 1 tablespoon mixed pickling spices.

Pickled watermelon rind: Peel rind and dice into 2-inch pieces, using 4 to 6 cups, or as much as can be covered with liquid given in basic recipe; after soaking, add 1 to 2 teaspoons cloves and 1 stick cinnamon bark, and simmer until rind is transparent. If a sweet pickle is preferred, increase sugar to 1¼ cups and omit salt.

SPICED FRUIT

Use about 4 quarts fruit. Wash quickly and drain.
Combine and simmer 10 minutes:

2 cups vinegar	2 teaspoons whole cloves
1 cup water	3 or 4 sticks cinnamon, or ½
1 cup white or brown sugar	ounce

Add the amount of fruit which can be covered by liquid; simmer until tender; pack firmly into clean jars, fill to the top with liquid, and seal. Turn upside down to sterilize lids.

Add more fresh fruit to liquid and continue until liquid is used.

VARIATIONS:

Pickled beets: Steam whole beets until tender; peel, slice, and reheat in pickling syrup containing ½ cup sugar and 2 teaspoons salt; put into jars and seal. Vary by omitting sugar and spices; add to each quart jar of pickles 1 teaspoon salt, 1 clove garlic, ½ bay leaf, 1 cayenne pepper, 2 tablespoons vegetable oil.

Spiced apricots, crabapples, figs, and plums: Leave fruit whole and unpeeled; pierce skins with fork to allow steam to escape; wash figs thoroughly but do not touch with soda.

Spiced peaches: Use peeled cling peaches and brown sugar instead of white. If crisp pickles are desired, add ¾ teaspoon calcium chloride to vinegar and water, and soak peeled peaches overnight. When peaches are out of season, use canned cling peaches, adding peach juice instead of water.

Spiced pears: If pears are large, cut in half and core; leave small pears whole without coring; do not peel.

Unlimited Vitamin C Free for the Extracting

A source of vitamin C, or ascorbic acid, which is fantastic in its concentration is that of wild rose hips, or rose apples. Rose hips are the seed pods left after roses bloom. The amount of vitamin C they contain varies with the species. Hips from cultivated roses contain relatively little of the vitamin, but those from wild roses have been found to average 1200 to 1800 milligrams per half cup, or about 24 to 36 times the vitamin-C potency of fresh orange juice. Some species have been found to contain 96 times the vitamin content of citrus juices. The amount of vitamin C which goes to waste annually from rose hips is estimated to be thousands of tons.

Just as people often go berrying, the nutrition-conscious person who lives in sections of Alaska or other states or Canada where wild roses grow in abundance goes "rose-hipping." The vitamin-C content is at its highest when the rose hips are red, or in the late fall, but gather them at any time when you have a chance. The vitamin can be extracted by boiling them until they are tender and letting them stand while the vitamin passes into the cooking water. Since the extract is very mild in flavor, lemon juice or vinegar must be added both to prevent enzymes from destroying the vitamin and to keep botulinus from developing.

If you cannot afford vitamin C from other sources, try to can enough rose-hip extract so that each member of your family may have at least one tablespoon daily. Add it as a routine procedure to the breakfast juice. Put a small amount into gelatin salads and desserts, appetizers, meat sauces, soups, fruit cups, and sherbets. Since vitamin C plays such an important role in maintaining the health of the teeth and gums, and in promoting resistance to infections, allergies, and diseases, the use of even a small amount of rose-hip extract throughout the winter months can contribute a great deal indeed. During a time of illness, such extract is invaluable.

ROSE-HIP EXTRACT

Gather rose hips; chill; remove blossom ends, stems, and leaves; wash quickly.

Meanwhile for each cup of rose hips bring to a rolling boil:

1½ cups water

Add:

1 cup rose hips

Cover utensil and simmer 15 minutes; mash with a fork or potato masher. Let stand 24 hours.

Strain off extract, bring to a rolling boil, add 2 tablespoons vinegar or lemon juice for each pint, pour into jars, and seal.

VARIATIONS:

If extract is not to be prepared immediately, chill rose hips quickly to inhibit enzyme action; when they are thoroughly chilled, wash and pass through the meat grinder before adding to water; simmer 5 to 10 minutes. Proceed as in basic recipe.

To make rose-hip jelly, substitute the extract for fruit juice and add sugar and commercial pectin; follow directions given for the specific pectin used.

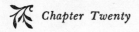

Chapter Twenty

Desserts Can Contribute to Health

One of the most encouraging trends of today is that many housewives serve fruit or yogurt with fruit rather than an oversweet
dessert which fills no nutritional needs.

The tremendous consumption of refined sugar in America has
caused untold ill health. The more refined sugar eaten, the
greater the need for several of the B vitamins; yet sugar satisfies
the appetite so rapidly that the more sugar eaten, the less vitamins obtained.

Almost every food contains sugar or starch which is changed
into sugar during digestion. A person who eats rather heartily
can obtain as much as 2 cups of sugar in the course of a single
day even though he does not taste refined sugar in any form.

The so-called breakfast problem which causes hundreds of
thousands of children to go to school and adults to go to work
without breakfast results from eating oversweet desserts at dinner.
Other factors enter, of course, but the person who is hungry in
the morning usually eats breakfast and enjoys it.

If a mother who customarily prepares oversweet desserts is
sincere in wishing to produce ideal health for her family, she can
serve a filling soup or a delicious salad before the dinner course
so that there will be little room left for dessert. Some simple dessert such as fruit cup or apricot sauce, which will not tempt one
to overeat, can then be offered without evoking complaints.

Fruits Make Ideal Desserts

Although fruits should be served daily for breakfast and mid-meals, and frequently in salads and appetizers, no recipes for these foods are needed. The dessert superior to all others is fresh fruit accompanied perhaps with nuts or cheese and whole-grain crackers.

In planning your dinner desserts, always think of fruits first. Glance through this section and see if you can pick up an idea which may not have occurred to you recently. When fresh fruits are not available, use canned or frozen ones, but dress them up a bit at least part of the time, perhaps by adding coconut or chopped nuts or by combining fruits of two or more attractive colors. Even for guest dinners—especially for guest dinners, which are usually too heavy—no dessert is so ideal as fruit.

If the nutritive value of fruits is to be retained during preparation, the same general rules must be followed as were given for preparing salads and cooking vegetables. Enzyme action should be kept to the minimum by refrigeration, by the exclusion of oxygen and light, by avoiding all contact with copper and iron, and by rapid heating in case the fruit is to be cooked. Fruit should be cooked in the shortest time possible.

The vitamin content of fruits increases until they are ripe. If fruits are gathered or purchased when underripe, leave them at room temperature, preferably in a dark place, until well ripened. With the exception of fruits having a heavy peel which protects the vitamins from oxygen, such as citrus fruits, bananas, and apples, put fruits into the refrigerator as soon as they have ripened. Purchase only the amount of ripe fruits which can be refrigerated, canned, or frozen immediately. If ripe fruits are left at room temperature, their vitamins A, B_2, and C are gradually destroyed. The destruction of these vitamins takes place rapidly when fruits are allowed to become overripe, especially if they are bruised. For example, guavas, one of the richest sources of vitamin C, contain 1600 to 2000 milligrams of this vitamin per pound when ripe but firm. If they are allowed to stand until overripe and soft, though only for a day, four-fifths of the vitamin is lost.

On the other hand, if citrus fruits, protected by a thick peeling, are stored in a cool place, almost no loss of vitamin C occurs even after several months, provided the fruit stays in good condition.

Soft fruits, such as berries, should be put into the refrigerator unwashed and unstemmed. Any handling causes bruises which result in increased enzyme action and vitamin loss. Just before being used, the chilled berries should be washed so quickly that they will not reach the temperature of the water. If they cannot be served immediately, they should again be put into the refrigerator. Fruits which are sufficiently firm not to bruise may be washed before being chilled. No fruit should be peeled or cut until shortly before it is to be used; any exposure to oxygen increases loss of vitamin C.

Wash all fruits rapidly. If they are allowed to stand in water, considerable amounts of sugars, vitamin C, and the B vitamins dissolve out and are lost. Avoid soaking any fresh fruit. Instead of loosening the skin of tomatoes or peaches by soaking them in hot water, steam them a few minutes until the peel can easily be slipped off. Before cutting apples chill them to prevent discoloration. Do not put them into water afterward. Avoid using any knife which contains copper; such a knife will cause almost instant discoloration and complete loss of vitamin C in the discolored portions. Since acid retards enzyme activity, discoloration can be prevented by mixing cut fruit with a little lemon juice.

Trim fruits as little as possible. When fruits are not chilled, leave them in large pieces; the less surface exposed, the less nutritive value lost. Since fruits are usually served in the liquid in which they are cooked, little or no loss of minerals or heat-stable vitamins occurs during cooking.

Keep oranges from which juice is to be extracted in the refrigerator until chilled; then extract the juice quickly to prevent unnecessary contact with air. If you use frozen juice, purchase the brands which have no sugar added. Oranges high in vitamin C are also rich in sugar and need no added sweetening. The vitamin is protected by citric acid; hence vitamin C is not lost in freezing.

There is some loss of nutrients when fruits are frozen or during the time they are stored after they are frozen. Losses may have occurred before the fruit was frozen unless scientific rules for food preparation were observed. When frozen foods are thawed, however, loss of vitamin C takes place rapidly.

Since certain unavoidable losses occur when fruits are cooked, serve raw fruits in preference to cooked, canned, or frozen ones whenever possible.

Fruits Are Ideal for Desserts

Adopt the Italian and French custom of serving a bowl or basket of assorted fresh fruits or raw apples for dessert, supplying each person with a fruit knife and small plate. Serve with any one of the following:

Camembert, Roquefort, Swiss, American, Jack, or other cheeses.

Unhulled walnuts, peanuts, or paper-shell almonds or pecans; heat nuts 10 minutes in moderate oven and serve hot; supply a nutcracker for each person.

Toasted and salted almonds, pecans, peanuts, or other nuts.

Salted and buttered popcorn or cheese popcorn (p. 530); have popcorn hot, apples chilled.

Caraway or poppy seeds; heat seeds in oven 10 minutes and serve hot; dip slices of fruit into the seeds.

Remove cores and cut chilled red apples into slices ½ inch thick; spread with Camembert or cream cheese; sprinkle with caraway or poppy seeds.

Since apples are often available the year round, I have used them in basic recipes to illustrate cooking methods which will retain the greatest nutritive value. These same methods may be used in cooking all fruits.

"BAKED" APPLES AND OTHER FRUITS

Wash quickly, dry, and core:

4 or more large chilled apples

Remove peel from upper fourth of apples; put peeled side down into:

½ cup boiling water

Heat through quickly; reduce heat and simmer until almost tender when pierced with a toothpick, or about 10 minutes; turn apples peeled side up and sprinkle with:

cinnamon, nutmeg, or grated   **¼ cup sugar**
   lemon rind

Brown in oven or under broiler and serve with top milk, sour cream, yogurt, whipped evaporated milk, or whipped cream. These apples appear to be baked, yet are cooked with much less nutritive loss.

VARIATIONS:

Before browning apples, fill centers with raisins or broken walnuts, pecans, almonds, or mincemeat.

If apples cook easily, heat through, then transfer to the oven and bake until tender.

Apricots, nectarines, peaches, and other fruit: Do not remove pits; put whole, unpeeled fruit into preheated utensil containing 1 or 2 tablespoons boiling water, or just enough to prevent sticking; steam until tender, or 6 to 10 minutes. Skins may be removed from peaches and apricots after steaming; sprinkle with ¼ cup sugar; chill. The less water used in cooking the fruit, the more delightful the flavor will be when they are served.

Cinnamon apples: Use 1 cup boiling water; add while stewing apples **6 cloves, small piece of cinnamon, ¼ cup sugar;** soak 2 teaspoons gelatin in ¼ cup water and dissolve in 1 cup hot liquid after apples are removed; chill until it starts to congeal, brush over apples, pour remainder into centers. Or instead of spices, add **2 tablespoons cinnamon drops.**

Fruit with custard sauce: Steam whole unpeeled peaches or unpeeled pears cut in half and cored; remove from heat, pit peaches, and sprinkle lightly with sugar; serve covered with soft custard (p. 484), pouring custard into centers.

Glazed fruit: Steam whole unpeeled pears or peaches; core pears from blossom end, leaving stems on; pit and peel peaches after steaming; prepare and apply a glaze as directed for cinnamon apples, omitting spices.

Stewed apples: Cut each piece into bite sizes; do not peel; use water-less-cooking utensil and 2 tablespoons boiling water; cool and sweeten to taste.

Spiced apples: While apples are cooking, add 4 to 6 cloves, a small piece of cinnamon or 3 tablespoons cinnamon drops.

Stewed whole pears: Stew whole unpeeled pears with cores removed from blossom end; stuff with **broken nuts or raisins or nuts and raisins mixed,** or with **chopped candied or preserved ginger.** Just before removing from heat sprinkle with **¼ cup sugar and 1 teaspoon grated lemon rind;** chill and serve. Vary by stewing without added seasonings; serve with apricot or plum sauce.

Pears with orange sauce: Cut unpeeled pears in half and remove cores; stew in **1 cup diluted frozen orange juice;** remove pears and sweeten juice with **½ cup sugar;** add **1 teaspoon grated orange rind;** pour syrup over pears and chill.

Stuffed peaches: Stew whole unpeeled peaches; cool, remove pits and skins; stuff with **broken walnuts or pecans;** or remove pits before stewing and stuff with **raisins or nuts and raisins mixed.**

Whole fruit with crumbs: Stew whole unpeeled apples, peaches, apricots, or pears as in basic recipe; sweeten and chill; roll in **graham-cracker crumbs** to which **1 or 2 drops almond extract** are added. Serve with whipped evaporated milk or cream.

APPLESAUCE AND OTHER FRUIT SAUCES

Wash quickly and quarter:

2 pounds tart cooking apples

Do not peel or remove cores if fruit is in good condition; put apples into saucepan containing:

½ cup boiling water

Heat quickly, then steam until soft, or about 15 minutes; press apples through colander or food mill.

Unless fruit is to be served immediately, chill thoroughly before sweetening to taste.

Season to taste with **dash of nutmeg, cinnamon, or small amount of lemon juice or grated lemon or orange rind.** If flavor of the apples is excellent, add no seasonings.

VARIATIONS:

While applesauce is still hot, add 3 or 4 tablespoons cinnamon candies.

Add 3 or 4 tablespoons uncooked or lightly toasted wheat germ to applesauce just before serving; add wheat germ to any fruit sauce.

Follow the procedure of the basic recipe and make fruit sauces of small pears, peaches, apricots, plums, or other fruit; if apricots or peaches are extremely small, do not remove pits before steaming.

Serve any fruit sauce as a sundae over yogurt.

Combine bananas with other fruits in fruit cup and compotes; or serve sliced, whole, or cut in half lengthwise and sprinkled lightly with powdered sugar and lemon or orange juice. Since baking is a slow process, broil bananas in preference to baking them.

BROILED BANANAS

Peel:

4 ripe bananas

Set in low oiled baking dish and broil with moderate heat until well browned, or about 6 minutes; turn and sprinkle with **coconut mixed with brown sugar**; brown and serve hot or cold.

VARIATIONS:

Omit coconut and serve with orange juice, grated lemon or orange rind, or stewed raisins seasoned with lemon rind; or sprinkle with nutmeg, cinnamon, or lemon juice.

Wash raspberries, youngberries, blackberries, strawberries, and similar soft berries not earlier than 1/2 hour before they are to be served. Sprinkle lightly with granulated or powdered sugar and serve with top milk. Larger berries may be sliced or cut in half. Serve firm, attractive strawberries without stemming them, especially if you desire to avoid the calories in cream and sugar.

When washing blueberries and huckleberries, discard those which come to the top of the water; worms have usually eaten

the center of such berries, making them light. Chill berries
thoroughly and serve with top milk and sugar. Stew berries by
adding 2 cups berries to ¼ cup boiling water; lower heat and
steam until berries are tender, or about 5 to 7 minutes. Chill
before adding sugar to taste. Serve frozen berries before they
have completely thawed.

Chill melons thoroughly before serving. Cut as desired. Serve
small melon halves in chopped ice but do not allow ice to touch
edible parts.

CANTALOUPE CUP

Cut cantaloupe or other small melon in half, making sawtooth edge;
remove seeds; cut thin slice from bottom of each half so that it will rest
securely on plate. Fill center with one of the following:

diced pineapple, sliced peaches, or other fruit	strawberries
unstemmed black cherries	mixed diced fruits
	ice cream

Garnish with **mint leaves.**

VARIATIONS:

Make rings of small melons by cutting center portion into 1-inch
slices; fill centers of rings with mixed diced fruits, strawberries, cherries,
or ice cream.

FESTIVE WATERMELON BOWL

Cut chilled watermelon in half lengthwise; remove pulp; dice into
1-inch cubes, discard seeds, and combine pulp with the following:

sliced peaches or apricots	diced honeydew or casaba melon
halved and seeded purple grapes	diced pineapple

Place mixed fruit in watermelon rind. Garnish with **fresh mint.**

Wash cherries quickly; chill and serve without stemming. If stewing is desirable, cook in 2 tablespoons water; chill before adding sugar to taste.

BLACK CHERRIES WITH BRANDY

Put into heat-resistant casserole or serving dish:

1 can black cherries

Heat quickly to boiling; add:

¼ cup brandy

Ignite brandy and bring to the table flaming; serve flaming cherries over vanilla ice cream.

VARIATIONS:

Instead of cherries use canned apricots, peaches, or pears.

DRIED FRUITS

Drop into 2 cups boiling water:

1 pound dried prunes, apricots, apples, raisins, peaches, pears, or figs

Cover utensil, reduce heat to simmering, and cook until fruit is tender, or about 12 to 15 minutes. Chill.

Let stewed fruit soak in cooking liquid overnight; sweeten to taste.

VARIATIONS:

Add bits of lemon or orange rind to prunes, apples, pears, or figs during cooking. Add to cooking water ½ teaspoon cloves and stick of cinnamon; use for prunes, pears, peaches, or apples.

Sweeten prunes and raisins with 2 or 3 tablespoons honey or molasses; add at the end of cooking.

Add to dried pears during cooking 2 tablespoons diced preserved or candied ginger.

Canned Fruits

Canned fruits are excellent to serve alone as desserts. If you wish to make them more festive, serve them with one or more of the following:

Whipped and sweetened evaporated milk or whipped cream.
Sour cream or thick yogurt.
Sprinkle generously with broken walnuts, pecans, crushed peanuts, or other nuts.
Sprinkle with moist shredded coconut.
Quarter 2 or 3 marshmallows and add to each serving of fruit.

Guavas are such a rich source of vitamin C that as many of them as possible should be used. Add them to appetizers, fruit cups, fruit salads, and gelatins containing mixed fruits. Slice chilled peeled guavas and serve with lemon sections or mix with lemon juice; sweeten to taste.

STEWED GUAVAS

Peel and slice:

2 cups chilled guavas

Heat to boiling:

2 tablespoons water   **1 tablespoon lemon juice**

Add the guavas, cover utensil, and steam 5 to 8 minutes. Chill and sweeten to taste.

VARIATIONS:

Omit water and lemon juice and stew guavas in ¼ cup orange juice; chill, sprinkle with grated orange rind and sugar to taste.
Stew guavas with an equal amount of sliced peaches, pears, or other fruit.

The large California persimmons are an excellent source of vitamin A. If you have facilities for quick freezing, obtain them in season and freeze enough to use throughout the year. Persimmons are delicious when served unthawed. Prepare persimmons and serve in any of the following ways:

Cut unpeeled persimmons petal-fashion, leaving base intact; separate the sections slightly, sprinkle with shredded coconut or lemon juice, or garnish center with mint leaves or grated lemon rind.

Cut either chilled or frozen unpeeled persimmons crosswise into ½-inch slices; serve alone garnished with mint or with sour cream or yogurt.

Cut chilled or frozen persimmons into thin slices; alternate with orange slices.

Freeze very ripe persimmons; immediately before serving shred and serve in sherbet glasses; garnish with fresh mint.

Shred frozen persimmons and mix with shredded coconut and broken walnuts, almonds, or pecans.

Add 1 cup mashed or shredded persimmon pulp to ice cream, custard (pp. 484–485), or Bavarian cream (p. 496).

Dice and mix with other fruits in preparing fruit cup, or slice and use in fruit compote.

Fresh uncooked pineapple contains protein-digesting enzymes. Persons whose digestion is below par often benefit by eating it uncooked. For festive occasions, one of my favorite desserts is filled pineapple halves.

FILLED PINEAPPLE HALVES

Cut off part of green top, leaving 3 or 4 inches; split in half lengthwise:

1 large chilled pineapple

Use grapefruit knife to remove core and pulp. Discard core and dice pulp; mix with diced pulp:

1 to 2 cups strawberries cut   ¼ cup sugar
in halves

Fill one or both halves, depending on number of people to be served. Keep chilled.

VARIATIONS:

Instead of strawberries, mix diced pineapple with fresh raspberries, melon cubes, sliced peaches, diced unpeeled apple, or other fruit; serve from half shell. Or mix diced pulp with slices of stoned dates and/or shredded coconut, or with walnuts, pecans, or almonds.

Slice fresh pineapple; pile slices, cut into quarters lengthwise and core; serve without removing the peeling. Eat with fingers, holding to peeling edge.

Spread slices of fresh or canned pineapple with sour cream or yogurt.

Alternate slices of orange or California persimmon with slices of pineapple.

Peel fresh pineapple, slice, and serve uncored with fruit knives and forks; sprinkle lightly with powdered sugar.

Remove pulp from whole pineapple by cutting off top 1 inch below leaves, inserting knife near bottom, revolving it without cutting edges, and cutting out entire center in one piece; slice, sprinkle with powdered sugar, return slices to shell; serve with leaves as if uncut; or dice pulp and mix with fresh fruit; sweeten to taste and serve from shell.

To make an elaborate fruit platter for a buffet, set in center of platter whole pineapple with pulp sliced as directed above; cut skin of oranges petal-fashion; pull back and separate the orange sections; sprinkle with powdered sugar; surround pineapple with oranges and lay chilled bananas around edge. Just before serving, remove skin from top of bananas, brush with lemon juice, and sprinkle with powdered sugar. Scatter unstemmed black cherries or strawberries over platter.

STEAMED RHUBARB

Cut into 1-inch pieces without peeling:

1½ pounds rhubarb

Add to:

1 or 2 tablespoons boiling water

Cover utensil, keep heat low, and steam 16 to 18 minutes. Chill thoroughly and add:

½ cup sugar

Stir well and let sugar dissolve before serving.

Cooked cranberries: Cook like rhubarb, using ¼ cup boiling water; chill thoroughly before sweetening.

FRUIT ASPICS

Soak 5 minutes in saucepan:

1 tablespoon gelatin in   ½ cup fruit juice

Heat gelatin slowly until dissolved. Prepare in liquefier and add to gelatin:

1½ cups plum, apricot, peach, loganberry,
or other berry purée

If fruit is not tart, add:

1 or 2 tablespoons lemon juice

Sweeten to taste. Pour into chilled mold; chill until firm, unmold. Serve with yogurt or whipped cream.

VARIATIONS:

Make aspic of prune or apple purée or 1 cup each prune purée and applesauce; when gelatin starts to congeal add a few chopped or broken walnuts, pecans, or almonds.

Make purées and juices of small fruits or fruits which are too soft to be attractive when cooked whole. Blend to purée in liquefier.

Chill aspic until it starts to congeal before putting into mold; whip 1 cup chilled evaporated milk, add 3 tablespoons lemon juice, ¼ cup each sugar and powdered milk; stir into aspic, pour into mold, chill, and serve.

Pour aspic into flat baking dish; chill, cut into cubes, and serve.

Fruit Compotes

A fruit compote is a combination of two or more fresh or canned fruits. The fruit is cut as little as possible and served from an attractive bowl at the table. Dark-colored juices should be drained before the fruits are combined. Use fresh fruits of contrasting colors or combine fresh with canned fruits. For additional vitamin C, add rose-hip extract or sliced guavas to compotes if they are available. Following are suggestions for compotes:

Canned apricots, fresh or frozen strawberries.
Apricot halves, preferably fresh, drained canned black cherries.
Large dices of casaba or honeydew melon, canned or stewed purple plums.
Pineapple cubes or slices, fresh or canned peach halves, fresh or frozen raspberries.
Canned unpeeled pear halves, orange slices; drain 1 cup canned black cherries and scatter over top of compote just before serving.
Cubes of chilled cantaloupe; layer in bowl with canned or fresh grapefruit sections, sliced pineapple, or fresh youngberries.
Canned figs, orange slices, seeded purple-grape halves.

Fruit cup makes an ideal dessert usually enjoyed by everyone. It is essentially the same as an appetizer of mixed fruits except that the fruit is diced in larger, or bite, sizes. When canned fruits are used, add them to oranges, grapefruit, diced unpeeled apples, or other fresh fruits. Combine the fruits, sweeten slightly, and allow to stand at least 15 minutes before serving so that the flavors blend. When rose-hip extract or fresh guavas are available, use them to supply additional vitamin C.

FRUIT CUP

Cut into fourths:

6 or 8 fresh or canned apricots

Add:

1 or 2 diced oranges   ½ cup strawberries or other fresh
1 sliced banana or 2 sliced peaches   or canned berries

Sweeten to taste, mix well, and set in refrigerator; serve in sherbet glasses.

VARIATIONS:

Use any combination of fresh and canned fruit.

Add ½ cup broken walnuts, pecans, chopped almonds, or other nuts.

Add ½ to 1 cup moist shredded coconut or 6 to 8 marshmallows cut into quarters with scissors.

Fruit cup with custard: Prepare fruit cup using 3 cups fruit, such as diced canned pineapple, fresh unpeeled pears or red apples, seedless grapes or canned cherries; add ¼ **pound quartered marshmallows;** put into a shallow dish, cover top with **soft custard** (p. 484), using half the recipe and seasoning custard with **2 tablespoons lemon juice;** let chill overnight until marshmallows absorb fruit juices; cut into cubes and serve.

Commercial gelatin desserts supply no vitamins or minerals; yet they readily satisfy the appetite. They contain coloring, flavoring, a small amount of inadequate protein, about 90 per cent water as they are usually prepared, and at least 100 calories of sugar per serving. Since both the synthetic coloring and flavoring may be harmful to health, they cannot be recommended. In order to make a dessert even of unflavored gelatin nutritionally valuable, generous amounts of fruits should be added. One package of gelatin will hold 2 cups or more of diced fruits and nuts.

FRUIT GELATIN

Heat to boiling:

> 1½ cups pineapple, apple, or grapefruit juice

Dissolve in ¼ cup cold water and add:

> 1 package or tablespoon unflavored gelatin

Stir well and chill until gelatin starts to congeal; add:

½ cup canned cherries, cut in half   1 cup sliced peaches
½ cup fresh seedless grapes   ¼ cup walnuts or pecans

Sweeten to taste, stir, pour into ring mold, and chill until firm; unmold and serve with center filled with yogurt, whipped evaporated milk flavored with vanilla, or whipped cream.

VARIATIONS:

Put gelatin in loaf bread pan, unmold, slice; or mold in flat baking dish, chill, cut into cubes.

Add guavas or 2 or 3 tablespoons rose-hip extract, using extract instead of equal amount of juice.

Use sliced or diced bananas, apricots, plums, fresh or frozen berries, pears, or other fruits instead of those suggested; the total amount of fruit should measure 2 to 2¼ cups.

FROZEN FRUIT PURÉES OR JUICES

Use canned puréed fruit or applesauce; or blend in liquefier soft fresh, stewed, or canned apricots, pitted plums, prunes, peaches, or other fruits until puréed; or use plum, loganberry, pineapple, grapefruit, or other fruit juices. If purées or juices are extremely tart, add sugar to taste; if they are too sweet, add 2 or 3 tablespoons lemon juice.

Put into freezing compartment:

2 or 3 cups fruit juice or purée

Stir or beat 3 or 4 times as juice or purée freezes; serve as dessert or with meat course. Serve frozen applesauce or pineapple juice with ham or pork; plum, peach, or apricot with beef; apricot, grapefruit juice, or loganberry juice with lamb.

VARIATIONS:

If frozen purée or juice is desired for dessert, sweeten to taste, using more sugar than for a meat accompaniment.

Season applesauce or prune purée with a dash of nutmeg or cinnamon; or add 3 tablespoons cinnamon candies to applesauce.

Before freezing, shake with juice or blend with purée ¼ cup powdered milk; sweeten to taste and serve for dessert.

FRUIT SNOW

Prepare in liquefier and heat to boiling:

1 cup apple, apricot, plum, prune, peach, or other fruit purée

Meanwhile beat until stiff:

2 egg whites

Fold egg whites into hot fruit; add **sugar and lemon juice** to taste. Cool slowly, then pour into serving dishes, chill, and serve.

VARIATIONS:

Add before folding in egg whites ½ cup broken or chopped walnuts, pecans, or other nuts.

Fruit whip: Chill ½ cup evaporated milk in ice tray until crystals form around edges; whip; add 4 tablespoons each lemon juice, powdered milk, and sugar, 1 teaspoon vanilla or ¼ teaspoon lemon extract; fold into 2 cups thick sweetened and chilled fruit purée, such as prune, plum, apple, apricot, or mashed chilled bananas; prepare no earlier than ½ hour before time to serve. Add diced candied ginger to pear whip.

Fruit sherbet: Freeze any fruit purée slowly to a soft mush and then fold in whipped evaporated milk; finish freezing until firm.

Make Desserts Particularly Nutritious

When you serve desserts other than fruits, they should be made particularly nutritious to compensate for the disadvantages they offer. Plan them to meet the individual needs of your family. If you have adolescent youngsters whose need for calcium has skyrocketed because of rapid growth, serve desserts crowded with evaporated and powdered milk. If your husband does hard physical work, make your desserts supply the B vitamins needed to give him energy and endurance. If you, like thousands of other women, are deficient in protein, make your desserts contribute to your protein intake. Even when you prepare desserts for special occasions such as holidays, birthdays, and guest dinners, take pride in making them contribute to health.

Persons frequently ask why I do not recommend that desserts be made with "raw" sugar. Anything which crystallizes is chemically pure. Sugar crystals, regardless of variety, contain no nutrients other than calories. The microscopic traces of vitamins and minerals found in so-called "raw" sugar come from unrefined molasses which adheres to the sugar crystals; the amounts are nutritionally insignificant. If one is sincere in wishing to eat the best food possible, why not use unrefined molasses or give up sugar entirely? Actually, I do not *recommend* any kind of sugar. I am convinced, however, that people will continue to use it; my purpose is merely to show how nutrients may be added to commonly eaten foods high in sugar. My observation has been that persons who believe "raw" sugar and honey to be nutritious foods usually eat far too much of them.

FIVE-MINUTE CUSTARD

Use a saucepan which does not develop hot spots or cause food to stick; combine and stir well:

¼ cup sugar   ⅛ teaspoon salt
½ cup powdered milk

Add and beat until smooth:

½ cup fresh milk   2 whole eggs or 4 egg yolks

Stir in after beating:
1½ cups fresh or reconstituted milk

Fasten cooking thermometer to side of saucepan; cook over moderate heat, stirring constantly until temperature reaches 180° F., or about 4 minutes; remove from heat and cool at room temperature before chilling.
Stir in 1 teaspoon vanilla and serve.

VARIATIONS:

Use 2½ cups fresh milk and add ¼ to ½ cup soy grits before cooking custard.
Add 2 to 8 tablespoons wheat germ before serving.
Before serving stir into custard ½ to 1 cup sliced canned or sweetened fresh apricots or peaches; well-drained crushed pineapple; sliced bananas or fresh, frozen, or canned berries; omit vanilla or decrease to ½ teaspoon; add ½ teaspoon lemon extract with bananas and pineapple.
Almond custard: Omit vanilla; add ¼ teaspoon almond extract and ¼ cup chopped toasted almonds or soy grits.
Caramel custard: Use 3 tablespoons sugar and add 1 tablespoon dark molasses, or use 2 tablespoons each sugar and molasses, or omit sugar and add ¼ cup molasses; flavor with ½ teaspoon maple flavoring.

Coconut custard: Add ½ cup shredded coconut or coconut meal to warm custard; garnish servings with coconut.

Date custard: Use 2 tablespoons sugar; add ½ to 1 cup chopped dates before serving.

Eggnog custard: Omit vanilla and add 1 tablespoon rum, brandy, or whiskey.

Floating island: Use 2 egg yolks and 1 whole egg in custard; beat 2 egg whites until stiff, add gradually 3 tablespoons sugar, ½ teaspoon vanilla. Drop meringue from large spoon onto surface of hot water in flat baking dish; bake in slow oven at 300° F. for 25 minutes. Put chilled custard in attractive bowl, transfer meringues on top. Floating island is easy to make and delightful to look at. It is one of my favorite desserts.

Lemon custard: Omit vanilla and ¼ cup fresh milk; increase sugar to ½ cup. When custard has chilled, add ¼ cup lemon juice and 1 teaspoon grated lemon rind.

Orange custard: Omit vanilla; add 1 teaspoon orange flavoring, and/ or grated rind of 1 or 2 oranges. This is a delicious custard.

Whenever I think of baked custards, I chuckle at a ridiculous scene which occurred when I was testing the following recipe. Three of us, all reasonably good cooks and certainly experienced ones, would pierce the custard with a knife, gaze at the knife earnestly and seriously, then argue violently about the degree of doneness. If we disagreed, surely other women would do likewise. When it dawned on me to let the meat thermometer solve the problem, we were unanimous in saying perfection had been attained. The custard continues to cook while it is cooling, and the texture is easily ruined by slight overbaking.

BAKED CUSTARD

Combine and beat slightly:

¼ cup sugar stirred with	3 whole eggs or 6 yolks
½ cup powdered milk	½ cup fresh milk
⅛ teaspoon salt	1 teaspoon vanilla

When mixture is smooth, add and stir:

1½ cups fresh or reconstituted milk

Pour into a shallow greased baking dish or custard cups; sprinkle with nutmeg; set meat thermometer in 1 cup or insert when custard is almost done. Bake in a slow oven at 300° F. for about 40 minutes, or until center of custard is 175° F. and margin is 190° F. If baking dish is used, cut into squares to serve.

VARIATIONS:

For fluffy custard use whole eggs, fold in stiffly beaten whites sweetened with 2 tablespoons sugar; serve hot.

To shorten baking time, heat 1½ cups milk to lukewarm; add to other ingredients.

Use 2 tablespoons each sugar and dark molasses; add 4 to 8 tablespoons wheat germ with ¼ teaspoon salt; or add ½ cup broken nuts, chopped dates, raisins, or shredded coconut.

Cover bottom of baking dish or custard cups with sweetened fresh or canned peaches, apricots, pears, or well-drained pineapple slices; decrease vanilla to ¾ teaspoon. Vary custard with pears by omitting vanilla and adding 3 tablespoons diced candied or preserved ginger.

Omit vanilla; use 2⅓ cups milk; add ½ teaspoon almond flavoring and ⅓ cup soy grits.

My sisters and I were brought up to be extremely thrifty (my mother's maiden name was McBroom). Whenever stale bread accumulated, bread pudding was served so inevitably that our name for it became "Duty." I suspect other families feel much the same about this somewhat plebeian but nevertheless delicious dish.

BREAD PUDDING

Combine and beat until smooth:

⅔ cup sugar stirred with	½ cup fresh milk
½ cup powdered milk	2 whole eggs or 4 egg yolks
⅛ teaspoon salt	1 teaspoon vanilla

When smooth, add:

4 cups diced stale whole-wheat bread	2 cups fresh or reconstituted milk

Pour into greased baking dish; sprinkle top with **nutmeg or cinnamon and sugar**. Bake at 325° F. for 45 minutes, or until temperature, taken by inserting meat thermometer in center, is 175° F.

VARIATIONS:

Stir into pudding before baking ½ cup of any of the following: raisins, chopped dates, shredded coconut, broken walnuts or pecans; or use 3½ cups fresh milk and add ½ cup soy grits.

Cottage-cheese bread pudding: Omit vanilla; beat **1 cup cottage cheese** with eggs; add **grated rind of 1 lemon, ¼ teaspoon lemon extract, 2 tablespoons lemon juice**; add other ingredients and proceed as in basic recipe.

Date-nut bread pudding: Add ½ cup each chopped dates and broken walnuts or pecans.

RICE PUDDING

Combine and beat until smooth:

½ cup sugar stirred with	½ cup fresh milk
½ cup powdered milk	2 whole eggs or 4 yolks
¼ teaspoon salt	½ teaspoon vanilla

Add and stir well:

2 cups fresh or reconstituted milk	2 cups cooked brown or converted rice

Pour into greased baking dish; sprinkle with **nutmeg**. Bake in slow oven at 325° F. for 30 minutes, or until temperature in center of pudding, taken with a meat thermometer, is 175° F. Stir once or twice during baking.

VARIATIONS:

Add ½ cup of one or more of the following: raisins, chopped dates, shredded coconut, broken walnuts or pecans; or add ¼ to ½ cup wheat germ or soy grits and use ½ teaspoons salt.

Use 3 tablespoons each sugar and dark molasses or omit sugar and sweeten with ⅓ cup molasses.

Poor man's rice pudding: Omit eggs; use ½ cup uncooked rice and 4 cups fresh or reconstituted milk; add other ingredients of basic recipe, sprinkle generously with **nutmeg**; bake in a slow oven at 300° F. for 3 hours. Stir occasionally during baking. Add **raisins or nuts** as desired.

APPLE BETTY

Mix thoroughly with fingertips:

1 cup wheat germ
2 teaspoons cinnamon
½ cup white or brown sugar

2 tablespoons partially hardened
  margarine or butter

Sprinkle half the above mixture over bottom of a greased 8- by 8-inch pan.

Wash, peel, and slice:

3 to 5 tart cooking apples

Add to apples and mix well:

⅓ cup sugar
pinch of salt

½ to 1 teaspoon cinnamon

Put apples over wheat-germ mixture and sprinkle remainder over top.

Bake in moderate oven at 375° F. for 30 minutes, or until apples are tender when tested with a fork. Be careful not to overbake. Serve with top milk.

VARIATIONS:

If apples are not tart, add 1 tablespoon lemon juice.

Omit or decrease cinnamon and sprinkle with nutmeg.

Add ½ cup raisins or broken walnuts, pecans, or roasted almonds.

Instead of apples use 1½ cups fresh or canned apricots, sliced peaches, pears, or pitted stewed prunes; add ¾ cup water or fruit juice; decrease sugar in filling to 2 tablespoons if sweetened canned fruit is used. Bake 20 minutes.

Use 2 cups sliced apples, 1 cup steamed pitted prunes, ½ cup prune juice; bake as in basic recipe.

Apple cobbler: See page 424.

Apple crisp: Spread sliced apples on a greased flat baking dish; add ¼ cup water; combine ¼ cup each white and brown sugar, whole-wheat-pastry flour, wheat germ, and fat; sprinkle over top of apples with 1 teaspoon cinnamon.

Apple pan-dowdy: Omit wheat-germ mixture; prepare apples as directed using ⅔ cup brown sugar; bake 20 minutes. Remove from oven and increase temperature to 450° F. Make **wheat-germ biscuits** (p. 424), roll dough thin, and cut; dip each in **melted partially hardened margarine or butter,** roll in ½ **cup sugar mixed with 2 teaspoons cinnamon,** and put over apples. Bake for 8 to 10 minutes.

The trick of whipping evaporated milk easily is to chill it in an ice tray until it is partially frozen. When lemon juice is added, the flavor can scarcely be detected.

MARSHMALLOW CREAM

Beat until stiff:

½ **cup chilled evaporated milk**

Add and beat slightly:

¼ **cup powdered milk**　　　　　　2 **tablespoons each sugar and**
1 **teaspoon vanilla**　　　　　　　　**lemon juice**

Cut into eighths with wet scissors and drop into whipped milk:

10 or 12 marshmallows

Add:

1 **cup drained crushed pineapple**　6 **quartered maraschino or candied**
½ **cup broken walnuts or pecans**　　**cherries**

Stir until all ingredients are combined; place in sherbet glasses; garnish each with a **whole cherry or nut meat.** Prepare no earlier than 2 hours before serving. This is an excellent dessert to prepare when time is limited.

VARIATIONS:

Omit cherries and add ¼ cup shredded coconut, toasted soy grits, raisins, chopped dates, or diced bananas.

Instead of pineapple use 1 cup of any of the following: diced bananas; fresh sliced or canned apricots or peaches; fresh or frozen berries; thick applesauce or prune pulp; use peanuts with applesauce or prune pulp; omit sugar if sweetened canned or frozen fruit is used.

Rice cream: Use ¼ cup sugar; instead of marshmallows add 1 cup cooked brown or converted rice to basic recipe or any variation.

JUNKET

Blend in liquefier or combine and beat or shake until smooth:

1 cup fresh milk
⅔ cup powdered milk
¼ cup white or brown sugar

1 teaspoon vanilla
pinch of salt

Add and heat until lukewarm, or 110° F.:

1 cup fresh or reconstituted milk

Meanwhile dissolve 1 rennet, or junket, tablet in 1 tablespoon water; add dissolved tablet to warm milk, stir no longer than 10 seconds, and pour immediately into sherbet glasses; do not move glasses until junket is firmly set, or about 10 minutes.

Chill; sprinkle with **shredded coconut, finely diced citron, or broken nuts.**

VARIATIONS:

Use 2 tablespoons each sugar and dark molasses; add ½ teaspoon maple, rum, brandy, or black-walnut flavoring; or omit sugar and sweeten to taste with molasses.

Omit vanilla and flavor to taste with almond extract or freshly shredded orange or lemon rind.

Before adding junket tablet stir into milk ½ cup toasted wheat germ, Grape Nuts, or graham-cracker crumbs.

The fillings for meringue-cream pies (p. 515), chiffon-cream pies (p. 517), and fresh-fruit pies (p. 518) can be served as puddings, and therefore only one pudding recipe is given here.

The less nutritious prepared puddings have gained popularity because of their simplicity and deliciousness. If you use these puddings, increase their nutritive value by adding powdered milk.

PREPARED PUDDINGS

Mix well in a cooking utensil:

1 package prepared pudding   ½ cup powdered milk

Add a small amount at a time and stir until smooth:

2½ cups fresh or reconstituted milk

Cook slowly over direct heat, stirring constantly until mixture is thick, or about 4 minutes; remove from heat, cool slightly, and add:

1 teaspoon vanilla (optional)

Pour into serving dishes and chill.

VARIATIONS:

Stir ½ cup broken walnuts, pecans, or other nuts into pudding after removing from heat.

Beat 1 or 2 eggs slightly with other ingredients before cooking; do not allow pudding to boil.

Fold ½ cup whipped evaporated milk into pudding when cooled.

Cake filling: Make pudding with 2 cups fresh milk; add **1 tablespoon each sugar and partially hardened margarine or butter.** Use as filling between layers of cake and/or as substitute for icing. Add **diced bananas, chopped dates, sweetened fresh fruit, or nuts** as desired.

Flaming puddings: For a festive winter evening (it is not effective except by candle light) top each serving with a **marshmallow** into which has been pushed a **cube of sugar.** Immediately before taking to the table, pour ½ teaspoon **lemon extract** over each cube of sugar and light. The flame caramelizes the sugar and toasts the marshmallow.

Fruit pudding: Prepare vanilla pudding with 1½ cups fresh milk; after cooling stir in ½ to 1 cup **drained crushed pineapple, sliced strawberries, or sweetened apricots or peaches.**

Pie filling: Add 2 egg yolks to pudding; do not boil; pour into crumb crust or baked pastry shell; make meringue (p. 516) of egg whites.

MARSHMALLOW SPONGE

Heat to simmering:

1 cup fresh or reconstituted milk   pinch of salt

Cut into quarters with wet scissors and drop into milk:

1 pound (about 40) marshmallows

Stir until marshmallows are dissolved, or about 2 minutes; remove from heat, *cover,* and cool, stirring occasionally; do not chill.

Meanwhile place **graham-cracker crumbs** ¼ inch deep in flat baking dish, ice tray, square mold, or 9-inch pie pan; sprinkle generously with **cinnamon.**

Whip until stiff:

1 cup chilled evaporated milk

Add and whip slightly:

½ cup powdered milk   **2 teaspoons vanilla**
2 tablespoons lemon juice

Fold whipped milk into cooled marshmallow mixture and pour into mold; sprinkle top with more **graham-cracker crumbs and cinnamon.**
Chill, cut into squares or wedges, and serve.

VARIATIONS:
Omit crumbs and cinnamon; use ring mold; before serving sponge fill center with fresh or frozen berries or mixed fresh fruit.

The following recipe is an Americanized version of English trifle, which is a delicious dessert having a most adaptable recipe. If you arrive home late, yet want to make a fancy dessert, it can be prepared in 5 to 8 minutes and served immediately. On the other hand, you can make it hours ahead and have it ready for guest dinners. Almost any combination of fresh or canned fruit, jam or jelly, or wines can be used. Should you wish to gild the lily, meringue or whipping cream may be put on top. I have yet to find anyone who did not like it.

AMERICANIZED TRIFLE

Line sides and bottom of an attractive serving dish with:

1 package lady fingers

Peel, slice, sweeten slightly, and add:

2 to 4 fresh peaches

Drop over peaches:

2 or 3 tablespoons strawberry jam   **2 tablespoons sherry (optional)**

Blend in liquefier in the order given:

2 cups fresh milk   **⅓ cup powdered milk (not in-
1 package instant vanilla pudding   stant)**

Pour pudding over peaches; sprinkle top with **coconut;** chill 5 minutes or longer and serve.

VARIATIONS:

Layer ingredients in 7- by 11-inch baking dish, using cooked or canned fruit. Combine ingredients of boiled custard (p. 484) with 4 egg yolks and pour over fruit. Beat egg whites stiff, add 2 tablespoons sugar, 1 teaspoon vanilla, and spread meringue over pudding. Bake in oven at 300° F. for 20 minutes.

Top with sweetened whipped cream flavored with vanilla or almond.

Instead of peaches, use fresh or frozen strawberries, fresh or canned pears, sliced oranges, pineapple chunks, black cherries, or fresh, canned, or frozen apricots; use or omit jam. Red currant jelly is delicious with pears.

Combine several fresh fruits and jam, jelly, or marmalade.

Instead of lady fingers, use slices of stale white or yellow cake.

The usual variety of sponges in which flavored gelatins are beaten after they have started to congeal offer almost no nutritive value. The sponges made by folding beaten uncooked egg whites into the whipped gelatin often cause egg allergies and probably skin rashes or unrecognized biotin deficiencies. If both evaporated and powdered milk are used in making sponges, the equivalent of a quart or more of fresh milk may be added, yet the flavor remains delicious.

A friend who "simply couldn't stand the taste of evaporated milk" acted as the final judge of all desserts containing this valuable product. She pronounced each final product delicious and the flavor of the milk completely disguised.

Although foods containing such large amounts of synthetic coloring and flavoring as flavored gelatins cannot be recommended, I am including the following recipe for housewives who nevertheless serve such gelatins.

STRAWBERRY SPONGE

Combine and stir well:

1 cup boiling water   1 package strawberry gelatin

Cool by adding:

¾ cup cold water

Chill until gelatin starts to congeal. Meanwhile beat until stiff:

½ cup chilled evaporated milk

Add and beat slightly:

2 tablespoons lemon juice   ¼ cup powdered milk

Fold whipped milk into gelatin with **1 cup sliced and sweetened fresh or frozen strawberries.** Pour into mold and chill until set.

VARIATIONS:

Omit strawberries from sponge; pour sponge into ring mold; unmold and fill center with sliced and sweetened or frozen strawberries.

Use raspberry gelatin; fold in fresh, canned, or frozen raspberries; if canned berries are used, substitute juice for part of the water.

Banana sponge: Use **lemon gelatin;** fold in with whipped milk **1 cup mashed bananas;** add **2 tablespoons sugar.**

Gelatin chiffon pies: Prepare basic recipe or any variation; pour into a 9-inch pie plate brushed with soft margarine or butter and sprinkle with **cereal, cracker, or cookie crumbs;** sprinkle top with crumbs. Or mold gelatin in a 9-inch baked crumb or pastry shell.

Lemon sponge: Use **lemon gelatin;** instead of ½ cup water, cool with **½ cup lemon juice;** sprinkle square mold or buttered 9-inch pie plate with **cereal, cookie, or cracker crumbs;** pour gelatin over crumbs and sprinkle top with crumbs; chill; cut into cubes or wedges and serve.

Lime-pineapple sponge: Use **lime gelatin;** stir in 1 cup well-drained crushed pineapple with whipped milk; use juice from pineapple to cool gelatin instead of part of the water.

Orange sponge: Use **orange gelatin;** add **grated rind of 1 orange and/ or 1 teaspoon orange flavoring;** fill center of ring mold with **sweetened orange sections.**

Yogurt sponge: Omit evaporated milk and lemon juice; fold into gelatin **1 cup thick yogurt;** prepare as in basic recipe or any variation. Yogurt is particularly delicious with the crushed-pineapple-and-lime gelatin.

ORANGE WHIP

Put into saucepan:

½ cup water   1 tablespoon unflavored gelatin

Soak 5 minutes, dissolve by heating slowly; cool slightly and add:

½ cup sugar   1¼ cups fresh or diluted frozen
2 tablespoons lemon juice   orange juice
grated rind 1 large orange

Chill until gelatin starts to congeal. Meanwhile beat until stiff:

¾ cup chilled evaporated milk

Add and beat slightly:

½ cup powdered milk

Fold milk into gelatin; pour into square mild, chill, cut into cubes and serve with sweetened diced oranges; or pour into ring mold and serve with center filled with sweetened orange sections or diced mixed fruits.

VARIATIONS:

Instead of adding powdered and evaporated milk, beat congealed gelatin before pouring into mold and serve with five-minute custard (p. 484).

Omit orange rind; just before folding in whipped milk add 1 cup of any of the following: diced bananas, sliced fresh and sweetened or canned peaches, pears, or apricots, diced fresh California persimmons, or drained crushed pineapple.

Instead of orange rind and juice use 1¾ cups of any of the following juices: canned pineapple, apricot, purple plum, Concord grape (this is my favorite), raspberry, or any berry juice. If sweetened juices are used, decrease or omit sugar.

Gelatin chiffon pies: Brush serving pie plate generously with partially hardened margarine, sprinkle liberally with crumbs; when gelatin starts to congeal, pour over crumbs, using basic recipe or any variation; sprinkle top with crumbs; or pour gelatin into a baked crumb or pastry shell.

Bavarian cream is often thought of as being difficult and expensive to prepare. The following Bavarian cream, which I think you'll agree is delicious, can be made in a few minutes at little cost. It supplies the equivalent of 2½ quarts fresh milk, no small amount when protein, riboflavin, and calcium requirements are often difficult to meet.

BAVARIAN CREAM

Make five-minute custard (p. 484) using 1½ cups fresh or reconstituted milk; add to hot custard:

1 tablespoon unflavored gelatin soaked in	½ cup cold milk

Chill custard until gelatin starts to congeal; whip:

½ cup chilled evaporated milk

Fold milk into custard after adding to it:

¼ cup sugar	2 teaspoons vanilla

Pour into greased mold; chill until firmly set.

VARIATIONS:

Line square baking dish with graham-cracker crumbs and sprinkle generously with cinnamon; pour Bavarian cream over crumbs; sprinkle top with crumbs and cinnamon. Cut in cubes to serve.

Before folding in whipped milk add 1 cup of any of the following: diced banana; fresh sliced and sweetened or canned and drained peaches, pears, or apricots; drained, crushed or sliced canned pineapple; frozen or sweetened fresh strawberries, raspberries, or boysenberries; canned black cherries; diced fresh California persimmons; leftover cooked rice.

Add ½ cup of any of the following: walnuts, pecans, or other nuts; shredded or ground coconut; raisins, chopped dates, diced drained pitted prunes, or soft figs; or add ¼ cup each nuts and coconut, dried fruit, or soy grits.

Almond cream: Omit vanilla and add 1 teaspoon almond extract and ¼ cup chopped toasted almonds or ¼ cup soy grits.

Caramel cream: Omit 2 tablespoons sugar and add 2 tablespoons dark molasses and ½ teaspoon maple, rum, or brandy flavoring. Add nuts and/or coconut as desired.

Eggnog pie: Omit vanilla and add 2 tablespoons rum or brandy; pour into 9-inch serving pie plate brushed with partially hardened margarine and sprinkled with wheat germ or crumbs; or into baked crumb or pastry shell; sprinkle with nutmeg. This pie is truly delicious.

Gelatin chiffon pies: Mold basic recipe or any variation in 9-inch baked crumb or pastry shell; sprinkle top with crumbs, coconut, or ground nuts.

Lemon cream: Omit vanilla and ¼ cup fresh milk, making custard with 1¼ cups fresh milk; add to chilled custard grated rind of 1 lemon and ¼ cup lemon juice.

Orange cream: Omit vanilla; add grated rind of 1 large orange and/ or 1 teaspoon orange flavoring.

ORANGE SHERBET

Soak for 5 minutes:

2 teaspoons gelatin in   **½ cup water**

Heat until the gelatin is dissolved; cool and add:

1½ cups fresh or diluted frozen orange juice

Freeze slowly to a soft mush, then beat until stiff:

1 cup chilled evaporated milk

Add and beat until velvety:

frozen juice   2 tablespoons lemon juice
grated rind of 1 orange

Sweeten to taste; return to freezing compartment; freeze only to a firm texture.

VARIATIONS:

Instead of orange juice use 2 cups of any of the following juices: purple plum; Concord grape; strawberry, raspberry, or other berry juice; pineapple; apricot; black cherry. Omit orange rind. When juices from heavily sweetened canned fruits are used, such as juice from commercially canned raspberries, dilute with any unsweetened juice; otherwise it is very difficult to freeze them.

It is unfortunate that commercial gingerbread mixes prepared with soda and refined flour have gained wide popularity, especially when gingerbread of outstanding nutritive value can be made in a few minutes.

GINGERBREAD

Combine and stir well:

⅓ cup vegetable oil   ⅓ cup sugar
½ cup wheat germ   ¾ cup sour milk, buttermilk, or
1 egg   yogurt
⅔ cup dark molasses

Sift into moist ingredients:

1 cup sifted whole-wheat-pastry   ¼ cup powdered milk
    flour   2 teaspoons ginger
3 teaspoons double-acting baking   1 teaspoon cinnamon
    powder   ½ teaspoon salt

Combine ingredients with no more than 20 strokes. Grease ring mold or 8-inch square loaf pan and dust with flour. Pour batter into pan and bake in moderate oven at 350° F. for 45 minutes; be particularly careful not to overbake. Remove from oven as soon as dough no longer adheres to toothpick or cake tester.

VARIATIONS:

Use 1½ cups nutritious mix instead of flour, wheat germ, salt, and baking powder.

Instead of ½ cup whole-wheat flour use ½ cup rice polish or soy flour. Since these products contain no gluten, they are excellent for making gingerbread.

Omit 2 tablespoons flour and add 2 tablespoons brewers' yeast; the yeast cannot be tasted.

PLUM PUDDING

Sift into mixing bowl:

⅔ cup sifted whole-wheat-pastry flour
¾ cup sugar
1½ teaspoons cinnamon
1 teaspoon nutmeg

2 teaspoons double-acting baking powder
½ cup powdered milk
¾ teaspoon salt
2 tablespoons brewers' yeast

Add and stir well:

½ cup wheat germ
2 tablespoons each oil and dark molasses
1½ cups finely shredded raw unpeeled carrots

1 cup raisins
½ cup broken pecans, walnuts, or toasted almonds
1 egg
½ cup milk or buttermilk

Grease 3 pint-sized tin cans; put pudding in cans and tie brown paper securely over tops; place on rack, jar lids, or crumpled foil in cooking utensil in water 3 or 4 inches deep; cover utensil and boil slowly 2 hours. Serve hot with hard sauce; reheat in oven.

VARIATIONS:

Instead of wheat germ use ½ cup rice polish or soy flour.

Add ½ cup of any one or more of the following: chopped dates; finely diced citron; dried currants; diced raw apple or persimmon; ground dried apricots or peaches; beat batter with 50 strokes if more than 2 cups fruit are to be added.

Date pudding: Omit raisins and nutmeg; add 2 cups chopped dates.

The usual varieties of hard sauce are so rich that only a few bites can be enjoyed without discomfort. The following sauce is not only more nutritious but extremely delicious. The powdered milk absorbs the brandy so readily that the sauce can have a great deal more flavor without becoming runny than it does when only powdered sugar is used. While it is delightfully sweet, it is not nauseously so.

HARD SAUCE FOR PLUM PUDDING

Sift together:

½ cup powdered sugar   ½ cup powdered milk

Add and mix well:

⅓ cup partially hardened marga-   3 tablespoons brandy, rum,
rine or butter   or whiskey

Serve chilled on steaming-hot plum pudding.

Few desserts surpass cheese cakes in nutritive value. Certainly they are delicious and easily prepared. Uncooked cheese cake, or pasha, is a modification of the famous Russian Easter cake.

UNCOOKED CHEESE CAKE, OR PASHA

Beat with electric mixer until smooth:

2 pounds hoop cheese, or dry,   ¼ pound sweet, or unsalted, butter
unsalted cottage cheese

Add and stir well:

¼ cup powdered milk sifted with
1¼ cups sugar
1 cup top milk or cream
1 cup chopped, blanched almonds

2 tablespoons vanilla or grated
 vanilla bean
½ small citron, finely chopped

Cover colander with clean cloth; pour cheese mixture over cloth and place a small inverted plate on top as weight; set colander on cake pan and let stand in refrigerator overnight.

Turn cake onto large plate, remove cloth, slice, and serve. Any left-over cheese cake may be frozen.

VARIATIONS:

Add any of the following: 1 cup seedless raisins, ¼ cup finely chopped candied orange peel or candied cherries cut into quarters; 1 tablespoon grated lemon rind.

If it is impossible to obtain hoop cheese, use farmer-style cottage cheese and omit top milk or cream.

BAKED CHEESE CAKE

Beat until smooth:

2 eggs
2 teaspoons vanilla
¾ teaspoon almond extract
¾ cup honey or sugar

1 cup cottage cheese
1 large package (8 ounces) cream
 cheese
¼ cup powdered milk

Spread a 7- or 8-inch pan generously with partially hardened margarine or butter; sprinkle with thick layer of cookie- or graham-cracker crumbs; pour cheese mixture over crumbs.

Set over jar lids or crumpled foil in a pan of boiling water and bake at 300° F. for 25 minutes.

Meanwhile mix together:

1 cup sour cream
1 teaspoon vanilla

⅓ cup honey or sugar

Take cheese cake from oven at end of 25 minutes and pour sweetened sour cream over top; return to oven and bake 10 minutes longer.

VARIATIONS:

To make really professional cheese cake, omit cottage cheese and use 2 packages (8 ounces each) cream cheese; to decrease calories use 2 cups cottage cheese and omit cream cheese. To decrease fat content still more, instead of cream cheese and cottage cheese, use 2 cups (16 ounces) hoop cheese, or dry cottage cheese; sprinkle top with crumbs and omit sour-cream topping.

Double recipe; bake in standard cake pan 1½ inches high for 35 minutes before adding cream topping. Freeze any cake not eaten.

Nuts are an excellent source of protein, unsaturated fatty acids, and the B vitamins. They should be used as much as a budget allows, particularly if there are growing children in the family. The quantity of nuts used in the following torte makes it of outstanding nutritive value. Aside from their contribution to health, walnut and almond tortes are both delicious desserts. Almost every person who has tested the ones I have made has asked me for the recipe.

WALNUT TORTE

Line bottoms of two 8-inch layer-cake pans with heavy paper; brush paper with soft **partially hardened margarine or butter.**

Stir together thoroughly:

1 cup sugar	2 cups ground walnuts
3 egg yolks	¾ cup wheat germ

Beat stiff and fold **6 egg whites** into above ingredients.

Pour batter into pans, spread evenly to edges, and bake in slow oven at 325° F. for 30 minutes. Turn out of pans and remove paper immediately.

Prepare filling by mixing thoroughly:

⅓ cup sugar	⅓ cup powdered milk

Add and stir well:

3 egg yolks   ½ cup top milk or cream

Cook slowly over direct heat until thick, stirring constantly; do not boil.

Remove from heat and add:

1 cup ground walnuts

Spread between layers of torte.

VARIATIONS:

Instead of walnuts use ground pecans or half black walnuts and half English walnuts.

Simmer ¾ cup soy grits in ¾ cup water for 8 minutes, or until all water is absorbed; turn out on paper towels; measure after cooking and use 1 cup cooked grits in torte instead of 1 cup walnuts; add 1 teaspoon black-walnut flavoring. Use remaining cooked grits in filling instead of ½ cup walnuts; cool and add ½ teaspoon black-walnut flavoring.

Almond torte: Use ground blanched almonds instead of walnuts in torte; add ½ teaspoon almond flavoring to torte, ¼ teaspoon to filling. Or use 1 cup ground almonds in torte, ½ cup in filling, and supplement nuts with soy grits cooked as directed above. Blanch almonds by steaming 3 minutes in 2 tablespoons boiling water; cool and remove skins. Instead of filling use a ¼-inch layer of marzipan paste (p. 538).

At least once in her lifetime every housewife who wishes to should serve crêpes suzette, if only to keep from being impressed by the three-to-ten-dollar variety offered in restaurants. They are not difficult to make and nutritionally they rank above many desserts. Since the liquors are added for flavor and the alcohol is evaporated off or burned, this dish should not offend temperance-minded persons. The following recipe is geared for entertaining and serves 6.

As I was testing this recipe, a neighbor remarked, "Health foods have taken a new turn. They've gone classy."

Why not?

CRÊPES SUZETTE

Prepare thin pancakes (p. 418) about 3 or 4 inches in diameter.
Make sauce by combining:

¼ cup partially hardened
  margarine or butter
½ cup sugar
½ cup frozen undiluted orange
  juice

½ cup water
¼ cup cognac, curaçao, or Coin-
  treau
1 tablespoon grated lemon rind

Heat sauce until sugar is melted.

Dip each pancake into sauce, making sure it is moist on both sides.
Roll and leave in sauce. When all pancakes have been rolled, set aside
until almost time to serve.

Cover utensil and simmer pancakes in sauce 5 minutes, or just long
enough to heat through. If not in chafing dish or attractive heat-resistant utensil, transfer to a heated platter.

Immediately before bringing to table, pour over hot pancakes:

¼ cup brandy

Light brandy. Serve crêpes with sauce as flames are dying.

Cakes and Cake Fillings and Icings

Frankly, I have never been good at baking cakes. For this reason
I asked a friend of mine, Ann Mihaylo, who I suspect could
make a delicious cake from a sack of cement, to supply and test
the cake recipes which appeared in the original edition of this
book. Her cakes were marvelous, even her angel foods and
"white" cakes which were made with whole-wheat flour and
powdered milk. It seems to me that being good at cake baking,
however, is similar to having a green thumb in gardening; some
people have the knack and others do not. Partly because more
housewives seem to have my talents at cake making than Ann's,
and partly because cake mixes are so widely used, I have deleted
the cake recipes from this edition.

Should you wish to improve your favorite cake recipes, Ann's advice is this: "Take any cake recipe and substitute for the white flour the same amount of whole-wheat-pastry flour; add 1 teaspoon more baking powder, 1 more egg (fold in stiffly beaten whites) and ⅓ cup powdered milk; follow whatever procedure the recipe calls for. Stir just till the batter is well mixed. Do not overbeat it. For a light cake I do not add wheat germ.

"If you want your cake to be moist and delicate and to have a soft, velvety texture, underbake it. The tendency of amateurs is to overbake cakes."

Since cake fillings require considerably less sugar and contain larger amounts of milk, eggs, and nuts than do most icings, they are nutritionally superior to icings. They offer the advantage of keeping the cake moist for many days. Puddings (p. 491) and fillings for meringue-cream pies may be used and even spread over the entire surface of a cake to be served with a fork. Lemon, banana, or date-nut filling can enhance any cake.

In my opinion cake icings can be tremendously improved nutritionally without sacrificing flavor by the addition of non-instant powdered milk. (Instant powdered milk gives an unpleasant gritty texture.) Neither the food coloring nor the chocolate or cocoa used in icings can be recommended, much less the sugar. I merely suggest a way to enrich icings in case you choose to make them.

When icings are made of powdered milk, they take only a few minutes to prepare and there is no problem of their being overcooked, sugary, too thick, or too thin. To facilitate even blending, it is important to stir in the flavoring and coloring before adding the powdered milk.

The quantities suggested in the following recipes are sufficient to cover a large loaf cake, a 9-inch cake baked in a tube pan, or two 8- or 9-inch layers.

The variations are the same regardless of the type of icing, and those on page 507 can be used with any of the three icings.

UNCOOKED ICING

Combine:

½ cup top milk or cream
1 teaspoon vanilla
2 or 3 drops food coloring
   (optional)

3 tablespoons partially hardened
   margarine or butter
dash of salt

Sift together into liquid:

1½ cups powdered sugar

¾ cup non-instant powdered milk

Beat until creamy. Add more powdered sugar or a combination of
powdered sugar and powdered milk if needed to give the texture you
wish. Spread between layers and over cake.

QUICK ICING

Combine:

1¼ cups sugar
½ cup top milk or cream

2 tablespoons partially hardened
   margarine or butter

Boil slowly for about 2 minutes, or enough to melt sugar. Cool completely and then beat in:

1 cup powdered milk
1 teaspoon vanilla

nuts or food coloring if desired

Add more powdered milk if needed to give desired texture.
Spread between layers and over cake.

DOUBLE-BOILER ICING

Combine in top of double boiler:

¾ cup sugar
2 tablespoons water
dash of salt

1 teaspoon vinegar
1 unbeaten egg white

Stir and set over boiling water; beat with rotary beater about 5 minutes or until stiff enough to stand in peaks; remove and chill; when cold, add:

1 teaspoon vanilla	**2 or 3 drops food coloring**
½ cup non-instant powdered milk	(optional)

Beat until smooth, and spread between layers and over cake.

VARIATIONS *for the three foregoing icing recipes:*

Just before spreading on cake add any one of the following: ½ cup finely chopped dates, figs, walnuts, pecans, or almonds; ¼ cup non-hydrogenated peanut butter; candied pineapple, or citron; ½ cup each chopped dried or candied fruits and chopped nuts.

Caramel icing: Use tightly packed brown sugar instead of white in quick icing; the sugar will cause the milk to curdle, but an even texture will result after beating.

Cheese filling: Blend with half the icing 1 package (3 ounces) cream cheese; add 2 teaspoons grated orange or lemon rind. Put between layers of cake; use remaining icing for top.

Chocolate icing: Melt 1 or 1½ squares unsweetened chocolate over low heat, add liquid ingredients, stir well, and proceed as in uncooked icing or quick icing. Or stir 2 or 3 tablespoons cocoa with sugar in quick icing.

Coconut icing: Spread icing on cake and sprinkle generously with fresh or slightly toasted coconut.

Icing for banana cake: Slice bananas lengthwise and spread over layers; brush bananas lightly with lemon juice; cover with icing.

Lemon icing: Instead of vanilla add grated rind of 1 lemon.

Maple icing: Use maple sugar in quick icing; or add 1 teaspoon maple flavoring to any icing. Maple is especially good with ½ cup walnuts.

Orange icing: Instead of vanilla add grated rind of 1 orange and orange coloring.

Peppermint icing: Add a few drops of oil of peppermint and pink coloring.

Pineapple icing: Use crushed pineapple and juice instead of milk in uncooked icing; or add ¼ cup diced candied pineapple to any icing.

Pies

When you must make your pie dough from mixes, at least add ¼ cup of wheat germ for each crust. It does not detract from tenderness and does give a rich, nutty flavor.

If pie crusts are to be tender, the dough must not be stirred, kneaded, or even handled any more than is absolutely necessary; and the flour used must be low in gluten.

Pie dough can be more easily handled if rolled on a lightly floured canvas with a rolling pin covered with a knitted stocking. The materials hold flour and prevent dough from sticking; and the canvas can be easily inverted over a pie tin.

Flaky pie crusts are made by carefully observing four rules: the fat must be chilled; it must be cut into the flour only until the pieces are the size of large peas; the water used must be cold, preferably ice water; and the oven temperature must be sufficiently high so that the crust will bake before the bits of fat have time to melt and penetrate evenly throughout the flour. The cold, firm fat, mashed into layers when the crust is rolled, prevents flour in one part of the crust from sticking to that in other parts of the crust, and flakiness results. If the fat is warm or soft before the dough is made, if it is warmed by mixing with the hands or by adding warm water, if the oven temperature is low, or if oil is used instead of a solid fat, a flaky crust cannot possibly be obtained.

Crusts made with oil, warm ingredients, or hot water can be delicious and crisp but they are never flaky. A crust can be made even more crisp by being thoroughly chilled or frozen after it has been rolled but before it is baked. If chilled, the water in the dough expands more when it is changed into steam during baking than if it is warm. If you have a freezer, you may wish to prepare several single-crust pie shells at one time, keep them frozen, and bake them as you need them.

To my way of thinking, no shortening can compare with natural lard for making flaky pie crusts, but most lard is now hydrogenated and cannot be recommended. Partially hardened margarine and butter are also satisfactory for making flaky crusts.

FLAKY PIE CRUST

To make two single-crust 9-inch pie shells or one double crust, sift into mixing bowl:

1½ cups whole-wheat-pastry flour   1 teaspoon salt

Add and stir well:

**½ cup wheat germ   ⅔ cup partially hardened marga-
½ cup chilled natural lard or   rine or butter**

Cut shortening into dry ingredients with pastry cutter or two knives until particles of fat are the size of large peas; do not touch with hands. Add:

¼ cup cold water, preferably ice water

Mix only enough to moisten ingredients. Turn dough onto floured canvas or other cloth; knead just enough to hold dough together. If crust is to be baked without filling, divide into two equal parts; for a two-crust pie, use a slightly larger amount of dough for lower crust. Pat dough quickly into a flat, round "ball," dust top lightly with flour, and roll ⅛ inch thick, using a circular motion of the rolling pin to give a perfect circle of dough; turn canvas during rolling and avoid touching dough if possible.

Turn pie tin over dough; pick up canvas, invert over pan, and remove cloth. If a single-crust shell is being prepared, put on bottom of pie tin; trim and flute edges and make perforations with a fork at ½-inch intervals.

See page 511 for preparing and baking double-crust pies.

If time permits, chill in refrigerator or freeze before baking.

Bake single crusts in hot, preheated oven at 425° F. for 8 to 10 minutes. Wheat germ burns quickly at this temperature; watch the baking time carefully.

VARIATIONS:

If crisp but not flaky crust is desired, all ingredients may be at room temperature; use 3 or 4 tablespoons water, depending on softness of fat, combine ingredients with fingertips if desired. Bake at 350° F. for 18 to 20 minutes.

Instead of wheat germ use ½ cup rice polish or soy flour; use 5 tablespoons water with soy flour.

If wheat germ is not available, use 2 cups whole-wheat-pastry flour; increase lard to ⅔ cup, other fats to 1 cup.

Boiling-water pie crust: Bring water to boiling; add and melt fat; remove from heat, stir in dry ingredients with no more than 15 strokes; chill thoroughly before rolling. Bake at 350° F. for 18 to 20 minutes. Use this method for basic recipe or any variation. This is an easy and foolproof procedure for making crisp crusts.

CRISP PIE CRUST

To make two single-crust 9-inch pie shells or one double-crust pie, sift together:

2 cups sifted whole-wheat-pastry flour	1 teaspoon salt

Combine, beat with a fork, then pour over flour:

½ cup vegetable oil	¼ cup ice water

Cut liquid into flour with fork, form into ball, and proceed as for flaky pie crust. Bake at 350° F. for 15 to 18 minutes.

VARIATION:

Use 1½ cups whole-wheat-pastry flour and ¾ cup wheat germ. Press against sides and bottom of greased pie tin as if making a crumb crust.

CRUMB CRUST

Toast and pass through the meat grinder, using smallest knife:

4 or 5 slices stale whole-wheat bread

Sift crumbs and measure; combine:

⅔ cup whole-wheat-bread crumbs	¼ cup powdered milk
¼ cup wheat germ	½ to ¾ teaspoon cinnamon

Stir dry ingredients together thoroughly; add:

⅓ cup melted butter or partially hardened margarine

Mix until fat is evenly distributed; add and blend well:

1 tablespoon dark molasses or syrup

Grease 9-inch serving pie pan, being particularly careful to grease the rim. Press crumbs firmly against pan to form crust ⅛ inch thick, making the margin first.

Bake in a moderate oven at 300° F. for 10 minutes, or add filling and bake as meringue cooks. This crust burns easily; watch it carefully.

VARIATIONS:

Use crumbs from any of the following: bran flakes; whole-wheat-cereal flakes; stale cookies of any kind; toasted slices of stale cake; whole-wheat zwieback; graham crackers.

FRUIT PIES

Prepare dough for two-crust pie; line 9-inch pie pan with dough; chill while filling is being prepared.

Mix together thoroughly:

½ to 1 cup sugar, depending on sweetness of fruit **pinch of salt**	**2 or 3 tablespoons whole-wheat-pastry flour**

Add and stir well:

3 to 4 cups fresh sliced fruit or	**2½ cups canned fruit and juice**

Spread filling over lower pie shell. Roll dough for top crust ⅛ inch thick; make attractive feather design in dough with blunt edge and end of silver knife, making holes through which steam can escape; moisten edges of lower shell with small amount of juice; pick up canvas upon which dough has been rolled, invert it over pie, and remove cloth; press dough firmly around edges; trim and flute edges by pinching with thumbs and forefingers.

If juicy uncooked fruit is used, such as cherries, rhubarb, or berries, make small cones of heavy paper 3 inches square; fasten together with paper clips; insert in holes in upper crust to prevent juice from spilling during baking.

Bake in hot oven at 425° F. for 8 minutes; lower heat to 325° F. and continue baking 30 to 35 minutes for uncooked fruit pies, or 20 minutes for mince pie or canned-fruit fillings.

VARIATIONS:

If flaky crust is not desired or if boiling-water crust is used, bake pie at 350° F. for 45 to 50 minutes.

Apple pie: Slice **4 to 6 tart apples;** mix **1 teaspoon nutmeg or cinnamon** with sugar and flour. If apples lack flavor, add **1 tablespoon each margarine and lemon juice, ½ teaspoon grated lemon rind;** if dry, add **2 to 4 tablespoons sweet or sour cream;** if apples are a variety which will not cook readily, slice and steam for 8 minutes in ½ cup water; chill before mixing with other ingredients.

Open-top apple pie: Select green apples when possible; mix with sugar, flour, salt, and cinnamon; sprinkle with nutmeg; omit upper crust but turn a pie tin over apples during the first 15 minutes of baking. This is a Pennsylvania Dutch recipe and my favorite.

Apricot or peach pie: Use sliced fresh, canned, or partially cooked dried fruit; decrease sugar to ⅓ cup if sweetened canned apricots or peaches are used; proceed as in basic recipe.

Berry pies: Use blackberries, raspberries, currants, gooseberries, blueberries, or other berries; sweeten fresh currants or gooseberries with 1 cup sugar; add **1 tablespoon lemon juice** to blueberries or loganberries; proceed as in basic recipe. Prepare paper cones as directed above and insert in upper crust to prevent juice from spilling.

Cherry or grape pie: Use pitted pie cherries or Concord grapes; increase sugar to 1 cup if uncooked fruit is used or decrease to ⅓ cup with sweetened canned grapes, pie cherries, or black cherries.

Mince pie: Omit sugar, flour, and salt; most prepared mincemeat is improved by adding **1 or 2 finely diced unpeeled apples;** prepare and bake as in basic recipe.

Pineapple pie: Use canned crushed pineapple, omitting sugar or decreasing to 2 tablespoons; prepare as in basic recipe or cook pineapple with flour until thick, pour into baked shell or crumb crust, and top with meringue (p. 516).

Rhubarb pie: Use diced fresh rhubarb; increase flour to 4 tablespoons, sugar to 1 cup. Insert paper cones in upper crust to prevent juice from spilling.

Prune or raisin pie: Use steamed raisins, steamed and pitted prunes; sweeten fruit to taste; if desired add 1 tablespoon lemon juice or ½ teaspoon grated rind; prepare and bake as in the basic recipe. Or mix flour, salt, and sugar with 1 cup prune or raisin juice, cook until thick, add lemon rind and ½ cup chopped nuts; pour into baked shell or crumb crust, cover with meringue (p. 516).

There are numerous suggestions for preventing the crust of a custard or pumpkin pie from becoming soggy: brush the crust with fat or egg white; bake the crust 10 minutes before pouring the filling into it; and many similar precautions. I spent an entire day testing every such recommendation I could find, and although there were degrees of sogginess, not by any stretch of the imagination could any crust be called crisp.

To my way of thinking there is only one way to make a custard-type pie. Bake the shell first; while it is baking, prepare the filling; remove the baked shell from the pan and pour the custard into the same pan; lower the oven temperature and bake the custard. Immediately before the pie is to be served, slip the custard onto the crust. This method can work like a charm. A properly baked custard settles into the crust so beautifully that only the closest observer would notice the two had not been baked together. The contrast between the soft yet firm custard and the crisp, flaky crust so delights the palate that to bake a custard pie by another method seems a gastronomic crime.

CUSTARD PIE

Prepare a 9-inch flaky pie crust (p. 509); bake in pan with circular knife; while it is baking, combine:

⅓ to ½ cup sugar   ¼ cup powdered milk

Stir well; add:

½ cup fresh milk   1 teaspoon vanilla
3 eggs   pinch of salt

Beat until smooth and add 1½ cups fresh or reconstituted milk.

Take baked pie shell from oven; slip shell onto serving plate; grease the pan generously and pour custard into it; sprinkle top with nutmeg.

Lower oven temperature to 325° F.; bake custard 25 to 30 minutes, or until barely firm; cooking will continue as custard cools.

Immediately before serving, loosen custard with spatula or knife attached to pie pan; slip carefully into crust. The crust can become soggy about 30 minutes after the custard is put into it; combine the two just before pie is to be eaten.

VARIATIONS:

Substitute for vanilla grated rind of 1 lemon or orange.

Bake shell 8 minutes at 425° F. while preparing custard; remove from oven and brush generously with fat. Pour custard into shell and bake as directed above.

Almond-custard pie: Omit vanilla and nutmeg; add ½ teaspoon almond flavoring, ¼ cup each soy grits and additional fresh milk.

Apple-custard pie: Use 1 cup each thick applesauce and fresh milk; omit vanilla; add grated rind of 1 lemon. This is a delicious pie.

Banana-custard pie: Omit vanilla; add ½ teaspoon lemon extract or grated rind of 1 lemon to custard; immediately before serving slice 2 bananas over crust; slip custard over bananas.

Coconut-custard pie: Add ¼ cup shredded coconut to custard; sprinkle top of filling with ¼ cup before baking.

Date-custard pie: Use ⅓ cup sugar in custard; sprinkle ½ cup chopped dates over bottom of pan before baking custard; use ½ cup broken walnuts or pecans with dates as desired.

Lemon-custard pie: Omit vanilla; use 1¾ cups fresh milk; stir gradually into custard ¼ cup lemon juice, grated rind of 1 lemon.

Orange-custard pie: Omit vanilla; add 1 teaspoon orange flavoring and grated rind of 1 orange. This is my favorite custard pie.

Pineapple-custard pie: Omit vanilla; add ½ teaspoon lemon extract to custard; put crushed pineapple in strainer, squeeze out as much juice as possible; immediately before serving sprinkle ½ to 1 cup drained crushed pineapple over pie crust, cover with custard.

Pecan pie: Add ¾ cup broken pecans to custard before baking.

Pumpkin or squash pie: Combine custard ingredients, using 1 cup fresh milk; add 1 cup steamed and mashed or canned pumpkin or squash, 3 tablespoons dark molasses, ½ teaspoon each ginger and cinnamon; increase salt to ¼ teaspoon. If fluffy pie is desired, beat egg whites until stiff and fold into custard just before baking.

Raisin-nut pie: Sprinkle ½ cup each raisins and broken walnuts or pecans over bottom of pan before pouring custard into it to bake.

You can consistently make beautiful meringue pies if you bear two facts in mind: first, that hard-cooked eggs are firm; second, that high heat causes protein to shrivel and become tough. If the meringue is baked long enough for the egg white to be hard-cooked, it cannot fall. It must be baked at a low temperature if it is to stay tender and mountainous. It is wise to check the oven temperature with a thermometer before putting a meringue in to bake.

When water is added to egg whites, the surface tension is increased and the eggs will whip to a much larger volume than if no water is used.

The taste and texture of a meringue are greatly improved if sugar is beaten into the egg whites. To prevent the pie from becoming too sweet, less sugar should be used in the filling. All meringues are more delicious when a small amount of flavoring is added to them.

Chiffon-cream pies in which the egg whites are stirred into the filling seem to me even more delicious and more easily prepared than are meringue pies. The success of this type of pie depends entirely upon having the sweetened cream sauce boiling slowly while the eggs are being folded into it. If the sauce is not boiling, the eggs remain undercooked and the filling is runny; if the sauce is allowed to boil too hard or too long, the egg whites overcook and the texture becomes curdly. The eggs are cooked largely by low heat during the cooling process. If the directions are followed, pitfalls can be avoided.

Chiffon-pie fillings make delicious puddings which, if properly cooked, will hold their shape when molded.

MERINGUE-CREAM PIE

Mix well in saucepan:

⅓ to ½ cup sugar	¼ cup whole-wheat-pastry flour
½ cup powdered milk	pinch of salt

Add and beat well:

½ cup fresh milk	2 egg yolks

When batter is smooth, add and stir:

1½ cups fresh or reconstituted milk

If utensil does not develop hot spots, cook over moderate heat, stirring constantly, for about 8 minutes, or until custard becomes quite firm; or cook in the top of a double boiler; remove from heat and add:

1 tablespoon margarine or butter	1 teaspoon vanilla

Pour into a 9-inch crumb crust or baked pastry shell; cover with meringue.

MERINGUE FOR PIES

Combine:

2 egg whites	½ teaspoon vanilla
2 tablespoons water	dash of salt

Beat until egg whites are stiff; add 2 tablespoons at a time:

¼ cup sugar

Spread meringue over pie and bake in a slow oven at 300° F. for 30 minutes.

VARIATIONS:

Omit vanilla and 2 tablespoons milk from filling; add 2 tablespoons rum or brandy just before pouring into crust.

Almond pie: Omit vanilla and 2 tablespoons flour from filling; add ½ cup slivered almonds, ¾ teaspoon almond flavoring.

Banana pie: Slice 2 or 3 bananas into crust; cover with filling and meringue; or add sliced bananas to filling before pouring into crust.

Cake filling: Increase sugar in filling to ½ cup; omit meringue; use the basic recipe or any variation for cake filling.

Coconut pie: Add ½ cup shredded or ground coconut to filling; sprinkle coconut over top of meringue before baking.

Chiffon-cream pies: Use a 2-quart saucepan; when filling boils, add flavoring, margarine, and nuts or fruit suggested under variations; lower heat and fold in meringue while filling continues to boil slowly for 1 minute. Pour immediately into baked crust; omit meringue. Use for basic recipe or any variation.

Date-nut pie: Just before pouring filling into crust add ½ cup each chopped dates and broken walnuts or pecans. Vary by cooking ½ cup raisins in filling or adding ½ cup drained prune pulp.

Fruit-cream pies: Prepare filling, using 2 tablespoons sugar, 1 cup fresh milk; just before pouring filling into crust or folding in meringue add 1 cup fresh sweetened or canned berries, sliced peaches, apricots, or crushed pineapple and juice.

Lemon pie: Omit vanilla; use ½ cup sugar, 1½ cups fresh milk in filling; before pouring filling into pie add ½ cup lemon juice, grated rind of 1 lemon; add 1 teaspoon grated rind to meringue.

Maple-nut pie: Add 1 tablespoon dark molasses, ½ teaspoon maple flavoring, ½ cup broken walnuts or pecans.

Puddings: Use ½ cup sugar, 3 tablespoons flour, 2 whole eggs, omitting meringue. Pour into sherbet glasses while warm. Serve the basic recipe or any variation as pudding.

Chiffon-cream pudding: Prepare as for chiffon-cream pie; pour into sherbet glasses or into wet ring mold. Unmold before serving.

Gelatin Chiffon Pies

A large variety of chiffon pies may be prepared by using as fillings any of the gelatin sponges (p. 494) or Bavarian creams (p. 496). Allow the gelatin to become sufficiently set to pile well. Brush a 9-inch serving pie plate generously with butter or partially hardened margarine, being careful to grease the rim;

sprinkle with ½ cup crumbs. Pour gelatin over crumbs or into a 9-inch baked crumb or pastry shell. Sprinkle top with crumbs if desired.

FRESH-FRUIT PIES

Mix in saucepan:

3 tablespoons whole-wheat-pastry flour

⅔ cup sugar
pinch of salt

Add:

1½ cups small fresh berries, sliced apricots, or diced peaches

Stir well; cook 10 minutes; chill.
Put into 9-inch baked crumb or pastry pie shell:

2 cups large berries or sliced apricots or peaches

Whip until stiff:

½ cup chilled evaporated milk

Stir into whipped milk:

¼ cup powdered milk

1 tablespoon lemon juice

Combine whipped milk with chilled cooked fruit; pour over uncooked fruit in crust. Keep chilled until served.

VARIATIONS:

Pour chilled cooked fruit over uncooked fruit; omit whipped milk; whip ½ cup heavy cream, add powdered milk, ½ teaspoon vanilla; sweeten to taste; spread over top of pie.

Use strawberries, boysenberries, raspberries, loganberries, youngberries, mulberries, or blueberries.

Cake filling: Omit evaporated milk; chill cooked fruit, blend in fresh fruit; use basic recipe or any variation as a cake filling.

Cookies

Since cookies are often eaten between meals or carried in box lunches, they should be made to contribute as many nutrients as possible. Cookies made with powdered milk, wheat germ, rice polish, and soy flour are more crisp and have a much higher vitamin, mineral, and protein content than those made with wheat flour only. When soy grits and walnut or almond flavoring are added to cookies, the taste and texture are much the same as when nuts are added.

Cookies made with oil quickly lose their crispness unless kept in the refrigerator or freezer.

DROP SUGAR COOKIES

Mix well together:

½ cup partially hardened margarine, natural lard, or butter
¾ cup sugar
2 eggs
½ cup wheat germ

2 teaspoons vanilla or grated lemon rind
3 tablespoons evaporated or fresh top milk

Sift in:

1 cup sifted whole-wheat-pastry flour
½ cup powdered milk

½ teaspoon salt
2 teaspoons doube-acting baking powder

Stir enough to mix well; drop from teaspoon onto baking sheet covered with foil or well-greased brown paper; sprinkle lightly with sugar.

Bake in a moderate oven at 350° F. no longer than 8 minutes. Remove from paper or foil after cooling or freeze and remove later.

VARIATIONS:

Instead of other fat, use ½ cup vegetable oil and omit milk.

Omit vanilla and add 1 or 2 tablespoons poppy, caraway, or anise seeds or the grated rind of 2 oranges.

Use ¾ cup whole-wheat flour and add 3 tablespoons brewers' yeast, 1 teaspoon each nutmeg and cinnamon, ½ teaspoon allspice.

Instead of ½ cup whole-wheat flour use ½ cup rice polish or soy flour.

Add ½ to 1 cup soy grits, 1 teaspoon black-walnut or almond flavoring; or add ½ cup each soy grits and chopped nuts with or without flavoring.

Sprinkle top of cookies with any of the following: raisins; chopped candied pineapple or citron; chopped or ground nuts; shredded coconut; anise, poppy, sesame, or caraway seeds; cinnamon and sugar; press lightly into dough with fork.

Apricot cookies: Omit vanilla; add ½ cup ground dried apricots.

Coconut cookies: Add ½ to 1 cup shredded coconut and/or drop dough from teaspoon into a dish of shredded coconut, toss coconut over top, and transfer to the baking sheet with a spatula.

Cream-cheese cookies: Instead of ¼ cup shortening use 1 package cream cheese; add 2 tablespoons lemon rind, ½ cup raisins, soy grits, or chopped nuts. Vary by dropping into **ground walnuts or pecans** before placing on baking sheet.

Lemon cookies: Omit vanilla; add **grated rind of 2 lemons.**

Mincemeat cookies: Omit fresh milk and add 1 cup mincemeat.

Oatmeal cookies: Omit ½ cup flour and add 1½ cups old-fashioned rolled oats, 1 teaspoon each cinnamon and nutmeg. Vary by adding ½ cup each raisins and soy grits; or add to basic recipe ½ cup each rolled oats and chopped nuts, soy grits, shredded coconut or raisins.

Peanut-butter cookies: Use 2 tablespoons shortening; cream ½ cup non-hydrogenated peanut butter with sugar and shortening. Proceed as in basic recipe. Flatten cookies with prongs of fork, crossing at right angles.

Pineapple cookies: Omit flavoring and fresh milk; add 1 cup very well-drained crushed pineapple; add more flour if needed.

WHEAT-GERM-AND-OATMEAL COOKIES

Combine and stir well:

¾ cup vegetable oil	1 cup raisins or ½ cup each
1¼ cups honey or dark molasses	chopped nuts and raisins
2 eggs	1½ cups wheat germ
2 teaspoons vanilla	2 cups old-fashioned rolled oats

Sift in:

¾ cup whole-wheat-pastry or soy flour or rice polish	1 teaspoon salt ½ cup powdered milk

Stir until mixture is smooth. Push from teaspoon onto baking sheet covered with foil or well-greased heavy brown paper.

Bake in moderate oven at 350° F. for 10 to 12 minutes; remove from paper after cooling or freeze and remove later.

VARIATIONS:

Omit vanilla and use 1 teaspoon almond flavoring or sift with flour 1 teaspoon cinnamon, ½ teaspoon nutmeg.

Oatmeal cookies: Mix well 1 cup tightly packed brown sugar, ¾ cup powdered milk, ½ teaspoon salt; add ½ cup oil, 2 eggs, 1½ teaspoons almond extract, and 2 cups old-fashioned rolled oats or 1 cup each rolled oats and wheat germ; mix again, and bake as in basic recipe. **One cup raisins** may be added and **vanilla or spices** used instead of almond flavoring.

MOLASSES DROP COOKIES

Cream together:

½ cup partially hardened margarine, natural lard, or butter	⅓ cup sugar

Add:

1 egg ½ cup wheat germ	½ cup dark molasses ¼ cup evaporated or fresh milk

Sift in:

1 cup whole-wheat-pastry flour 2 teaspoons double-acting baking powder ½ cup powdered milk	½ teaspoon salt ½ teaspoon each cinnamon, ginger, and nutmeg

Stir only enough to mix well, or about 25 strokes; drop from a teaspoon onto baking sheet covered with foil or well-greased heavy paper.

Bake in moderate oven at 350° F. for 12 to 15 minutes. Remove from paper or foil after cooling or freeze and remove later.

VARIATIONS:

Omit liquid milk and use ½ cup oil instead of other fat.

Instead of ½ cup wheat flour use ½ cup soy flour or rice polish.

Substitute 3 tablespoons brewers' yeast for an equal amount of flour; increase spices to 1 teaspoon each.

Coconut-molasses cookies: Add **1 cup shredded coconut**; sprinkle coconut over top.

Fruit cookies: Add **½ to 1 cup raisins or chopped dates or figs.**

Gingersnaps: Increase ginger to 1½ teaspoons, omitting other spices; add ½ cup more whole-wheat flour, turn onto floured pastry cloth, make into small rolls, and chill overnight; slice ⅛ inch thick and bake 8 minutes.

Gingerbread men: Use gingersnap dough; chill overnight; roll ¼ inch thick, cut with figure cutter; use **raisins** for buttons and eyes.

Maple-nut cookies: Omit spices, add **1 teaspoon maple flavoring, ½ cup each walnuts or pecans and soy grits.**

Mock nut cookies: Omit spices; add **1 teaspoon black-walnut flavoring, 1 cup soy grits.**

Nut cookies: Add **1 cup broken English or black walnuts, pecans, almonds, or peanuts;** or drop dough from teaspoon into a dish of ground nuts before transferring to baking sheet.

Refrigerator cookies: Add ½ cup more whole-wheat or soy flour to the basic recipe or any variation; turn onto floured canvas, make into a roll 2 inches in diameter, wrap in wax paper; chill overnight; slice ⅛ inch thick and bake 8 to 10 minutes at 350° F.; or bake half the recipe as drop cookies; stir ¼ cup flour into the other half and bake later as refrigerator cookies.

Spice cookies: Increase spices to 1 teaspoon each ginger, cinnamon, and nutmeg and ¼ teaspoon each cloves and allspice.

I have purposely made the recipe for refrigerator cookies unusually large. After the dough is prepared, it may be divided and nuts, fruits, bran, oatmeal, soy grits, and flavorings added, thus making a wide variety of cookies at one time. The dough can be kept frozen and baked at any time you are in the cookie mood.

REFRIGERATOR COOKIES

Cream together:

1 cup partially hardened margarine, natural lard, or butter	1½ cups sugar

Add and mix well:

2 eggs	1 tablespoon vanilla
1 cup wheat germ	

Combine in sifter and add:

1 cup whole-wheat-pastry flour	2 teaspoons double-acting baking
1 cup rice polish or soy flour	powder
½ cup powdered milk	½ teaspoon salt

Stir only enough to mix well, or about 30 strokes. Turn out on floured board or canvas, form into a roll; slice and bake immediately or wrap in wax paper and chill or freeze overnight or longer.

Cut into ¼-inch slices and place on baking sheet covered with foil or well-greased heavy brown paper; bake in moderate oven at 350° F. for 8 to 10 minutes; remove from foil or paper after cooling or freeze and remove later.

VARIATIONS:

Instead of wheat germ, increase rice polish or soy flour to 2 cups; or substitute an additional cup of wheat germ for rice polish or soy flour.

Omit vanilla and add 1 or 2 tablespoons poppy, caraway, or anise seeds.

Instead of white sugar use 1½ cups tightly packed brown sugar or 1 cup brown sugar with ½ cup white; add 1 teaspoon cinnamon.

Add ½ to 1 cup of any of the following: soy grits; coconut meal; ground walnuts, pecans, almonds, peanuts, raisins, currants, dates, or figs. Add 1 teaspoon maple flavoring with walnuts or pecans, ½ teaspoon each almond and lemon extracts with almonds, 1 teaspoon black-walnut or almond flavoring with soy grits; or divide dough and add different nuts or fruits to each portion.

Bran cookies: Add 1 cup bran flakes, 1 tablespoon grated orange rind; omit or use vanilla.

Butterscotch cookies: Use tightly packed brown sugar instead of white; add 1 cup ground walnuts or pecans as desired.

Lemon cookies: Omit vanilla; add grated rind of 1 lemon.

Peanut-butter cookies: Use ½ cup shortening and ¾ cup each white and tightly packed brown sugar; cream 1 cup non-hydrogenated peanut butter with shortening and sugar; proceed as in basic recipe.

Spice cookies: Add 1½ teaspoons ginger or 1 teaspoon cinnamon and ½ teaspoon each nutmeg and allspice; add ground nuts, soy grits, and raisins as desired.

BUTTERSCOTCH BROWNIES

Combine and stir:

¼ cup vegetable oil	2 eggs
1 tablespoon dark molasses	2 teaspoons vanilla
⅞ cup sugar	1 cup wheat germ
½ cup broken walnuts or pecans	¼ teaspoon salt

Sift in:

½ cup powdered milk	½ teaspoon baking powder

Stir well. Spread in 8- by 8-inch pan lined with heavy, greased paper. Bake in moderate oven at 350° F. for 30 minutes, being careful not to overbake. Turn out of pan; remove paper immediately. Cut into squares or bars while hot.

VARIATIONS:

Instead of vanilla add 1 teaspoon cinnamon or use ½ teaspoon maple or rum flavoring or ground coriander or cardamon with vanilla.

Add 1 teaspoon black-walnut flavoring, ½ cup soy grits; bake 25 minutes.

Chocolate brownies: Melt 2 squares (2 ounces) unsweetened cooking chocolate before adding other ingredients; or sift ¼ cup cocoa with dry ingredients; prepare as in basic recipe; 1 tablespoon brewers' yeast may be added.

Coconut-fruit brownies: Add ½ cup coconut and ¼ cup each diced candied pineapple and citron.

Date-nut brownies: Add ½ cup chopped dates with 1 cup walnuts or pecans; or add with dates ½ cup soy grits and bake 25 minutes.

Spice brownies: Use ¾ cup sugar and add ¼ cup dark molasses, 2 teaspoons cinnamon, ¼ teaspoon each allspice and nutmeg, 2 table-spoons brewers' yeast, 1 cup raisins or ½ cup each raisins and shredded coconut or soy grits.

COCONUT CHEWS

Combine:

⅔ cup sweetened condensed milk	¼ cup powdered milk
2 teaspoons vanilla	¼ cup wheat germ
⅛ teaspoon salt	

Stir until thoroughly blended; add:

1½ cups shredded coconut

Mix well. Drop from a teaspoon onto baking sheet lined with aluminum foil or greased heavy paper. Bake in moderate oven at 325° F. for 12 to 15 minutes. Remove from paper while hot, from foil after cooling.

VARIATIONS:

Instead of ¾ cup coconut add ¾ cup broken walnuts, pecans, or other nuts; bran flakes; ground dried apricots or chopped dates; or ⅓ cup soy grits. If soy grits are used, let batter stand 20 minutes before dropping onto baking sheet.

Omit coconut in the following variations:

Almond chews: Omit vanilla; add 1½ cups ground blanched almonds, ½ teaspoon almond extract. Vary by using 1 cup ground almonds, ⅓ cup soy grits, ¾ teaspoon almond extract. If soy grits are used, let batter stand 20 minutes before dropping on baking sheet.

Apricot chews: Omit vanilla; add 1 cup ground dried apricots, ½ cup chopped or broken peanuts, walnuts, or other nuts.

Date chews: Add 1½ cups chopped dates or ¾ cup each chopped dates and broken walnuts or pecans; increase wheat germ to ⅓ cup.

Fruit chews: Add 1½ cups seedless raisins or ground seeded raisins, currants, or ground dried figs; or use 1 cup dried fruit, ½ cup broken nuts or soy grits.

Nut chews: Add 1½ cups broken walnuts, pecans, coarsely chopped peanuts, or other nuts. Vary by using ¾ cup nuts, ⅓ cup soy grits.

Soy chews: Add ⅔ cup soy grits; omit vanilla and add 1 teaspoon almond flavoring. Before dropping onto baking sheet let batter stand 20 minutes or longer so that grits will become soft. Soy chews are the most inexpensive and most nutritious of all chews.

Oatmeal chews: Add ⅓ cup steel-cut oats, ½ cup raisins; let batter stand 20 minutes or longer for oats to soften before dropping onto baking sheet.

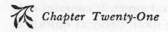

Chapter Twenty-One

Candies and Candy Substitutes

Few foods cause so much indirect harm as do the usual varieties of candy. Since most candies are made principally of refined sugar which contains no nutrients except calories, they cannot build health. Any concentrated sweet destroys the appetite to such an extent that the person who eats many sweets rarely eats sufficient other foods to meet his body needs. Furthermore, a type of bacteria, known as bacillus acidophilus, thrives in the mouth on sugar, breaking it down into lactic and pyruvic acids. These acids combine with the calcium in the teeth and cause them to decay or erode. Tooth decay has been produced in children who were formerly immune to decay in as short a time as six weeks when a single piece of candy was given to them daily.

Candy, honey, molasses, desserts, and other concentrated sweets will probably always be eaten, however, despite tooth decay. To our unconscious minds, sweet foods are symbols of the sweets of life, or love. The solace brought by eating such foods when one feels unloved may do more good psychologically than harm nutritionally. The following recipes have been included in this book for housewives who may wish to serve candy with the greatest nutritive value possible.

The candy recipes have been kept particularly simple in case children will be allowed to make them. A few recipes do call for food colorings, which cannot be recommended. It is hoped, however, that candies will be made too rarely for the colorings to be detrimental to health.

Despite the fact that honey is a natural sweet, it contains only traces of nutrients and appears to cause tooth decay as quickly as does refined sugar. Persons who are convinced that honey is "good for them" often eat large amounts, gain unwanted pounds, and spoil their appetite for more nutritious foods. If you do use honey, purchase the natural, uncooked varieties sold at health-food stores. Commercial honey is often produced by bees fed only refined-sugar water; it lacks flavor. Anyone who wishes to substitute honey or molasses for sugar in making the following candies may do so; either work well when powdered milk is used.

The detrimental effect of sweets upon the teeth can be partly overcome by incorporating generous amounts of calcium in candy and other foods containing much sugar. For this reason I have included powdered milk in many candy recipes. Only non-instant powdered milk of the best quality should be used; instant milk causes a gritty texture. Candies made of powdered milk, however, dry out quickly and should not be held for several days.

Sunflower seeds, popcorn, salted soybeans, or soy nuts, peanuts, and other nuts are excellent candy substitutes. Nuts are rich in protein, unsaturated fatty acids, and the B vitamins and tend to destroy the appetite far less readily than do candies. If candies are to be made, generous amounts of nuts added to them greatly improve their nutritive value.

Unfortunately, dried fruits have been found to cause tooth decay almost as quickly as does refined sugar. Most dried fruits are by weight 75 per cent or more natural sugar, and they adhere to the teeth far more tenaciously than does an easily dissolved candy. Dried fruits, however, offer nutrients which refined sugar lacks.

STUFFED DRIED FRUIT

Wash and dry fruit; stone dates; cut opening in figs which have not been pressed; use soft uncooked prunes or steam until tender before stoning; press halves of soft uncooked dried apricots or peaches together with filling between. Fill with any of the following:

Broken pecans, English or black walnuts, butternuts
Salted peanuts or almonds
Hulled sunflower seeds
Whole or chopped Brazil nuts
Marshmallows halved or quartered
Candied cherries, pineapple, or citron
Peanut-butter candy, fondant, or any soft candy

FRUITIES

Put through the meat grinder, using medium knife, and measure after grinding:

1 cup dates	½ cup walnuts or pecans
½ cup graham-cracker crumbs	

Add and stir well:

3 tablespoons orange or pineapple juice	¼ cup powdered milk
	8 chopped marshmallows

Press firmly on wax paper or buttered pan to thickness of ¾ inch; cut into squares or mold into balls or rolls. Chill. After chilling, roll in **ground nuts, powdered sugar, coconut, or graham-cracker crumbs.**

VARIATIONS:

Instead of dates use 1 cup ground dried figs or ¾ cup soft uncooked or partly steamed dried apricots; if fruit is moist, add more graham crackers or powdered milk.

Omit marshmallows and cracker crumbs. Combine the following groups of ingredients with powdered milk and juice: ½ cup each dates and figs, 1 cup English walnuts; ¾ cup each raisins and walnuts; ¾ cup each pecans and dried apricots; ½ cup each pecans, walnuts, dates, and figs or apricots; ½ cup each dried apricots, dates, walnuts; add ½ cup coconut to any variation.

Fruit-filled bars: Prepare fondant (p. 535); roll ⅛ inch thick, cover with ground fruit pressed ½ inch thick; cover fruit with another layer of fondant; press together, chill, and cut into bars.

Fruit rolls: Form fruit into small rolls 2½ inches long, ¾ inch thick; cover surface with **whole pecans or large peanut halves.**

Spiced fruit bars: Add to basic recipe or any variation 1 teaspoon cinnamon, ⅛ teaspoon nutmeg.

POPPING CORN THE EASY WAY

Use large utensil with tight-fitting lid. Keep heat high; combine:

½ to 1 cup popcorn   2 to 4 tablespoons vegetable oil

Stir until each kernel is coated with oil; cover utensil. As soon as corn starts to pop, turn heat as low as possible. Do not shake or lift lid. When popping has stopped, sprinkle with salt.

Cheese popcorn: Sprinkle hot popcorn with Parmesan cheese; salt to taste. If popcorn is cold, put in flat pan, sprinkle with cheese, and set in a slow oven until cheese melts; stir well and salt.

POPCORN BALLS

Combine:

1 cup dark molasses   1 tablespoon vinegar
½ cup sugar   ⅛ teaspoon salt

Boil to 270° F., or until brittle when tried in cold water; add:

1 tablespoon butter or partially hardened margarine

Pour over:

6 cups popcorn   ½ to 1 cup salted peanuts

Stir gently until evenly coated; when popcorn is cool enough to handle, press into balls.

VARIATIONS:

Use 4 cups popcorn and 2 cups large peanuts or 1 cup each peanuts and puffed wheat.

Taffy: Prepare basic recipe, cooking to 260° F.; pour on sheets of aluminum foil or well-buttered heavy paper; when taffy is cool enough to handle, pull until light brown.

Peanut brittle: Cook molasses slowly to 280° F., being extremely careful not to burn it; add **2 cups unsalted peanuts;** use aluminum foil or cover heavy paper generously with butter and lay over flat pan; pour brittle on paper; when candy is cool enough to handle, break into small pieces; set in refrigerator to keep candy from becoming sticky.

Puffed-wheat bars: Add to basic recipe with butter **3 cups puffed wheat, ½ to 1 cup peanuts;** stir until wheat is well coated; pour puffed wheat onto buttered baking pan; press firmly, cool slightly, and cut into bars.

The texture of soy nuts varies so widely with the age and variety of the beans used that it is impossible to give a recipe which will be equally successful with all types of beans. Some beans need only to be soaked, then browned, and salted; others require varying amounts of precooking. When the beans have soaked or cooked until their texture is that of fresh peanuts, care must be taken that they are not dried out as they are fried. Since few foods are so excellent for growing children as are soy nuts, a little experimentation with the type of beans you have is worthwhile. When preparing soybeans as a meat substitute, add 1 cup to be made into soy nuts.

SOY NUTS

Soak in ice tray for 2 hours or longer:

1 cup soybeans   **1 cup water**

Freeze for 2 hours or preferably overnight. Drop into:

½ cup hot water

Simmer for 30 minutes; taste and cook longer if soybeans are not as tender as salted peanuts; remove lid of utensil and let water evaporate. Cool beans.

Heat:

¼ cup vegetable oil

Add beans and cook quickly to a delicate brown, or about 1 or 2 minutes; remove from heat at once; sprinkle with:

1 teaspoon salt

VARIATIONS:

When fresh green soybeans are available, omit soaking and precooking; fry as in basic recipe; salt to taste.

Fry a few beans after soaking 1 or 2 hours or after soaking and freezing; if moisture content of the beans is high, they do not require precooking.

PINEAPPLE KISSES

Combine and stir well:

2 tablespoons partially hardened   ½ cup well-drained crushed pine-
   margarine or butter   apple
1 cup tightly packed brown sugar

Boil slowly 2 minutes, or until sugar is melted; remove from heat, cool thoroughly, and add:

¾ to 1 cup powdered milk, or enough to give firm, creamy consistency

Beat until smooth; drop from teaspoon onto buttered wax paper; chill 1 hour or longer, or until easily handled.

VARIATIONS:

Add any one of the following before adding powdered milk: 1 to 3 tablespoons finely chopped candied ginger; dash of salt, 4 tablespoons each wheat germ and chopped nuts; ½ to 1 cup shredded or ground coconut; ½ to 1 cup chopped walnuts, almonds, pecans, or other nuts.

Use white sugar instead of brown in basic recipe or any variation; add ⅛ teaspoon lemon extract. This candy is particularly delicious with chopped candied cherries or preserved ginger.

Coconut drops: Prepare candy as in basic recipe; drop from teaspoon into dish of **shredded coconut,** toss coconut over top, and transfer to aluminum foil; before adding powdered milk add ½ cup coconut if desired.

Pecan roll: Chill candy 1 or 2 hours after powdered milk is added; flour hands with powdered milk, form candy into rolls 4 inches long and ¾ inch thick; cover entire surface with **pecan halves;** serve whole or cut into slices.

Wheat-germ fudge: Stir in ½ cup each wheat germ and walnuts, ¼ teaspoon salt, 1 teaspoon vanilla, adding only enough powdered milk to make candy firm; press ¾ inch thick on buttered pan; cut into cubes.

FUDGE

Stir together:

⅓ cup fresh milk	2 tablespoons partially hardened
1 cup sugar	margarine or butter

Boil 2 minutes; begin to count time when bubbles cover entire surface. Remove from heat, cool thoroughly, and add:

2 teaspoons vanilla	½ to 1 cup walnuts
2 or 3 drops food coloring	⅔ to ¾ cup powdered milk
(optional)	

Stir until smooth and creamy; turn onto buttered paper or pan; cut into squares.

VARIATIONS:

Instead of walnuts add ½ cup or more shredded coconut, broken pecans, hickory nuts, hazelnuts, peanuts, or other nuts; or add shredded coconut or chopped candied cherries with nuts.

Omit vanilla and nuts; add 1 teaspoon maple, almond, orange, or lemon flavoring or a few drops clove or peppermint oil.

Use any fudge recipe; boil ingredients 2 or 3 minutes, chill, and add powdered milk to give consistency desired.

Add 2 tablespoon peanut butter, or omit fat and add 4 tablespoons peanut butter; omit vanilla; add ½ to 1 cup broken peanuts if desired.

Maple fudge: Boil 1 or 2 cups maple syrup 5 to 8 minutes; add 2 to 4 tablespoons partially hardened margarine or butter; chill; stir in enough powdered milk to give consistency desired; turn onto buttered pan and cut into squares; add walnuts or pecans as desired.

Panocha fudge: Instead of white sugar use 1 cup tightly packed brown sugar; prepare as in basic recipe. Vary by adding 2 to 4 tablespoons peanut butter or ½ cup coconut, pecans, or other nuts.

DIVINITY

Beat until stiff:

1 egg white

Set egg aside; combine and stir:

3 tablespoons water   1 cup sugar
1 teaspoon vinegar

Boil slowly 2 minutes, or until sugar is melted; begin to count time when bubbles cover entire surface. Pour boiling syrup over egg white and beat 2 or 3 minutes; cool.

When egg mixture is cold, add:

2 or 3 teaspoons vanilla   1 to 1¼ cups powdered milk, or
½ to 1 cup broken walnuts   enough to give consistency de-
  or pecans   sired

Push from teaspoon onto aluminum foil; cool 1 hour or longer.

VARIATIONS:

If candy is to be held a week or longer, add only ¾ cup powdered milk; chill 2 hours before dropping onto paper.

Use brown sugar instead of white; decrease or omit vanilla.

Add ½ to 1 cup of one or more of the following: raisins; chopped dates; ground dried apricots; or add ¼ cup quartered candied cherries or chopped candied pineapple.

Since children enjoy making their own candies, it seemed wise to stress uncooked varieties. Although the sugar must be melted in nut creams and the potato cooked for the modeling fondant, the procedure in each case is that of uncooked candy.

Cooked potato holds moisture in candy, keeping it fresh, and is used commercially in many delicious imported candies. The potato used in the modeling fondant gives it a wonderfully smooth texture, making it easy to handle without being sticky.

If you want to give a children's party which I'll guarantee will be a success, prepare a supply of modeling candy. Your guests may start by timidly making carrots and pears, and end up not only by making pigs, giraffes, and caricatures of each other but also by forgetting to go home.

MODELING FONDANT

Peel, quarter, steam, and mash through a sieve or wire strainer:

1 medium potato

Measure carefully:

¼ cup mashed potatoes

Add and stir well while potato is still warm:

1 teaspoon almond flavoring	2 tablespoons partially hardened margarine or butter

Sift together and add:

1 cup powdered sugar	½ cup powdered milk

Stir well and chill. After chilling, knead in enough powdered milk to handle well.

Shape into tiny melons, fruits, and vegetables. Use cloves for apple and pear stems, green-tinted coconut for other stems; paint with food colorings. Use cinnamon or cocoa for potatoes and bananas; roll strawberries in tinted sugar; model and paint leaves on strawberries, peaches, plums, and ears of corn. Knead orange coloring into a portion of the fondant to be used for oranges, carrots, pumpkins; red for radishes, apples, tomatoes, strawberries; yellow coloring for lemons, pears, and bananas. Use toothpick to make depression on cantaloupes and pumpkins.

VARIATIONS:

Omit almond flavoring, divide into portions, and add vanilla, lemon, banana, orange, or oil of peppermint, clove, or wintergreen to taste.

Use different food colorings for each portion; blend colorings to give colors desired.

Shape candy into balls, roll in cinnamon, crushed nuts, colored coconut, or colored sugar. Color sugar or coconut by mixing food coloring with ½ teaspoon water; moisten coconut or sugar, spread on paper, and let dry.

Use fondant for stuffing dates, figs, prunes; or press between halves of walnuts, pecans, apricots, or dried peaches; or surround pieces of nuts or candied fruits with fondant and roll in colored sugar.

NUT CREAMS

Combine in top of double boiler:

½ cup brown sugar	2 tablespoons partially hardened
½ cup sweetened condensed milk	margarine or butter

Heat over boiling water for about 10 minutes, or until sugar is melted. Remove from heat, cool thoroughly, and stir in:

⅔ to ¾ cup powdered milk, or enough to give consistency desired

Drop from teaspoon onto aluminum foil or buttered cookie sheet; put a walnut half on top of each cream.

VARIATIONS:

Stir in any of the following before adding powdered milk: ½ to 1 cup coconut, broken walnuts, pecans, almonds, hickory nuts, or other nuts; ¼ cup diced candied cherries and/or candied pineapple; 2 tablespoons peanut butter; press to thickness of ½ inch.

Pecan fudge: Before adding powdered milk stir in 1 cup broken pecans; spread on wax paper and cut into squares.

Pecan pralines: Drop candy from tablespoon onto wax paper; press 6 or 8 pecan halves into each praline.

Walnut-date creams: Stir in ½ cup each broken walnuts and ground or finely chopped dates; vary by using pecans, hickory nuts, or almonds.

UNCOOKED FONDANT

Combine and stir thoroughly:

⅔ cup sweetened condensed milk   2 teaspoons vanilla

Sift together and add:

1 cup powdered milk   ½ cup powdered sugar

Turn on bread board or canvas sprinkled with powdered sugar and knead gently until firm enough to handle, adding more powdered sugar if needed.

Divide into portions and add a different food coloring to each portion; flavor to taste with peppermint, orange, almond, black walnut, vanilla, or lemon.

Use for stuffing dates, figs, prunes; or press between nut or apricot halves; or surround pieces of nuts or fruit with fondant.

Shape into balls, roll in cinnamon, coconut, or ground nuts.

VARIATIONS:

Add any of the following: 1 cup coconut meal or shredded coconut; ½ cup peanut butter, chopped walnuts, pecans, or other nuts; ½ cup each nuts or peanut butter and coconut; press to thickness of ½ inch and cut into squares or rectangles.

Roll fondant ⅛ inch thick; put between two similar layers a third layer of contrasting color and flavor; press together firmly and cut into rectangles.

UNCOOKED PEANUT-BUTTER CANDY

Combine and stir enough to blend:

½ cup non-hydrogenated peanut   ½ cup natural honey
butter

Add and stir thoroughly:

¾ to 1 cup powdered milk

Turn on buttered wax paper and press to thickness of ¾ inch; cut into cubes.

VARIATIONS:

Add any of the following: ½ cup broken walnuts, small peanuts, chopped blanched almonds, pecans, hazelnuts, or Brazil nuts.

Add ½ to 1 cup shredded coconut and 1 teaspoon vanilla; make into balls, roll in coconut, powdered sugar, or crushed nuts.

Use for stuffing prunes, dates, figs; or press between halves of dried apricots, peaches, or nuts.

Make into rolls; chill and cut into slices.

MARZIPANS, OR UNCOOKED ALMOND CANDIES

Run through meat grinder 3 or 4 times, using finest knives:

1 pound bleached almonds

Add and stir well:

1 cup top milk   **1 teaspoon almond flavoring**

Sift in and stir until creamy:

1 cup powdered sugar   **½ cup powdered milk**

Turn onto bread board sprinkled generously with powdered sugar; knead until smooth and easy to handle.

Store in refrigerator until chilled.

Shape into tiny apples, peaches, bananas, carrots, potatoes, strawberries, and other fruits and vegetables; use whole cloves for stems; color by painting with food colorings; use cinnamon for potatoes and bananas; roll strawberries in tinted sugar.

VARIATIONS:

Roll ¼ inch thick and cut into fancy shapes with small cookie cutters; or use to stuff dates, figs, prunes, or apricots.

Omit kneading; use for filling between cookies, layers of cake, or almond torte.

Mock marzipans: Use uncooked fondant or modeling fondant; add 1 teaspoon almond extract; shape into miniature fruits and vegetables.

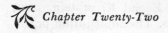

Chapter Twenty-Two

Revising and Creating Recipes

The chefs who share their famous recipes advising "melt ½ cup butter, add 1 cup heavy cream" are unmindful of the suffering your husband may have to endure for months before a coronary claims him or of the loneliness you may experience as a widow. The refiners of foods, the manufacturers of devitalized package products, and the authors of cookbooks recommending the destruction of nutritional value are not the ones who keep night-long vigil by the bedside of your sick child or who pay your medical and dental bills. Yet the aggregate use of faulty recipes and nutrient-robbed ingredients can bring about severe personal tragedy.

Science has shown that health is not a matter of chance; and that, to a large extent, health must come from the kitchen if it comes at all. For this reason, each housewife is personally responsible for the degree of well-being her family enjoys.

One of the principal purposes of this book is to show the homemaker not only how nutrients may be retained but also how she can improve her own pet recipes. Almost every recipe can be made more healthful by changing the method of preparation and by substituting or adding more nutritious ingredients than those called for. Often only slight revisions bring about tremendous improvements. For example, if you wish to substitute wheat germ for part of the flour called for in a recipe in order to increase your family's intake of vitamin B_1, you also increase the supply of ten or more B vitamins, vitamins E and K, protein, iron, copper, and a variety of other minerals. The substitution or addition of any nutritious food likewise brings multiple improvements. Should you alter a cooking procedure slightly in order to retain vitamin C, you probably retain larger amounts of some fifteen minerals and other vitamins. Make it a rule, therefore, to try to improve each recipe you use.

Learn to be critical of recipes you read or about which you hear. This morning, for example, my newspaper gave a recipe for stuffing bell peppers, excerpts from which are as follows: "Wash 6 green peppers and remove seeds; soak peppers in water half an hour and drain off water; cover with cold water and bring to a boil; drain well; stuff peppers . . . bake 1 hour."

This recipe advises one to extract and throw away as much vitamin C alone as could be obtained from 3 glasses of fresh orange juice, to say nothing of other vitamin and mineral losses. By substituting ripe peppers for green ones and by revising the recipe, the amount of vitamin C equal to that in 6 glasses of fresh orange juice could probably be retained, a saving by any standard.

Study each recipe carefully before you use it. Could procedures of handling and cooking be improved to retain nutritive value? Could less sugar be added? Could milk, fruit juice, or soup stock be used in place of water? Could undiluted canned milk be used instead of fresh milk, or could powdered milk be added? Could baking powder be substituted for soda, or yeast for baking powder? Might the cooking time be shortened, or might an entirely different method of cooking be used in order to shorten the cooking time? Could the temperature be lowered to protect the B vitamins, or could the initial heating be speeded up to increase the retention of vitamin C? Could wheat germ, rice polish, or high-protein soy flour be substituted for part of the flour called for? Could cheese be added to improve both taste and nutritive value? If, with these questions in mind, you revise each and every recipe you use, you will find not only that you produce greater health in yourself and your family but that you will enjoy cooking more than before. You will have discovered that cooking is truly a creative art.

If at times you find it expedient to use commercial mixes, fortify them as much as you can. A half cup of wheat germ and ¼ cup of powdered milk may be added to mixes for muffins, cookies, biscuits, cornbread, applesauce and spice cakes, and nut breads; in some cases the liquid must be increased slightly. Such foods cannot compare nutritionally to home-made ones, but their health-building value is improved, and the protein neutralizes some of the large amounts of soda which dominates the taste of foods made from mixes. A friend, telling me of fortifying a mix, remarked, "At first I was worried for fear the stuff wouldn't rise, but there was enough soda in the mix to raise a pan of iron ore. Actually, the flavor was greatly improved."

After you have learned the general rules for scientific cookery, originate your own recipes. This habit will bring delight and will satisfy your creative impulses. Since refrigerated ships and quick-freezing units are now realities, new foods frequently appear on the market. Sometimes there are no recipes to guide you in preparing such foods. In general, follow recipes of a familiar food which is similar to the new food in variety and texture. For example, if you plan to cook a new tuber, try preparing it in all the ways you would cook potatoes; if you wish to serve a new type of greens, add them to salads and cook them as you would spinach or chard; add a tropical fruit to fruit appetizers, fruit cup, fruit salads, ice cream, and gelatin desserts. When you arrive at an especially successful recipe, send it on to your newspaper or to a women's magazine and let others enjoy it.

The woman who follows recipes blindly, without revision or creation, has not yet discovered the fun of cooking.

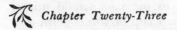

Chapter Twenty-Three

Where to Buy Foods of High Nutritive Value

Aside from yogurt, instant powdered milk, and, in some cases, wheat germ, the most nutritious foods are not often available at regular markets. If whole-wheat flour is carried, it is rarely stone ground or free from preservatives; and the turnover may be so slow that it is often rancid when purchased. Eggs are not fertile. Little can be said for the fruits and vegetables. It is to your nearest health-food store that you must turn for really nutritious products.

Many health-food stores now carry fertile eggs and a limited supply of fruits and vegetables grown without chemical fertilizers and poison sprays; a few handle meats from animals whose growth has not been forced by stilbesterol, tranquilizers, and other chemicals. All carry natural honey, non-hydrogenated peanut butter, wheat germ from which the oil (and vitamin E and unsaturated fatty acids) has not been removed, and a wide variety of stone-ground flours and cereals.

If there is no health-food store in your community, you can purchase stone-ground products and many other nutritious foods from El Molino Mills, Alhambra, California; Paule Keene, Walnut Acres, Penn's Creek, Pennsylvania; Great Valley Mills, Ivyland, Bucks County, Pennsylvania; Elam Mills, Chicago, Illinois; Wight's Grist Mill, Old Sturbridge Village, Sturbridge, Massachusetts; Stone Buhr Milling Company, 3509 Evanston Street, Seattle, Washington; Whole Grain Flour Mills, 2611 North Jones

Street, Chicago 47, Illinois; Huni Health Products, 207 East 87th Street, New York City; and The Vermont Country Store, Weston, Vermont.

Lindberg's Nutrition Service, 3945 Crenshaw Boulevard, Los Angeles 8, California, will ship health products to any part of the United States and Canada. Since the postage may exceed the purchase price, however, it is more practical to locate a health-food store near you.

Following are a list of jobbers who carry the products I have used in testing the recipes. These jobbers do not sell retail, but if you care to write them, they can give you the address of your nearest health-food store: Kahan and Lessin Company, 2425 Hunter Street, Los Angeles 21, California, and 200 Davis Street, San Francisco 11, California; Health Food Sales Company, 1523 Nineteenth Street, Denver, Colorado; Health Food Distributors, 7657 West McNichols Road, Detroit 21, Michigan; Sherman Foods, Incorporated, 276 Jackson Avenue, New York 54, New York; Balanced Foods Incorporated, 700 Broadway, New York 3, New York; Akin Distributors, Box 2658, Tulsa, Oklahoma, and Box 515, Jacksonville, Florida; Vital Foods Distributors, 314 Second Avenue South, Seattle 4, Washington; Health Food Jobbers, Incorporated, 216-226 North Clinton, Chicago 6, Illinois; Nu Vita Foods, 1325 South East 9th Avenue, Portland, Oregon; Food, Incorporated, 292 Main Street, Cambridge, Massachusetts; and Collegedale Distributors, Collegedale, Tennessee.

If you locate a health-food store but find it does not carry an item you want, ask that the item be ordered for you. Many nutritious foods are available. If you persist, you can locate them not only for yourself but also for your community.

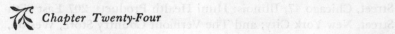

Chapter Twenty-Four

Your Reward

The health of yourself and your family is a mirror which reflects your intelligence, your efficiency, and your cooking methods. If you purchase your foods wisely, plan your menus carefully, prepare meals with minimum nutritive loss, and see that each body requirement is supplied to every member of your family daily, then you, your children, and your husband can probably possess as vibrant and buoyant health as it is possible for good nutrition to give. Sound nutrition can increase alertness, beauty, co-operativeness, and cheerfulness, and it can decrease bickering and quarreling as well as illnesses and infections.

To the mother of such a family come pride of accomplishment and deep satisfaction of a job well done. To her comes ego-gratification infinitely more satisfying than she may once have obtained from preparing fluffy-textured cake or devitalized white bread. When she hears her physician praise the beauty of her children, when she sees her husband, young beyond his years, succeeding because of his energies, when she feels the surge of vibrant health in her own body, she will realize that she is largely responsible. She has shouldered her tasks and has seen to it that good health has come from good cooking.

Notes and Other Recipes

Notes and Other Recipes

Notes and Other Recipes

Notes and Other Recipes

Notes and Other Recipes

Notes and Other Recipes

Notes and Other Recipes

Notes and Other Recipes

Notes and Other Recipes

Notes and Other Recipes

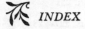 *INDEX*

Acids, value in cooking cabbage, 368; in cooking meats, 21, 53, 117–118; in dissolving calcium, 117–118; in making soups, 294–295; in preventing discoloration of food, 263, 469
  See also vinegar
Acorn squash, browned, 401
  stuffed, 401–402
  See squash, winter
Additives, 8–12
  carcinogenic, 8–9, 11–12
  cellulose, 10
  how to avoid, 11, 12
  increase in use, 8–9
  "safety" levels, 8–9
  varieties of, 8
  See also carcinogens
Age of animal, relation to tenderness, juiciness, and flavor of meat, 26–28
Albumen, 236
Almond, Bavarian cream, 497
  bread, 427
  chews, 525
  custard, 484
  -custard pie, 514
  pie, 517
  roll, 413–414
  sauce, 143
Aluminum cooking utensils, 6, 7
American potato salad, 386
Amino acids, effect of high temperatures, 20
  in cheese, 235; eggs, 235; fish, 145; soufflés, 193; soybeans, 171
  lack of, in meat substitutes, 171, 314
Ammonia, in kidneys, 83
Appetizers, 251–259
  apple juice with decorative juice cubes, 257
  citrus fruit, 252–254; grapefruit halves with oysters, 252–253; orange-apricot, 253; orange, 253–254; orange-pear, 254; persimmon-grapefruit, 254

Appetizers (*cont'd*)
  contribution to health, 251
  fish, 258; clams, crab, fish, lobster, oysters, or shrimp, 258
  frozen fruit or vegetable purées, 256; applesauce, 256; apricot, 256; pear or peach, 256; persimmon, 256; strawberry, 256; tomato, 256; youngberry, 256
  glandular meats, brain, 259; sweetbread, 259
  melon, 254; cantaloupe baskets, 254; cantaloupe-raspberry, 254; mixed melon, 254
  mixed fruit, 255; apricot-grape, 255; black raspberry-peach, 255; guava, 255; loquat, 255; papaya, 255; persimmon-pear, 255
  nutritive value, 251
  sea food, clams, crab, fish, lobster, oysters, or shrimp, 258
  tomato juice, 252; with grapefruit juice, 252; sauerkraut juice, 252
Apple, Betty, 488
  crisp, 488
  -custard pie, 514
  dressing, 133
  juice, with decorative cubes, 257; directions for canning, 458–459; freezing, 454
  pancakes, 200
  pan-dowdy, 489
  pie, 512; open-top, 512
  salads, carrot, 273; carrot and orange, 270
Apples, "baked," 470–471
  cinnamon, 471
  directions for canning, 457
  dried, cooked, 475
  fried, 390
  stewed, 472; spiced, 472
  with crumbs, 472; heart, 96; liver, 90; pork tongue, 115–116; sauerkraut, 373–374; sausage and sauerkraut, 114; spareribs, 120

Applesauce, 472–473
  appetizer, frozen, 256
  directions for canning, 458–459;
    freezing, 454
Apricot, appetizer, frozen purée, 256;
    -grape, 255; -orange, 253
  aspic, -cheese, 286; -grape, 284; and
    prune, 286
  chews, 525
  cookies, 520
  juice and purée, directions for can-
    ning, 458–459; for freezing, 454
  -nut bread, 427
  pie, 512, 518
  sauce, 473
  stuffing, 133
Apricots, "baked," 470
  directions for canning, 456; freez-
    ing, 453–454
  dried, cooked, 475
  spiced, 464
  with brandy, 475; crumbs, 472
Arm steaks of veal, definition of, 25
Artichokes, globe, cooked in milk,
    327
  filled, with cheese sauce, 327;
    creamed chicken, crab, or lobster,
    327; chicken, fish, or shrimp
    salad, 327
  French-fried, 327
  jellied ring, 282
  steamed, 327
Artichokes, Jerusalem, 327
  broiled, 328
  creamed, 328
  fried, 328
  simmered in milk, 328
  steamed, 328
Ascorbic acid, *see* vitamin C
Asparagus, aspic, 282
  cooked in milk, 329
  creamed, 329; with cheese, 329
  directions for freezing, 454
  patties, 329
  sautéed, 329
  soufflé, 329
  steamed, 329
Aspics, beef stock for, 300
  cheese loaf, 228
  chicken loaf, 226–227; with noodles
    or rice, 228
  cooking water, use in, 281
  cottage-cheese loaf, 228
  fish, 225–226
  fish loaf, 228; with lobster or
    shrimp, 228
  fish salads, 230–233
  flaked fish loaf, 226

Aspics (*cont'd*)
  for fruit salads, 285
  for vegetable salads, 282
  fruit, as dessert, 479
  fruit-juice, for meat, 231
  fruit salads, 284–286
  glaze for meat or fish, 231
  ham loaf, 227–228
  loaf of leftover meats, 227–228
  meat salads, 230–234
  mint, for lamb or mutton, 231
  pressed tongue, 227
  tomato, I, 283; II, 283
  veal loaf, 227
  vegetable, 282–283, 284–285
  whole fish in, 226
  See also gelatin salads
Avidin, in egg white, 236
Avocado, -pineapple aspic, 284
  salads, 271–272; with shrimp, 271–
    272
  soup, 310

B vitamins, *see* vitamin B complex
Backbones, pork, pickled, 118; stewed,
    120–121
Bacon, broiled, 34
  definition of, 26
  pan-broiled, 37
  with beans, 342; brains, 78; liver,
    41; rolled tongue, 116
Bacteria in yogurt, 441–442
Baked beans, 175
  lima beans, dried, 177
  navy, 177; with tomatoes, 177
  soybeans, 173
Baked fish, 152
"Baked" fruits, 470–471
Baked meats, 51
Baking, definition of, 59
Baking powder, biscuits, 424–425
  pancakes, 417
  waffles, 419
Banana, aspic, 286
  icing, 507
  -nut bread, 427
  pie, 517; -custard, 514
  salad dressing, 290
  sponge, 495
Bananas, baked, 390
  broiled, 390, 473
  fried in batter, 390
  glazed, 390
  sautéed, 389–390
Barbecue sauce, 140
  for canning, 460
  spiced, 460
  when to apply, 50

Barbecued, beef, 51
  chicken, 51
  duck, 51
  ham, 51
  lamb, leg of, 50–51; stuffed, 51
  pork, 51
  spareribs, 47, 119–120
  veal, chilled, 221
Barbecuing, advantages of, 49
  cooking times and temperatures
    for, 43–44
  method of, 49–50
  sauce, when to apply, 50
  thermometer, need for, 50
Barley, hulled, simmered, 391
  steamed, 392
  sweet-sour, 397
  stuffing, 132
Basting meat, effect of, 20
Batter for French-fried foods, 158
Bavarian cream, 496
  almond, 497
  caramel, 497
  eggnog, 497
  lemon, 497
  orange, 497
Beans, dry, "baking" method, 175
  black-eyed, 176; with ham, 176;
    onions, 176–177; sausage, 177
  effect of fat, 175; of molasses, 175;
    of salt, 175; of soda, 175
  how to prepare, 175, 176
  kidney beans, Creole, 177; fried,
    Mexican style, 177; with chives,
    177; shell macaroni, 182–183
  lima beans, "baked," 177; creamed,
    177; with lentils, 177; vegetables,
    177
  navy beans, "baked," 177; savory,
    178; with bacon, 178; ham, 178;
    shell macaroni, 182–183; toma-
    toes, 177
  protein in, 171, 313–314
  red, Mexican style, 392
  soaking, 175
  soups, 314–316
Beans, green, chilled, 343
  creamed, 343
  directions for freezing, 454–455
  shredded, 342
  simmered in milk, 343
  steamed, 342
  succotash, 343
  sweet-sour, 343
  with bacon, 342; sour cream, 343;
    tomatoes and cheese, 343
Beans, lima, *see* lima beans

Bean soups, 314–316
  black, 315
  chili, 315
  kidney, 315
  leftover beans, 315
  lima, 315
  minestrone, 316
  navy, 314–315
  pinto, 316
  without bones, 315
Bean sprouts, 329–330
  cooked in milk, 330
  steamed, 330
  with tomatoes, 330
Bear meat, chicken-fried, 40
  loaf, 110
  pan-broiled, 38
  roast, 47
Beef, and kidney pie, 71
  and kidney stew, 208
  barbecued, 51
  brisket, braised, 64, 67; with wheat,
    64
  chipped, creamed, 104
  chow mein, 201
  cold roast, 222
  corned, braised, 54; cold, 221; hash,
    209
  creole, 215–216
  croquettes, 207
  curried, 75
  cuts of, 22–25
  dressing for, 130
  dried, creamed, 104; curry, 104–105;
    rolls, 221; sautéed, 105; with to-
    mato sauce, 105
  flank, braised, 64–65
  flank steak, marinated, 101; skew-
    ered, 102; with fruit, 103
  gravy, 126
  hash, 208–209; baked, 209–210
  heart, pot roast of, 65; stew, 71
  Hungarian goulash, 71
  Italian meat loaf, 109
  marinated, cold, 217
  meat loaf, 108–109; with other
    meats, 109
  New England boiled dinner, 71
  oxtail, braised, 67; pickled, 118
  paprika, 40, 71
  pot roast of, 63–64; with cherries,
    65; sour cream, 65
  roast, less tender cuts, 45; tender
    cuts, 45; stuffed, 45
  rump roast, braised, 65
  short ribs of, braised, 67
  steaks, broiled, 33, 35; chicken-

Beef *(cont'd)*
    fried, 40; pan-broiled, 38; stuffed, 38
    stew, 70–71; with dumplings, 71–72; fruit, 71; wheat, 71
    Stroganoff, 40
    Swiss steak, 65; broiled, 35; quick, 41
    top sirloin, skewered, 102
    with noodles, 187; spaghetti, 184–185, 186; soybeans, 174
    See also brains, ground meats, heart, kidney, leftover meats, liver, tongue, tripe, steaks
Beef soups, bouillon, 302
    consommé, 301–302; jellied, 302; with egg, 302
    stock for, 300; jellied soups, 300
    ground meat and vegetable, 303–304
    with meat balls, 305
Beet, aspic, 283; -celery, 285
    soup, Russian (Borsch), 307
Beets, baked, 331
    pickled, 464
    sautéed, 331
    shredded, crisp, 330–331
    simmered in milk, 331; with herbs, 331; with sour cream, 331
    spiced, 331
    steamed with tops, 362
Beet tops, steamed, with roots, 362
    vitamin A in, 355
    See also leafy vegetables
Bell peppers, *see* peppers
Berries, as dessert, 473–474
    directions for canning, 456–457; freezing, 453–454
    how to handle, 469; prepare, 473–474
Berry, juice or purée, directions for canning, 458–459; freezing, 454
    pies, 512, 518
Bioflavonoids, in green salads, 261
    solubility of, 76, 263, 295
Biotin, 236
    solubility of, 295
Biscuits, baking-powder, 424
    cheese, 424
    cobblers, 424–425
    drop, 425
    from mix, 430
    fruit or nut, 425
    peanut butter, 425
    sour cream, 425
Bisques, fish, 312–313; of canned salmon, 313

Bisques *(cont'd)*
    shellfish, 313
    stock for, 312–313
    tomato, 313
    with mushrooms, 313
Black-bean soup, 315
Black-eyed beans, how to prepare, 176
    with ham, 176; onions, 176; sausage, 176
Blade steaks of veal, definition of, 25
Blintzes, 199–200
Blueberries, as dessert, 473–474
    how to handle, 469; prepare, 473–474
Blueberry, muffins, 423
    pie, 512, 518
Boiling, fish, disadvantages of, 148; meat, 21, 22, 53; vegetables, 317–318
Bologna crisps, 105
Bones, *see* meat bones
Borsch, or Russian beet soup, 307
Botulinus, danger of, 453
    effect of lye, 452–453
    lack of warning of, 455
Bouillon, beef, 302
    calorie content of, 301
    chicken, 302; jellied, 302
    stock for, 301
    tomato, jellied, 302
    value of, 301
Brains, appetizer, 259
    baked in bacon rings, 78; broiled, 78
    broiled, 34
    casserole, 80–81; with other meats or fish, 80; with rice, 89
    chilled, 221
    cholesterol in, 77
    cholin in, 76
    creamed, 79; with other meats or fish, 79
    croquettes, 81
    fried in batter, 80
    how to prepare, 77
    in Spanish sauce, 78; with kidney or garbanzo beans, 78
    lecithin in, 77
    loaf, 81; with liver, 92
    mock oysters, 80
    Newburg, 167
    nutritional importance of, 76–77
    patties, 85
    peppers stuffed with, 81; **other** vegetables, 81

Brains (*cont'd*)
  salad, 81–82, 232; with sour cream or yogurt, 82
  sandwich spread, 82
  sausage, 82
  sautéed, with chives, 40; eggplant, 80; lemon sauce, 79; scrambled eggs, 80; sour cream, 80; tomatoes, 80; vegetables, 80; yogurt, 80
  soufflé, 196
Braised beef, brisket, 64, 67; with wheat, 64
  corned, 54
  flank, 64
  heart, pot roast of, 65
  oxtail, 67
  pot roast, 63–64; with cherries, 65; sour cream, 65
  rump roast, 64
  short ribs, 67
  Swiss steak, 65
Braised chicken, 54
  browned by frying, 59–60; with cream sauce, 61; fruit, 60; sour cream, 60–61; spinach, 60; tomato sauce, 61
  See also fried chicken
Braised duck, 61
  with sauerkraut, 61
Braised goose, 61
Braised guinea hen, 61
Braised ham, 54
Braised heart, 54; stuffed, 54–55
  pot roast of, beef, 65
Braised lamb, breast, 67; stuffed, 65
  riblets, 67
  shanks, 66
  shoulder, 65
  stew, 67–68
  tongues, creamed, 55
Braised liver, 55
Braised mutton, breast, 67
  shoulder, 65
Braised pork, pigs' feet, 118–119
  roast, 65
  spareribs, 120
Braised squab, 61
Braised rabbit, 61
Braised tongue, 55; creamed, lamb. 55
Braised veal, breast, stuffed, 65
  riblets, 102
  rump or shoulder roast, 65
  shanks, 66
  stew, 67–68

Braised sweetbreads, 99
Braising, definition of, 52
  in oven, disadvantages of, 59
Braising meats, browned by frying, 55–57, 59; by sautéing, 61–63
  method, 52–53
  temperature for, 52–53
  use of bones in, 53
  See also stewing
Bran, cookies, 524
  muffins, 423
Bread, bakers' yeast, how to buy, 406–407; use, 407
  calorie content, 404
  commercial, disadvantages of, 403–404
  "enriched" flour, 403–404
  gluten, value of, 405–406
  how to keep fresh, 407
  ingredients, freshness of, 405
  kneading, instructions for, 410–411; purpose of, 405–406
  nutritive value of, 403–404
  powdered milk in, 404, 406, 408
  preparing dough, instructions for, 410–411
  protein in, how to increase, 403
  soda, effect of, 415; substitute for, 415–416
  souring, causes of, 407
  soy flour in, 403, 406
  wheat germ in, 404
  whole-grain flours in, 404–405
  vitamin B complex in, 403, 404; vitamin E, 403, 404
Bread-and-butter pickles, 463
Bread pudding, 487
  cottage cheese, 487
  date-nut, 487
Breads, almond, 427
  apricot-nut, 427
  banana-nut, 427
  brown, steamed, 425; raised, 426
  date-nut, 427
  nut, 426
  orange-nut, 427
  peanut-butter, 427
  pineapple-nut, 427
  prune-nut, 427
  quick, 415–416
  raised brown, 426
  rye, 412
  spiced honey nut, 427
  steamed brown, 425–426
  sticks, for soup, 298
  wheat-germ, 412
  whole-wheat, 408–411

Breads *(cont'd)*
  whole-wheat mix, 406
  See also biscuits, cornbread, muffins, nut breads, pancakes, rolls, waffles
Breast of veal, definition of, 25
Brisket, braised, 64, 67; with wheat, 64
  definition of, 24
  New England boiled dinner, 71
Broccoli, baked in casserole, 366
  cooking methods, 365
  directions for freezing, 454–455
  quick-cooked, 366
  simmered in deep milk, 366
  soufflé, 196, 366
  steamed, 366; with herb butter, 366
  with cream sauce, 365–366; herb butter, 366
Broiled, bacon, 34
  beefsteak, 33
  brains, 34; in bacon rings, 78
  chicken, 34
  fish, 155
  ground beef on toast, 111
  hamburger steaks, 34
  heart, 93, 95
  kidney, 34
  lamb chops, patties, or steaks, 34
  liver, 34–35
  liver sausage, 105
  meat patties, 34
  pork chops or steaks, 35; stuffed, 35
  pounded steaks, 35
  sweetbreads, 35, 97
  tenderized steaks, 35
  tripe, 116–117
  veal cutlets, 35
  wieners, 35
Broiling meats, meat thermometer, need for, 31
  method, 30–31
  time and temperature tables, 32
Brown bread, equipment for steaming, 425
  raised, 426
  steamed, 425–426
Brownies, butterscotch, 524
  chocolate, 524
  coconut-fruit, 525
  date-nut, 525
  spice, 525
Brown sauce, 136
Brussels sprouts, 366
  cooking methods, 365
  creamed with celery, 367
  directions for freezing, 454–455
  sautéed, 367

Brussels sprouts *(cont'd)*
  simmered in milk, 367
  steamed, 367
  with mushroom sauce, 366–367; sour cream, 367
  See also broccoli, cabbage, cauliflower
Buckwheat, pancakes, 417, 420
  waffles, 420
  stuffing, 132
  -tomato purée, soup of, 306
Buckwheat groats, simmered, 391
  steamed, 392–393
  sweet-sour, 397
Buffalo, meat loaf, 110
  roast, 47
Buns, cinnamon, 414
Butter, garlic, 142
  herb, 142
  lemon, 142
Butterhorns, 415
Buttermilk, 450–451
  cultured, 451
  fat content, 450–451
Butterscotch, brownies, 524
  cookies, 524

Cabbage, green, aspic, 283; -carrot, 284; -cucumber, 283
  chop suey, 368
  cole slaw, 272–273
  cooked in milk, 367
  cooking methods, 365
  creamed, 368
  relish, 461
  sautéed, 368; with bacon, 368
  scalloped, 368
  steamed, 367–368
  with bacon, 368; pork chops, 37; purple cabbage, 368; sauerkraut, 368, 373; sausage, 114; wieners, 106–107
Cabbage, purple, 368
  cole slaw, 272–273
  cooking methods, 365
  sweet-sour, 368–369
  with green cabbage, 368; onion, 369; sour cream, 369; wieners, 107
Cake, cheese, cooked, 501–502; uncooked, 500–501
  spice, from mix, 432–433
Cake baking, 504–505
  powdered milk in, 505
  whole-wheat-pastry flour in, 505
Cake fillings, cheese, 507
  fresh fruit, 518
  meringue cream, 517

Cake fillings (*cont'd*)
  prepared puddings, 491
  puddings and meringue creams, use
    of, 505
Cake icings, caramel, 507
  chocolate, 507
  coconut, 507
  double-boiler, 506–507
  for banana cake, 507
  lemon, 507
  maple, 507
  orange, 507
  peppermint, 507
  pineapple, 507
  powdered milk in, 505; non-instant,
    505
  quick, 506
  uncooked, 506
Calcium, and chocolate, 442
  in bones, 21, 53, 69, 117; cheese,
    235, 248; milk, 438; pigs' feet,
    21, 117; salad greens, 261; soups,
    294, 296; soybeans, 171; spareribs,
    117
  radioactive fallout, relation to, 7
  trichinosis, relation to, 29
Calcium chloride, use of, 460–461
  where to buy, 461
Canadian bacon, definition of, 26
Cancer, danger from additives and
  contaminants, 8–12
  danger from charred meats and
    overheated fats, 10, 12
  nutrition, relation to, 11
  prevention, 10–11
  produced in animals from additives
    and contaminants, 8–11
Candies, coconut drops, 532
  divinity, 534
  fondant, modeling, 535–536; un-
    cooked, 537
  fudge, 533; maple, 533; panocha,
    533; pecan, 536; wheat-germ, 533
  marzipans or uncooked almond
    candies, 538; mock marzipans,
    538
  nut creams, 536
  peanut brittle, 530–531
  peanut-butter, uncooked, 536–538
  pecan, fudge, 536; roll, 532; pra-
    lines, 536
  pineapple kisses, 532
  potato in, 534
  puffed-wheat bars, 531
  taffy, 530
  walnut-date creams, 536
  wheat-germ fudge, 533

Candy, deficiencies of, 527
  disadvantages of use, 527–528
  honey as ingredient of, 528
  tooth decay, relation to, 527–528
  powdered milk in, value of, 528
Candy substitutes, fruit-filled bars,
    529; spiced, 530
  fruities, 529
  fruit rolls, 529
  popcorn, 530; cheese, 530
  popcorn balls, 530
  soy nuts, 531–532
  spiced fruit bars, 530
  stuffed dried fruit, 528–529
Canned fruits, as desserts, 476
Canning, 455–460
  advantages of, 452
  botulism, dangers of, 452–453, 455
  cold-pack method, 455–457
  cooking times for, 456
  discoloration, reason for, 455
  fruits, whole, 456–457
  fruit juices and purées, 457–459
  open-kettle method, 457–458
  rose-hip extract, 465–466
  sauces, 459–460
  thickness of syrup for, 455–456
  tomatoes, 457
  tomato juice and purée, 458
  vitamins, preserving, 453
  See also freezing, pickling
Cantaloupe, appetizers, 254; baskets,
    254; mixed melon, 254; -rasp-
    berry, 254
  cup, 474
Caper sauce, 136
Caramel, Bavarian cream, 497
  custard, 484
  icing, 507
Carotene, in beef fat, 27–28; leafy
    vegetables, 261, 355
  See also vitamin A
Caraway sauce, 136
Carcinogens, 8–12
  additives, 8–12; varieties of, 8
  animal-growth stimulants, 10
  charred meats, 10, 12
  contaminants, 8–12
  how to avoid, 11, 12
  non-food, 12
  overheated fats, 10, 12, 110, 296
  plant sprays, 9–10, 11
  waxes, 8, 11, 12
Carrot, aspic, 283; -cabbage, 284;
    -pineapple, 286
  salads, 273; and apple, 273; apple
    and orange, 270
  soufflé, 195

Carrots, "baked" with apples, 333
  broiled, 334
  creamed, 334
  deviled, 334
  sautéed, 332; with mixed vegetables, 333
  shredded, 334
  simmered in milk, 334
  steamed, 333
  to be served with roast, 332
Casserole dishes, brains, 80–81; with rice, 89
  corn, baked in milk, 395; pudding, 396; scalloped, 396
  eggplant with clams, 340
  fish, 165–166; with brains, 80; corn and tomatoes, 166; eggplant, 166; mixed vegetables, 166–167; potato chips, 165; rice, 166
  heart, 94
  how to prepare, 204
  kidneys with rice, 89
  liver with rice, 88–89; macaroni, noodles, or spaghetti, 89
  lamb and peas in, 205
  leftover meats, 205–206
  need to revise recipes for, 204
  onion, 372
  overcooking, 204
  potatoes, scalloped, 384–385
  sweet potato or yam, 385; with apples, 385
  use of cheese, powdered milk, wheat germ, 204
Catsup, tomato, 460
Cauliflower, 369
  cooking methods, 365
  creamed, 370
  directions for freezing, 454–455
  pickles, 463
  relish, 461
  simmered in milk, 370
  steamed, 370
  with cheese sauce, 369–370; tomatoes, 370
Celery, -beet aspic, 285
  broiled, 335
  cooked in soup stock, 335
  creamed, 335
  dressing, 131
  finger salads, 269; stuffed rings, 269; stuffed stalks, 269
  green, with leaves, 334
  -horseradish relish, 461
  marinated, 335
  sauce, 136
  sautéed, 335

Celery (cont'd)
  simmered in milk, 334
  with cheese, 335; tomatoes, 335
Celery root (celeriac), 336
  baked, 336
  chilled, 336
  creamed, 336
  mashed, 336
  sautéed, 337
  simmered in milk, 336
  steamed, 337
Cereals, adding powdered milk, 435–436; soy grits, 435
  effect of reheating, 435
  "enriched," 434
  how to cook, 436
  nutritive value, 434; how to increase, 434–435
  protein, inadequacy of, 434
  steel-cut oats, 435
  use of wheat germ in, 435
  wheat germ and middlings, 436
  whole-grain, advantages of, 434, 435
Chayote, 337
  baked, 338
  broiled, 338
  creamed, 338
  fried, 337
  sautéed, 337
  steamed, 337–338
  with cheese, 338
Cheese, -apricot aspic, 286
  baked rarebit, 250
  biscuits, 424
  blintzes, 199–200
  cake, baked, 501–502; uncooked, or pasha, 500–501
  cake filling, 506
  calcium in, 235
  digestibility of, 235–236
  chili relleno, or stuffed chili peppers, 192–193
  croquettes, and rice, 207; and vegetable, 207
  croutons, 299
  cutlets, 200–201
  enchiladas, 198–199
  -filled pancakes, 200
  fondue, 250
  fried kidney beans, Mexican style, 177
  loaf, 228
  muffins, 423
  mushroom rarebit, 250
  natural, advantages of, 235
  nutritive value of, 235
  omelet, 245
  oyster rarebit, 250

Cheese (*cont'd*)
popcorn, 530
processed, disadvantages of, 235
pizza, 188–190
puffs, 427
rarebit, Swiss-style, 250
salad dressing, 289, 290, 291
salads, 230, 231, 232
sauce, 136; -pimento, 136
storage of, 236–237
soufflés, 194–196
stuffed pepper rings, 275–276
stuffed pimentos, 193
temperatures, effect on, 236
tomato rarebit, 250
uses, 248
vitamin B₂ in, 235; destruction by
light, 236–237
Welsh rarebit, 249
with lasagne, 182; lentils or split
peas, 179; macaroni, noodles, rice,
or spaghetti, 182
See also cream cheese, cottage
cheese
Cherries, directions for canning, 456–
457; freezing, 453–454
with brandy, 475
Cherry, juice or purée, directions for
canning, 458–459; freezing, 454
pie, 512
Chestnut dressing, 130
Chews, almond, 525
apricot, 525
coconut, 525
date, 525
fruit, 526
nut, 526
oatmeal, 526
soy, 526
Chicken, barbecued, 51
braised, 54; browned by frying, 59–
60; with cream sauce, 61; fruit,
60; sour cream, 60–61; spinach,
60; tomato sauce, 61
broiled, 34
buying, 56–57
casserole with brains, 80
chow mein, 201
cold roast, 222
creamed, with brains, 79
croquettes, 207
curry, 74–75, 105; with tuna, 75
dressing, 130
fried, Indiana style, 57–58; in batter, 58; in crumbs, 58
fried roasting, 58
gravy, 126–127
Hawaiian, 75–76

Chicken (*cont'd*)
in blankets, 108
loaf, chilled, 226–227; with noodles,
227; rice, 227
marinated, 101; with orange rind,
102
-noodle ring, 187
paprika, 58
pie, 72
roast, 45–46
salads, 232
soufflé, 195
Spanish, 72
Spanish style, 58
stew, 72; with dumplings, 73; mushrooms and olives, 73; noodles,
73; paprika, 73; pineapple, 73;
rice, 73; vegetables, 73
with baked sweetbreads, 97; currant jelly, 76; lentils or split peas,
179; macaroni, noodles, rice, or
spaghetti, 183; noodles, 187; soybeans, 174
See also leftover meat
Chicken bouillon, 302; jellied, 302
Chicken-fried, bear, 40
elk, 40
heart, 92
steak, 40
venison, 40
Chicken soup, cream of, 308
-cucumber, 308
gumbo, 304
-mushroom, 309
stock for, 300
vegetable, 304
Chiffon-cream, pie, 517
pudding, 517
Chili, relleno, 192–193
sauce, 140; for canning, 459–460
soup, 315
soybean, 173
with heart, 94; heart and kidney,
94; meat and beans, 179–180
Chilling vegetables, importance of,
262, 263, 319, 320, 321, 322, 365,
376
Chinese soybeans, 173
Chipped beef, creamed, 104
how to buy, 103
Chocolate, brownies, 524
detrimental effect of, 442
icing, 507
Cholesterol, 7–8, 11–12, 77, 236, 326
B vitamins, effect of, 12
fats, effect of, 7–8, 11–12
in brains, 77; eggs, 236
lecithin, relation to, 77, 236

Cholin, in brains, 76
  relation to cholesterol, 12
  solubility of, 295
  See vitamin B complex
Chop suey, cabbage, 368
  pork, 201
Chops, of lamb, definition of, 25;
  pork, 26; veal, 25
Chowder, clam, with milk, 309; potatoes, 310; tomatoes, 304
  corn, 310
  oyster, 311
Chow mein, 201
  chicken, 201
Chuck of beef, definition of, 23
Chutney, imitation, 75
Cider, directions for canning, 459
  with decorative juice cubes, 257
Cinnamon, apples, 471
  buns, 414
  rolls, 414
Citron-cherry sauce, 143
Clam, appetizer, 258
  chowder, with milk, 309; potatoes,
  310; tomatoes, 304
Clams, creamed with dill, 164
  in casserole with eggplant, 340
  steamed, 163
  with macaroni, noodles, rice, or
  spaghetti, 183
Clod of beef, definition of, 23
Club steaks, definition of, 24
Cobblers, berry or fruit, 424–425
Cocoa, 445
  effect on calcium, 442
Coconut, chews, 525
  cookies, 520; molasses, 522
  custard, 485
  drops, 532
  -fruit brownies, 525
  icing, 507
  pie, 517; -custard, 514
Coffee cake, 414
  from mix, 432
Collards, *see* cabbage, "strong-flavored" vegetables
Compotes, fruit, 479–480
Connective tissue, effect of acids on,
  21; grinding, 18; heat, 16–18, 22,
  52–53, 147–148; slow braising,
  52–53; roasting, 49
  gelatin, relation to, 16, 17–18
  in fish, 146–147; meat, 16–18
  tenderness, relation to, 16
  thickness of, in meat, 16
Consommé, beef, 301
  jellied, 302
  with egg, 302

Contaminants, danger from, 8–12
  how to avoid, 11, 12
  insecticides, 8, 10, 11
  packaging, 8
  "safety" levels, 8–9
  See also carcinogens
Cooked salad dressing, 291–292
Cookies, from mix, 431
  peanut-butter, 431
  spice, 431
Cookies, molasses, 521–522
  coconut-molasses, 522
  fruit, 522
  gingersnaps, 522
  gingerbread men, 522
  maple-nut, 522
  mock nut, 522
  nut, 522
  refrigerator, 522
  spice, 522
Cookies, refrigerator, 523–524
  bran, 524
  butterscotch, 524
  lemon, 524
  peanut-butter, 524
  spice, 524
Cookies, sugar, 519–520
  apricot, 520
  coconut, 520
  cream-cheese, 520
  drop, 519–520
  lemon, 520
  mincemeat, 520
  oatmeal, 520
  peanut-butter, 520
  pineapple, 520
Cookies, wheat-germ-and-oatmeal,
  520–521
  oatmeal, 521
  See also brownies, chews
Cooking methods, four fundamental
  recipes, 4
  importance to nutrition, 3–4, 13
  See eggs, fish cookery, meat cookery,
  vegetable cooking methods
Cooking times and temperatures for
  broiling, pan-broiling, and sautéing meats, 32; roasting and barbecuing, 43–44
Cooking utensils, 6–7
  aluminum, 6–7
  for braising, 52; pan-broiling, 35,
  36; roasting, 41–42; sautéing, 39;
  waterless cooking, 322
  glassware, 6; disadvantage of, 6
  stainless steel, 6–7; disadvantages of
  6–7

Cooking water, hard, 320–321
losses in, 53, 295, 318, 322, 364, 375–376
value of, 21, 180, 251, 281
vegetable, preparation of, 301; amount, 321
Copper, in salad greens, 261; meats, 21
losses during soaking, 77
vitamin C, effect on, 263
Corn, baked, in milk, 395; with cheese, 395
broiled, 394
chowder, 310
cooked in milk, 395
creamed, 396
directions for freezing, 454–455
fritters, 395; and pepper fritters, 395
leftover, 394
omelet, 245
on the cob, 394; broiled, 394; leftover, 394; steamed, 394
patties, 396
pudding, 396
relish, 461
scalloped, 396
smothered, 396
soufflé, 195, 396
soup, 307; cream of, 320
steamed, 394
Cornbread, dressing, 130
quick, 421–422
raised, 422
Corn meal, muffins, 423
mush, 198
pancakes, 417
waffles, 420
Corned beef, braised, 54
cold, 221
hash, 209
New England boiled dinner, 71
salad, 233
Coronary disease, 7, 8, 11–12, 77, 110
Cottage cheese, bread pudding, 487
calcium, retention of, 248
loaf, 228
made with rennet, 248–249
methods of making, 248
salads, 232, 278–279
stuffed pepper rings, 275–276
Cottonseed oil, disadvantage of, 287
Crab, appetizer, 258
bisque, 313
creamed with dill, 164
croquettes, 207
deviled, 169–170

Crab (cont'd)
fish loaf, chilled, 228
how to clean, 151
omelet, 246
salad, 232
sea food Newburg, 167
soufflé, 195
steamed, 163
with creamed eggs, 243
Crabapples, spiced, 464
Cranberries, cooked, 479
Cranberry, -pineapple aspic, 286
Crawfish, steamed, 163
Cream cheese, balls, 269; rainbow, 269
cake filling, 506
cookies, 520
dried-beef rolls, 221
scrolls, 269
stuffed-prune salad, 281
Cream puffs, 427
Cream salad dressing, 289, 291, 292
Cream sauce, 135; variations, 135–138
Cream soups, 308–312
avocado, 310
chicken, 308; -cucumber, 308; -mushroom, 309
chowder, clam, 309, 310; corn, 310; oyster, 311
leek and potato, 310–311
mixed vegetable, 311
mock oyster, 311
mushroom, 311
oyster, 311
pea, 311
potato, 311
split-pea, 311
tomato, 311
turkey, 309
watercress, 312
Creamed, brains, 79; with other meats or fish, 79
chipped beef, 104
dried beef, 105
fish, 164; with dill, 164–165
heart, 95
kidney, 85–86
lamb tongues, 55
lentils or split peas, 179
lima beans, dry, 177
soybeans, 173
sweetbreads, 98
tripe, 116
with dill, clams, crab, lobster, mussels, oysters, or shrimp, 164
Creole, beef, 215–216
eggplant, 340

Creole (cont'd)
  kidney, 84
  omelet, 245
Creole sauce, 140; uncooked, 141
Crêpes suzette, 504
Croquettes, beef, 207
  brain, 81
  cheese and rice, 207; and vegetables, 207
  chicken, 207
  crab, 207
  fish, 160, 207; potato, 160
  ham, 206–207
  lamb, 207
  lobster, 207
  oyster, 207
  veal, 207
Croutons, soup, 299
  "buttered," 299
  cheese, 299
  garlic, 299
Crown roast, definition of, 23
Cucumber, aspic, 283; -cabbage, 283;
    -pineapple, 286; -tomato, 285;
    with sour cream, 283
  pickles, 462–463
  relish, 461
  salad, 274–275
Cucumbers, peeling, 274
  stuffed with brains, 81
Curry, accompaniments for, 74–75
  chicken, 74–75; and tuna, 75
  dried-beef, 104
  how to season, 73–74
  lamb, 75
  lobster, 75
  method, 73–74
  sauce, 137; pineapple, 144
  shrimp, 75, 165
  turkey, 75
  veal, 75
  with lentils or split peas, 75
Custards, almond, 484
  baked, 485–486
  caramel, 484
  coconut, 485
  date, 485
  eggnog, 485
  five-minute, 484
  floating island, 485
  lemon, 485
  orange, 485
  pies, 513–515
Cutlets of veal, definition of, 25
Cuts of meat, for stew, 69
  how to learn, 22–26

Cuts of meat (cont'd)
  of beef, 22–25; lamb, 25; pork, 25–
    26; veal, 25

Date, chews, 525
  custard, 485
  -custard pie, 514
  -nut bread, 427
  -nut bread pudding, 487
  -nut brownies, 525
  -nut pie, 517
  -walnut creams, 536
Desserts, criticism of, 467
  fruit as, 468, 470
  meeting health needs by, 483
  relation to breakfast problem, 467
  sugar in, 483–484
  See brownies, cakes, chews, cob-
    blers, cookies, cream puffs, crêpes
    suzette, custards, fruits, junket,
    pies, puddings, sherbets, sponges,
    tortes
Deviled sea food, 169–170
Dill pickles, 463
Dill sauce, 137
Divinity, 534
Dressings, see stuffings
Dried beans, see beans, dry
Dried beef, creamed, 105
  curry, 104–105
  in tomato sauce, 105
  rolls, 221
  sautéed, 105
Dried fruits, as candy substitutes, 528
  cooked, 475
  stuffed, 547
  sugar content, 528
Drop biscuits, 425
Duck, barbecued, 51
  braised, 61; with sauerkraut, 61
  dressing, 130
  fried, 58
  gravy, 127
  roast, 46; wild, 47
Dumplings, soup, 299

Edible-pod peas, see peas, edible-pod
Egg, foo yung, 202
  salads, 230
  sauce, 137
  white, uncooked, effect of, 236,
    439, 494
Eggnog, 444
  custard, 485
  pie, 497

Eggs, age of, how to determine, 238
  allergies from, 236
  baked, 241; in bacon rings, 241;
    meat cups, 241; with leftover
    meat, 241; rice or noodles, 241;
    sausage, 241; sauce, 241
  baking, method, 240
  Benedictine, 239
  boiled, 242
  boiling, method, 242
  creamed, 243
  digestibility of, 235–236
  cholesterol in, 236; effect on blood
    levels, 236
  fertile, superiority of, 235
  French toast, 247
  "fried," 240
  frying, method, 240
  hard-cooked, with chilled fish, 224
  iron in, 235
  lecithin in, 236
  need for cooking, 236
  nutritive value of, 235
  omelets, 244–247; fluffy, 244–245;
    quick egg, 246; thin, 247
  poached, 239; with tomato sauce,
    239
  poaching, method, 238
  protein in, 235, 236; undigested,
    effect of, 236
  scrambled, 237–238; with brains,
    80; leftover fish or meat, 238;
    sausage or wieners, 238
  soufflés, 194–196
  Spanish style, 238
  steamed, 239
  steaming, method, 238–239
  stuffed, hard-cooked, 244
  temperatures, effect on, 236
  vitamins A and B₂ in, 235; de-
    struction by light, 236–237
Eggplant, baked, 339
  broiled, 341–342
  casserole, 341; with clams, 340; fish,
    166
  chilled, 339
  creole, 340
  dressing, 131
  grill, 342
  leftover, 339
  sautéed, 341; with brains, 80
  steamed, 339
  stuffed, 217–218
  with bacon, 339; onion, 339; rice,
    341
Elk, chicken-fried, 40

Elk (*cont'd*)
  pan-broiled, 38
  roast, 47
Enchiladas, 198–199
"Enriched" flour, 403–404
Enzymes, destruction, 319
  effect of acids on, 262; light, 262;
    temperatures, 262
  in kidneys, 83; in "strong-flavored"
    vegetables, 364
  preventing action of, 262, 319
  relation to vitamin destruction,
    262, 319–320
Evaporated milk, how to whip, 489

Fats, carotene in, 27–28
  color of, 27–28
  content in buttermilk, milk, and
    skim milk, 450–451
  effect in cooking dry beans, lentils,
    split peas, 175
  effect on flavor of meat, 26–27;
    juiciness, 27; tenderness, 26
  fish, 146
  hydrogenated, 7, 235
  in cheese, 235
  marbling, 27
  overheated, danger from, 8, 10, 110
  saturated, 7, 11–12; effect of cholin,
    12
  solid, 7
  unsaturated, 7–8; in nuts, 502, 528;
    wheat germ, 437
  vitamin A from, 27–28
Fertilizers, effect on fresh food, 9;
  on proteins, vitamins, minerals, 9
Figs, directions for canning, 456–457
  dried cooked, 475
  spiced, 464
Filet mignon, definition of, 25
Filled pancakes, blintzes, 199–200
  with apples, 200; cheese, 200; spin-
    ach, 200
Finger salads, 267–269
  cream-cheese balls, 269; rainbow
    cheese balls, 269; scrolls, 269
  stuffed celery, 269; celery-stalk
    rings, 269; cucumbers, 269
  with French dressing, 268; other
    foods, 269
Fish, amino acids in, 145
  connective tissue in, 146–147
  fat content, 146; unsaturated, 146
  frozen, disadvantages of, 148
  iodine in, 145

Fish (*cont'd*)
moisture in, 147
phosphorus in, 145
protein, value of, 145, 146
salted fish, disadvantage of, 146
salt in, 147
wholesomeness of, 145
Fish, chilled, appetizer, 258; in
grapefruit halves, 252–253
aspic, 225–226; aspic salads, 230,
232, 236; whole fish in, 226
baked ring, 223
glazed with aspic cubes, 224
fillets rolled with pimentos, 224
flaked fish loaf, 226
flakes, spiced, 224–225; with mushrooms, 223; radishes, 223
glaze for, 231
loaf, 226, 228
platter, 224
roe with capers and olives, 224;
egg sauce, 224; onion sauce, 224
salads, 230, 232, 233
whole, in aspic, 226
with beet pickles, 223; cucumber
sauce, 224; hard-cooked eggs, 224;
pickles, parsley, eggs, 223; sour-
cream and capers, 223
See also crab, lobster, scallops,
shrimp, roe
Fish cookery, 145–151
amount to buy, 149
B vitamins, retention of, 145–146
baking, 152
basic methods, 148–149
boiling, disadvantages of, 148
broiling, 155
browning, 148
cooking temperatures, 147–148, 151;
time, 146
comparison with meat, 146–148
connective tissue, retention of, 146–
147
cooking without odor, 151–152
deep-fat frying, 157–158; cooking
time and temperatures, 157–158;
use of meat thermometer, 157;
vegetable oils, 157; vitamin E,
157
frying, 160
glycogen, retention of, 146
how to clean, 150–151; prepare fillets, 150–151; steaks, 151
overcooking, 147–148
protein in, 147
salt, effect of, 147
sautéing, 161

Fish cookery (*cont'd*)
seasoning, 147
steaming, 162
stewing, disadvantages of, 148
tests for doneness, 148
thermometer, use of, 147–148, 152,
157
varieties for cooking, 150
washing, 146
Fish, hot, baked fillets, 153; browned,
153; in sauce, 154; stuffed, 153;
with barbecue sauce, 153; pickles
and onions, 154; with fried rice,
155; mushrooms, 154; oysters,
154–155
baked, stuffed, 152–153
baked roe, 155
bisque, 312–313; how to prepare,
312; salmon, 313; shellfish, 313;
tomato, 313; with mushrooms,
313
broiled, 155–156; seasoned fillets or
steaks, 157; with herbs, 157
casserole, 165–166; with brains,
80; corn and tomatoes, 166; eggplant, 166; mixed vegetables,
166–167; potato chips, 165; rice,
166
creamed, 164; with dill, 164–165;
brains, 79
croquettes, 160, 207; with potato,
160
deviled sea food, 169–170
French-fried, 159; mock scallops,
160
fried, 160–161; skate and roe, 161;
squid, stuffed, 161
in egg foo yung, 202
leftover with creamed eggs, 243;
scrambled eggs, 238
loaf, 168
omelet, 245
patties, 168
sautéed, 161
sea food Newburg, 167
soufflé, 195
steamed, 162–163; fillets, 163; in
paper bag, 163
stuffing for, 131
with macaroni, noodles, rice, or
spaghetti, 183; seasoned lentils or
split peas, 178–179
Flank of beef, braised, 64–65
definition of, 24
marinated, 101
Flavor, in meat, how to determine,
22–23, 26–28; to develop, 16, 17,

Flavor (cont'd)
  19, 20; relation to age, 26; to
  fat content, 26–27, 28
  seasonings, use of, 5
Floating island, 485
Flours, where to buy, 542–543
Folic acid, destruction by heat, 295,
  320
  in green leaves, 261
  solubility, 295
Fondant, modeling, 535–536
  uncooked, 537
Fondue, cheese, 250
Food, effect of additives, 8–12; animal growth stimulants, 10; cellulose, 10; contaminants, 8–12;
  fertilizers, 9; insecticides, 8, 10;
  weed killers, 10
  where to buy, brewers' yeast, 542–
  543; calcium chloride, 461; eggs,
  fertile, 542–543; flours, 542–543;
  little-known, 542–543; peanut
  butter, non-hydrogenated, 542–
  543; powdered milk, 542–543;
  tiger's milk, instant, 447; wheat
  germ, 542–543; whole-wheat
  bread mix, 406; yogurt, 542–543
Freezing, 453–455
  advantages of, 452
  botulism, dangers of, 452–453
  buying produce for, 452, 453
  fruits, 454; cooked, 454; juices, 454;
  purées, 454
  leftover meats, 203–204
  shepherd's pie, 214
  vegetables, 454; purées, 455
  vitamins, preserving, 453
French dressing, 288–289
French-fried foods, batter for, 158
French toast, 247
Fricasseed meats, see braised meats
Fried meats, brains, in batter, 80
  chicken, in batter, 58; crumbs, 58;
  Indiana style, 57–58; paprika, 58;
  Spanish style, 58; roasting chick-
  en, 58
  duck, 58
  goose, 58
  guinea hen, 58
  mock oysters, 80
  rabbit, 58
  rice, 191–192
  turkey, 58–59
  wieners, French-fried, 106
Frozen appetizers, 256
Fructose, in vegetables, 262
  losses in soaking, 262

Fruities, 529
Fruit, appetizers, 252–257; frozen
  purées, 256; juice with decorative
  cubes, 257; mixed fruits, 253–255
  aspics, 231, 479
  biscuits, 425
  chews, 526
  -coconut brownies, 525
  compotes, 479–480
  cookies, 522
  -cream pies, 517
  cups, 480–481; with custard, 481
  fresh, cake filling, 518
  fresh, pies, 518
  -filled bars, 529; spiced, 530
  gelatins, 481–482
  glazed, 471
  pies, 511–513, 518
  pudding, 491
  purées, canning, 457–459; freezing,
  454
  purées, frozen, 482
  rolls, 529
  salad dressing, 292
  salads, 279–280; bowl, 280–281
  sauces, 472–473
  sherbet, 483, 497–498
  snow, 482–483
  spiced, 464
  whip, 483
  whole, with crumbs, 472
  with custard sauce, 471
  See also individual fruits, as apples,
  apricots, bananas
Fruits, as dessert, 468, 470; accompaniments for, 470
  "baked," 470–471
  canned, as dessert, 476
  discoloration, 469
  enzyme action, retarding, 468
  handling, 468–469
  how to peel, 469; store, 468–469;
  wash, 469
  losses during freezing, 469–470
  skins, loosening, 469
  superiority as desserts, 468
  vitamins, how to preserve, 468–470
  vitamins, relation to ripeness, 468
Fruit juices, decorative cubes of, 257
  directions for canning, 458–459; se-
  lection of fruit for, 452; value of,
  452
  directions for freezing, 454
  freezing, effect of, 256–257
  frozen, 482
  how to preserve vitamin C in, 256

Fruit juices (*cont'd*)
  orange juice, how to prepare, 469
Frying, braised meats, browned by, 55–57
  chicken, method, 55–57
  definition of, 22
  disadvantages of, 22, 157
  fish, 157–158, 160
  mature rabbits, chickens, method, 59
Fudge, 533
  maple, 533
  panocha, 533
  wheat-germ, 533

Game, gravy, 127
  loaf, 110
  pan-broiled steaks, 38
  patties, 111
  roast, 47
Garbanzo beans, with brains, in Spanish sauce, 78; shell macaroni, 182–183
Garlic, croutons, 299
Gelatin, chiffon pies, 494–497, 517–518
  connective tissue, relation to, 16–18
  fruit, 481, 482
  inadequacy of, 493
  protein in, 282
  raw pineapple and papaya, effect on, 282
Gelatin salads, apricot-grape aspic, 284
  apricot-prune aspic, 286
  artichoke jellied ring, 282
  asparagus aspic, 282
  banana aspic, 286
  beet aspic, 283
  cabbage aspic, 283; -cucumber, 283
  carrot aspic, 283
  carrot-cabbage aspic, 284–285
  carrot-pineapple aspic, 286
  celery-beet aspic, 285
  cheese-apricot aspic, 286
  cranberry-pineapple aspic, 286
  cucumber aspic, 283; with sour cream, 283
  cucumber-pineapple aspic, 286
  green-pepper aspic, 283
  mixed fruit aspic, 286
  mixed greens in aspic, 283
  mustard greens in aspic, 283
  pineapple-avocado aspic, 285
  pineapple-watercress aspic, 284
  tomato aspic I, 283; II, 283

Gelatin salads (*cont'd*)
  tomato-cucumber, 285
  watercress aspic, 283
  watercress and grapefruit aspic, 286
German potato salad, 386–387
Gherkins, 463
Gingerbread, 498–499
  men, 522
  waffles, 420
Gingersnaps, 522
Glandular meats, nutritional importance of, 76–77
  See brains, heart, kidney, liver, sweetbreads
Glass cooking utensils, 6
Glaze for meat or fish, 231
Glazed chicken, 222
  fish with aspic cubes, 224
  ham, 222
  lamb, 222
  mutton, 222
  tongue, 222
  veal, barbecued, 221
Glazing meat, 221
Globe artichokes, *see* artichokes, globe
Glucose, losses in soaking, 262
Gluten, effect of, 406
  relation to size of loaf, 406
  value in bread making, 405–406
Glycogen in fish, 146
Goose, braised, 61
  fried, 58
  gravy, 127
  roast, 46
Gooseberries, directions for freezing, 453–454
Goulash, Hungarian, 71
  of leftover meats, 216
  veal, 216
Grape, -apricot aspic, 284
  juice or purée, directions for canning, 458–459; freezing, 454
  pie, 412
Grapes, directions for canning, 456–457
Grapefruit, and watercress aspic, 286
  appetizers, 252–254; halves with oysters, or shrimp, 252–253; persimmon-grapefruit, 254; -tomato juice, 252
  directions for canning, 456–457
  juice, directions for freezing, 454
  salad, 281
Gravy, color of, 123
  extracting meat juices for, 19–20
  fat, proportion of, 124
  flour, proportion of, 124

Gravy (cont'd)
how to season beef, 126; chicken, 126–127; duck, goose, or game, 127; lamb, 127; mutton, 127; pork or ham, 127; tomato, 127; turkey, 127; veal, 127
how to thicken, 123–124
made with flour added to fat, 125; with thickening added to liquid, 126
milk in, 124
nutritive value of, 124
seasoning, 125
Green beans, see beans, green
Green peppers, see peppers
Green tomato relish, 461
Greens, salad, drying of, 260–261
effect of soaking, 262–263
handling of, 260–263
minerals in, 261
nutritive value, 261
vitamins in, 261
washing of, 260
See leafy vegetables
Ground meats, beef broiled on toast, 111; in blankets, 107–108; pepper rings, 111
economy of, 110
chili, with heart, 94; heart and kidney, 94
chili with meat and beans, 179–180
croquettes, 206–207
enchiladas, 198–199
hamburger, fat content of, 110
hamburger steaks, broiled, 34; pan-broiled, 38
hamburger or heart with liver loaf, 92
hash, 208–209; baked, 209–210
head cheese, 121–122
heartburgers, 94
lamb in blankets, 108
lasagne with meat and mushrooms, 185–186
meat balls, 112
patties, broiled, 34
patties, beef, 111; game, 111; ham, 112; heart, 112; lamb, 111, 112; mutton, 111; veal, 111, 112
patties, lamb, broiled, 34; pan-broiled, 38
peppers stuffed with heart, 94; liver, 92
pizza, 188–190
scrapple, 122
soup, and vegetable, 303; with meat balls, 305

Ground meats (cont'd)
spaghetti with beef, 184–185; meat balls, 186
Spanish rice with meat, 190–191
storage of, 107
stuffed peppers, 112–113, 215
tamale loaf, 198; pie, 197–198
veal in blankets, 108
which to buy, 110
See also loaves, patties, sausage
Grouse, roast, 47
Guavas, appetizer, 255
as dessert, 476
directions for canning, 456–457; freezing, 453–454
stewed, 476–477
vitamin C content of, 468, 476
Guinea hen, braised, 61
fried, 58

Ham, and veal with sage, 38
baked, 46
barbecued, 51
braised, 54
cold, 221
creamed with brains, 79
croquettes, 206–207
definition of, 26; butt end, 26; picnic, 26; shank end, 26
glazed, 222
gravy, 127
jambalaya, 212–213
loaf, 110; chilled, 227–228
on skewers with yams, 379
pan-broiled, 38
patties, 112
roast, 46
salads, 233
soufflé, 195
steak, marinated, 101; with orange rind, 102
steaks, pan-broiled, 38
with beans, 176, 178; baked sweetbreads, 97; macaroni, noodles, rice, or spaghetti, 182; noodles, 187; sautéed sweetbreads, 99; soybeans, 174
See also leftover meats
Hamburger, see ground meats
Hard sauce, 500; use of powdered milk in, 500
Hash, baked, 209–210
beef, 208–209
corn-beef, 209
kidney, 84
of leftover meat, 208–210

Hawaiian, chicken, 75–76
  lamb, 76
  turkey, 76
  veal, 76
Head cheese, 121–122
Health, additives and contaminants, effect on, 8–12
  fats, effect on, 7–8
  importance of choice of foods, 3, 13; cooking methods, 3–4
Heart, B vitamins in, 77
  braised, 54; stuffed, 54–55
  broiled, 95
  burgers, 94
  casserole, 94
  chicken-fried, 92
  cold sliced, 222
  creamed, 95
  cutlets, 94
  loaf, 93–110
  nutritional importance of, 76–77
  patties, 93–112
  peppers, stuffed with, 94
  pie, 96
  pot roast, 65
  precooked in soup stock, 95–96
  salads, 233
  sautéed, 95
  soup, 304
  stew, 71
  stuffed, 54–55
  with apples and prunes, 96; chili, 94; fruit, 94–95; liver loaf, 92; raisin sauce, 96; soy beans, 174
  See also leftover meats
Hollandaise sauce, 138–139; mock, 137
Honey, overemphasis of, 528; relation to tooth decay, 528
Hot-weather dinners, 219–220
  aspics, 225–228
  chilled fish entrées for, 222–227
  cold meats for, 220–222
  salads, 229–234
Hotcakes, *see* pancakes
Horseradish sauce, 137; mustard, 143–144
Huckleberries, as dessert, 473, 474
  how to handle, 469; prepare, 473–474
Hulled barley, *see* barley, hulled
Hungarian goulash, 71
Hydrogenated fats, 7
  in cheese, 235

Icings, cake, *see* cake icings
Inositol, solubility of, 295

Iodine, in fish or sea food, 145, 251
Iron, in bread, 404; cereal, 434; eggs, 235; meats, 21; salad greens, 261; wheat germ, 437; white potatoes, 375
  losses during soaking, 77
Italian, meat loaf, 109
  meat soup, 304, 305
  sauce, 140; for canning, 460
  soup, 316

Jambalaya, 212, 213
Jellied, bouillon, chicken, 302; tomato, 302; stock for, 300
  consommé, 302; stock for, 300
  meats, *see* aspics
  salads, *see* gelatin salads
Juiciness of meat, how to maintain, 15–20; relation to age of animal, 27; to fat content, 27; to moisture content, 27
Junket, 490

Kale, and radish tops with sour cream, 360–361
  See also leafy vegetables
Kidney, ammonia in, 83
  and beef stew, 208
  B vitamins in, 77
  beef and kidney pie, 71
  broiled, 34
  capillaries in, 82
  casserole with rice, 89
  connective tissue in, 82
  cooking in sauce, 83
  cortex, 82
  creamed, 85–86
  creole, 84
  flaming in brandy, 86
  hash, 84
  how to prepare, 82–83
  nitrogen, conversion by, 83
  nutritional importance of, 76–77
  omelet, 246
  patties, 84–85
  powdered milk, use of, 83
  salads, 233
  sauce, kind to use, 83
  sautéed, 83
  vinegar, use in cooking, 83
  with chili, 94; onion, 86; sour cream, 85–86; tomato sauce, 86
Kidney beans, chili with meat and, 179–180
  creole, 177
  enchiladas, 198–199
  fried, Mexican style, 177

Kidney beans (*cont'd*)
how to prepare, 176
red beans, Mexican style, 392
soup, 315
with brains, in Spanish sauce, 78; chives, 177
See also beans, dry, meat substitutes
Kidney chops of veal, definition of, 25
Kitchen equipment, 6–7
cooking utensils, 6–7
essential equipment, 6
Kohlrabi, 343
baked, 344
broiled, 344
chilled, 344
sautéed, 344
simmered in milk, 344
steamed, 344
vitamin C in, 343
with cheese sauce, 344; tomatoes, 344

Lamb, barbecued leg of, 50–51; stuffed, 51
breast, braised, 67; stuffed, 65
casserole with brains, 80
casserole with peas, 205
chops, broiled, 34; pan-broiled, 38
cold, 222
cold braised shoulder, 222
croquettes, 207
curried, 75, 105
cuts of, 25
dressing for, 130
gravy, 127
Hawaiian, 76
in blankets, 108
loaf, 110
marinated, cold, 217
mint aspic for, 231
on skewers with yams, 379
patties, 112; broiled, 34; pan-broiled, 38
riblets, braised, 67
roast breast, leg, loin, rack, or shoulder, 46; stuffed, 46
salads, 233–234
shepherd's pie, 214
shish kebab, 103
shoulder roast, braised, 65
shanks, braised, 66–67
steaks, broiled, 34; pan-broiled, 38; sautéed, 40
skewered, 103; with fruit, 103
steaks, 40; marinated, 101
stew, 67–68

Lamb (*cont'd*)
tongues, creamed, 55
with baked sweetbreads, 97; noodles, 187
See also brains, ground meats, heart, kidney, leftover meats, liver, tongue, tripe
Lasagne with cheese, 182
Leafy vegetables, chilled greens, 361
cooking methods, 356
cooking, use of protein in, 356; value of, 355–356
creamed, 357–358
directions for freezing, 454–455
drying, importance of, 356
flavor of, 356
French-fried, 359
list of, 357
nutritive value, 355
mixed garden greens, with salt pork, 358–359
oxalic and phytic acids in, 356
sautéed, 361; in batter, 359
shredding, 356
simmered in milk, 362
steamed, 363; with vinegar sauce, 364
steamed tops and roots, 362
vitamin A in, 355
wild greens, with salt pork, 359
with bacon and garlic, 360; cheese, 361; mushroom sauce, 363; salt pork, 358; sour cream, 360–361; vinegar sauce, 364
Lecithin, in brains, 77; eggs, 236
relation to cholesterol, 77, 236
Leek and potato soup, cream of, 310
Leeks, 370
See also onions
Leftover meats, casseroles, 205, 206
casserole, with brains, 80
chop suey, 201
chow mein, 201
cold, diced, 222
corn, 394
creole, 215–216
croquettes, 206–207
curry, 105; beef, 75; lamb, 75; turkey, 75; veal, 75; with lentils or split peas, 75
egg foo yung, 202
enchiladas, 198–199
eggplant, stuffed, 217–218
freezing, 203, 204
goulash, 216
hash, 208–209

Leftover meats (*cont'd*)
Hawaiian lamb, 76; turkey, 76; veal, 76
in blankets, 108
Jambalaya, 212–213
kidney and beef stew, 208
loaves, chilled, 227–228; with liver, 92
marinated, cold, 217
peppers, stuffed, 113, 215
quick egg omelet, 246
salads, 230–234
shepherd's pie, 214
soufflés, 194–196
spinach-filled pancakes, 200
squash, winter, 402
tamale pie, 197–198
vegetable soup, 304
with baked eggs, 241; baked sweetbreads, 97; creamed eggs, 243; fried rice, 192; lentils, 213, 214; noodles, 187; scrambled eggs, 237–238; seasoned lentils or split peas, 178–179; spaghetti, 185; Spanish rice, 190–191
Leftover vegetables, bean soup of, 315
potatoes, 378, 381, 383–384, 388–389
rutabagas, 373
TV dinners from, 326
Leg of lamb, definition of, 25
Lemon, Bavarian cream, 497
cookies, 520, 524
custard, 485
icing, 507
pie, -custard, 514; -meringue, 517
sauce, 139, 143
sponge, 495
Lemon juice, to prevent fruit discoloration, 469
Lentils, creamed, 179
effect of fat, 175; molasses, 175; salt, 175; soda, 175
how to prepare, 175
protein in, 171
seasoned, with meat or fish, 178–179
soaking, 175
soup, 315
steamed, 393
sweet-sour, 396–397
with bacon, 397; cheese, 179; chicken, 179; curry, 75; lima beans, 177; leftover pork, 213; other meats, 214
Lima beans, dry, "baked," 177
creamed, 177
how to prepare, 176
soup, 315

Lima beans (*cont'd*)
with lentils, 177; vegetables, 177
Lima beans, fresh, chilled, 400
creamed, 400
directions for freezing, 454–455
simmered in milk, 400
steamed, 400
Lime-pineapple sponge, 495
Liquefier, use in preparing soups, 305, 309
Liver, and onions, 87; bacon, 87; celery and pepper, 87
baked with cherry juice or tomato purée, 88; sour cream, 89; wine, 88
braised, 55
broiled, 34–35
broiling, disadvantages of, 87
casserole with brains, 80; macaroni, noodles, or spaghetti, 89; rice, 88–89
chilled, 221
how to prepare, 87
loaf, 91–92; with other meats, 92
marinated, 101
nutritional importance of, 76–77
paste, or mock liverwurst, 228–229
patties, 85
peppers, stuffed with, 92
roast, 46; stuffed, 46
salads, 233
sautéed, 40–41; with bacon, 41; onions, 41
sautéing, advantages of, 87
soufflé, 195
stew, 90–91
with apples, 90; carrots, 90; macaroni, noodles, rice, or spaghetti, 183; tomatoes, 90
See also leftover meats
Liver sausage, broiled, 105
crisps, 105
mock liverwurst, 228–229
nutritional value of, 105
Liverwurst, *see* liver sausage
Loaves, brain, 81
cheese, 228; cottage cheese, 228
chicken, chilled, 226–227; with noodles or rice, 227
fish, 168; chilled, 226, 228
ham, 109; chilled, 227
heart, 93, 110
Italian meat loaf, 109
lamb, 109–110
liver, 91–92; with other meats, 92
mutton, 110
pork, 110

Loaves (cont'd)
  soybean, 173
  stuffed meat loaf, 110
  tamale, 198
  thermometer, use of, 108
  veal, chilled, 227
  vegetables in, how to heat, 108
Lobster, appetizer, 258
  bisque, 313
  broiled, 156
  creamed with dill, 164
  croquettes, 207
  curried, 75
  fish loaf, chilled, 228
  how to clean, 151
  Newburg, 167
  omelet, 246
  salad, 232
  soufflé, 195
  steamed, 163
  with creamed eggs, 243
Loin of beef, definition of, 24; lamb, 25; pork, 26; veal, 25
Loquat appetizers, 255
Low calorie salad dressing, 290-291
  cheese, 291
  "cream," 291
Low-temperature cooking, advantages of, 15, 16
  slow roasting, 47-49
  value in fish cookery, 147-148, 151; meat cookery, 15, 16, 47-49, 68-69
· Luncheon-loaf crisps, 105
Luncheon meats, bologna crisps, 105
  broiled liver sausage, 105
  disadvantage of, 103
  liver-sausage crisps, 105
  luncheon-loaf crisps, 105
  eggs in meat cups, 241

Macaroni, noodles, or spaghetti, casserole with liver, 89
  chicken-noodle ring, 187
  composition of, 180
  cooked in milk, 181
  cooking water, amount to use, 181
  gluten-flour, 180
  how to cook, 181
  lasagne, with cheese, 182; meat and mushrooms, 185-186
  macaroni, with cheese, 182; chicken, 183; clams, 183; fish, 183; ham, 183; lamb, 183; liver, 183; mushrooms, 183; oysters, 183; peas,

Macaroni (cont'd)
  183; salmon, 183; seeds, 183; shrimp, 184; veal, 183; vegetables, 184
  noodle pudding, 186-187
  noodles, with beef, lamb, or veal, 187; chicken, 187; ham, 187; shrimp or tuna, 187
  shell macaroni, with beans, 182-183; cheese, 182
  soy or whole-wheat, 180
  spaghetti pie, 198
  spaghetti, with beef, 184-185; leftover meats, 185, 186; meat balls, 186
  stuffed rigatoni, 186
  with cheese, 182; chicken, 183; clams, 183; fish, 183; ham, 183; lamb, 183; liver, 183; mushrooms, 183; oysters, 183; peas, 183; salmon, 183; seeds, 183; shrimp, 184; veal, 183; vegetables, 184
Magnesium, in salad greens, 261
Malted milk, 444
Maple, fudge, 533
  icing, 507
  -nut cookies, 522
  -nut pie, 517
Margarine, unsaturated fat content, 7
Marinades, how to use, 100
  seasoned, 100
  sweet, 101
Marinated meats, chicken, 101
  cold leftover beef, lamb, or pork, 217
  flank steak, 101
  ham steaks with orange rind, 102
  Hawaiian chicken, 76
  kidneys, sautéed, 83
  liver, 101
  method, 100
  shish kebab, 103
  skewered beef, 102-103; lamb, 103; veal, 103
  skewered meat with fruit, 103
  steaks, ham, lamb, round, or veal, 101
Marshmallow, cream, 489
  sponge, 492
Marzipans, 538; mock, 538
Mayonnaise, 289
  peanut butter and banana, 290
  cheese, 290
  thousand island, 290
  See also salad dressings

Meat, age of animal, how to determine, 27–28
  B vitamins in, 21
  browning, 20
  butchering of, 23–26
  color of, 27–28; relation to age, 27–28
  color of fat, 27–28
  connective tissue in, 16–18, 52–53
  cooking methods, how to choose, 28; four basic methods, 30
  cuts, how to learn, 22–26
  extracting juices from, 19, 20
  fibers, 15–16; size of, 27
  flavor, how to judge, 22–23, 26–28; to develop and maintain, 16, 17, 19, 20
  gelatin in, 16–18
  glandular meats, 76–77
  grinding, effect of, 18
  how to buy, 26–28
  inexpensive, 103
  juiciness, how to judge, 26–28; to maintain, 15–20
  marbling, 27–28
  minerals in, 21
  muscle meats, definition of, 77
  nutritive value of, 20
  pounding, effect of, 18
  salting, effect on, 19, 39, 53
  seasonings, ineffectiveness of, 19; use of, 19
  shrinkage, 14–15, 17
  tenderness, how to judge, 22–23, 26–28; to develop, 14–18
Meat balls, *see* ground meats
Meat bones, acid, effect on, 21
  appearance of, 27
  calcium in, 21, 53, 69, 116, 117, 294
  use in braising meats, 53; in cooking tripe, 116; in soups, 294–295; in stews, 69
Meat cookery, acids, use of, 21
  barbecuing, 49–50
  basting, effect of, 20
  boiling, disadvantages of, 21–22
  braising, 52–53; browned by frying, 55–57, 59; by sautéing, 61–63; slow braising, 68–69
  broiling, 30–31
  dry-heat methods, names for, 51
  evaporation of juices, how to prevent, 19–20
  frying, 55–57; browning by, 55–57, 59; disadvantages of, 22
  glazing, 221, 231
  low-temperature cooking, 15, 16, 47–49

Meat cookery (*cont'd*)
  marinating, 100
  method, how to choose, 28
  moist-heat methods, 51–52; names for, 51; variations of, 51–52; *see* braising, stewing
  origin of many recipes, 51
  pan-broiling, 35–36
  roasting, 41–43
  sautéing, 39
  scoring, effect of, 62; methods, 62–63
  searing, disadvantages of, 62; effect of, 20; method, 36
  skewering, 102
  slow braising, 68–69; roasting, 47–49
  steaming, *see* braising
  stewing, 69
  stuffings, 128–129
  tables of cooking times and temperatures for broiling, pan-broiling, and sautéing, 32; roasting and barbecuing, 44
Meat loaf, *see* loaves
Meat substitutes, cheese blintzes, 199; croquettes, 207; cutlets, 200–201; fondue, 250; loaf, 228; rarebits, 249–250; soufflés, 194–196
  chili with meat and beans, 179–180
  chow mein, 201
  dry beans, 175–178
  egg foo yung, 202
  enchiladas, 198–199
  filled pancakes, 199–200
  inadequacy of, 171
  lentils, 175, 178–179
  macaroni, noodles, or spaghetti, 180–188
  pizza, 188–190
  protein in, 171
  rice, 180–184, 190–192
  soufflés, 193–196
  stuffed peppers, 192–193
  soybeans, 171–174; value of, 171
  soy grits, 172–175
  split peas, 175, 178–179
  tamale pie, 197–198
  wheat, whole, 196–197
Melon, cup, 474
  salads, 281
Menu planning, need for variety, 5–6
Meringue, cause of falling, 515; of shriveling, 515
  -cream cake filling, 517
  -cream pies, 516–517
  for pies, 516
Mexican sauce, 141; for canning, 460

Mexican-style kidney beans, 177
Milk, amount needed, 438
  certified raw, 438
  chocolate, effect of, 442
  cocoa, effect of, 442
  eggnog, disadvantage of, 439
  evaporated, advantages of, 440
  fresh, importance of, 440
  heat, effect of, 440
  light, effect of, 439
  nutritive value of, 438–439
  pasteurization, effect of, 438
  powdered skim, 440; instant, 440–
    441; non-instant or spray-process,
    440–441
  reconstituted, 450
  skim milk, 439
  tiger's, 446–447
  uses in cooking, 439–440
  value against cancer, 11; radioactive
    fallout, 7
  yogurt, 441–442
Milk drinks, buttermilk, cultured,
    451
  cocoa, 445–446
  eggnog, 444
  float, 443; pineapple, 443
  malted milk, 444
  milkshakes, 443; vanilla, 443
  Postum, 446
  reconstituted milk, 450
  shakes, 445; orange, 445
  tiger's milk, 446–447
  yogurt, 444–445; popsicles, 449;
    raspberry, 444–445
  yogurt-fruit, 444
Milk, powdered, instant, disadvan-
    tages for cooking, 7, 440, 505
  non-instant, or spray-process, 440–
    441; how to store, 441; use in
    recipes, 7, 440, 505
Milk, powdered skim, amount equiva-
    lent to fresh, 440
  how to keep, 441
  problems in using, 440, 505
  reconstituted milk, 450
  types of, 440–441
  value of, 440
  where to buy, 542–543
Milkshakes, 443
Millet, simmered, 391
  steamed, 392
  stuffing, 132
  sweet-sour, 396–397
Mincemeat cookies, 520
Mince pie, 512
Minerals, in meat bones, 294; salad
    greens, 261; soups, 294, 295

Minerals (*cont'd*)
  losses from soaking foods, 77, 295–
    296, 317–318
  solubility of, 263, 317
  See also copper, iron, phosphorus
Minestrone, 316
Mint sauce, 143
Mixed fruit, aspic, 286
Mixed greens, garden, 358–359
  in aspic, 283; tossed salads, 266–268
  wild, 359
Mixed vegetables, sautéed, 332
  soup, cream of, 311
  soup purée, 305–306
Mixes, commercial, how to fortify, 541
Mock, Hollandaise, 137
  liverwurst, 228–229
  marzipans, 538
  -nut cookies, 522
  oysters, of brains, 80; of oyster
    plant, 347
  oyster soup, cream of, 311
  poached eggs, 239
Modeling fondant, 535–536
Moist-heat methods of meat cookery,
    51–52
  multiplicity of, 51
  names for, 51
  seasoning, need for, 51
  variations of, 51–52
  See braising, stewing
Molasses, cookies, 521–522
  effect in cooking dry beans, 175
Molasses recipes:
  acorn squash, 401
  "baked" beans, lima, 177; navy, 177;
    soybeans, 173
  barbecue sauce, 140
  barbecued spareribs, 119–120
  beef stew, 70
  braised pigs' feet, 118–119; spare-
    ribs, 120
  bread, 409, 426; steamed brown, 425
  brownies, 524–525
  chili sauce, 140
  cookies, 520–522
  custard, baked, 486; caramel, 484
  gingerbread, 498–499
  heart in casserole, 94; with raisin
    sauce, 96
  junket, 490
  pancakes, 417, 418
  parsnips, baked, 347–348; sautéed,
    347
  peanut brittle, 530–531
  pepper-pot stew, 117
  pie crust, 510–511

Molasses recipes (cont'd)
  pies, maple-nut, 517; **pumpkin or squash**, 515
  plum pudding, 499–500
  popcorn balls, 530
  puffed-wheat bars, 531
  rolls, 412–413
  sautéed carrots, 332
  soybeans, "baked," 173; Chinese, 173; with tomatoes, 174; with vegetables, 174
  spaghetti with beef, 186; leftover meat, 185, 186; meat balls, 186
  spareribs, with apples, 120
  spiced red onions, 372
  stewed backbones, 120–121; pigs' feet, 119; spareribs, 121
  stuffed rigatoni, 186
  sweet potato and yam casserole, 385
  taffy, 530
  tamale loaf, 198
  tomatoes, with green onions, 352
  tomato gravy, 127
  waffles, 419, 420
Moose, meat loaf, 110
  roast, 47
Mornay sauce, 137
Muffins, blueberry, 423
  bran, 423
  cheese, 423
  corn-meal, 423
  from mix, 430–431
  oatmeal, 423
  orange, 423
  rice, 424
  rye, 424
  yeast, 424
Muscle meats, definition of, 77
Mush, corn-meal, 198
Mushroom, dressing, 131
  omelet, 245
  sauce, 136
  soufflé, 195
  soup, cream of, 311
Mushrooms, baked, 345
  sautéed, 345
  with fish bisque, 313
Mussels, creamed with dill, 164
  steamed, 163
Mustard greens, in aspic, 283
  with salt pork, 358
  See also leafy vegetables
Mustard sauce, 137; -horseradish, 143–144
Mustard-spinach, sautéed, 361
  See also leafy vegetables

Mutton, breast, braised, **67**
  chops, pan-broiled, **38**
  cold, 222
  cuts of, 25
  dressing for, 130
  gravy, 127
  loaf, 110
  mint aspic for, 231
  patties, 111
  shoulder, braised, 65
  roast leg, loin, rack, or shoulder, 46

Navy beans, "baked," **177**; with tomatoes, 177
  how to prepare, 176
  savory, 178
  soup, 314–315
  with bacon, 178; ham, 178
Nectarine juice or purée, directions for freezing, 454; canning, 458–459
Nectarines, "baked," 471
  directions for canning, 456–457; freezing, 453–454
Newburg, brains, 167
  lobster, 167
  sea food, 167
  shrimp, 167
  sweetbreads, 168
New England boiled dinner, 71
New York cut, definition of, 25
New Zealand spinach, French-fried, 359
  sautéed in batter, 359
  See also leafy vegetables
Niacin, solubility of, 295
Nitrogen, converted by kidneys, 83
Noodles, *see* macaroni, noodles, or spaghetti
Nut, biscuits, 425
  chews, 526
  cookies, 522
  creams, 536
  salad dressing, 289
  torte, 502–503
Nut breads, 426–427
  almond, 427
  apricot, 427
  banana, 427
  date, 427
  orange, 427
  peanut-butter, 427
  pineapple, 427
  prune, 427
  spiced honey, 427
Nut loaf, from mix, 431

Nutritious quick-bread mix, 428–429
Nuts, nutritive value, 502, 528
   See also candy substitutes

Oatmeal, chews, 526
   cookies, 520, 521; and wheat germ,
      520
   muffins, 423
Oats, steel-cut, 435
Okra, fried, 346
   sautéed, 345
   soup, 307
   with tomatoes, 346
Olive, salad dressing, 289
   sauce, 137
Omelets, fluffy, 244–245
   bacon and bean sprouts with, 245
   cheese, 245
   corn, 245
   creole, 245
   fish, 245
   mushroom, 245
   parsley-anchovy, 245
   rice, 245
   tomato, 245
Omelets, quick egg, 246
   crab, 246
   kidney, 246
   lobster, 246
   oyster, 246
   Spanish, 246
Omelets, thin, or Pfannkuchen, 247
   Swedish pancakes, 247
Onion, dressing, 131
   sauce, 137, 144
   soup, 302
Onions, baked, 371
   broiled, 371; slices, 371
   casserole, 372
   cooked in sour cream, 372
   cooking methods, 365, 370
   creamed, 371; green, 371
   French-fried rings, 371–372
   pickled, 463
   sautéed, 372
   scalloped, 371
   spiced red, 372
   steamed, 372
   stuffed, 372; with brains, 81
Orange, appetizers, 253–254; -apricot,
      253; -pear, 254
   Bavarian cream, 497
   custard, 485
   icing, 507
   juice, 469; frozen, 469; how to
      prepare, 469
   muffins, 423

Orange (*cont'd*)
   -nut bread, 427
   pie, custard, 514
   roll, 414
   salad, 281; apple and carrot, 270
   sherbet, 497–498
   sponge, 495
   whip, 495–496
"Organic" gardens, 11
Overcooking, casserole dishes, 204
   fish, 147–148
   meats, effect of, 20
   pork, 29
   vegetables, 320, 321–322, 364
Oxalic acid, in leafy vegetables, 356;
      spinach, 356
Oxtail, braised, 67
   definition of, 24
   Italian meat soup, 304–305
   pickled, 118
Oyster, appetizer, 258; in grapefruit
      halves, 252–253
   dressing, 131
Oysters, baked with fish, 154–155
   bisque, 313
   chowder, 311
   creamed with dill, 164
   croquettes, 207
   in stuffed eggplant, 217–218
   omelet, 246
   rarebit, 250
   sea food Newburg, 167
   soup, cream of, 311
   with fried rice, 192; macaroni,
      noodles, rice, or spaghetti, 183
Oyster plant (salsify), 346
   chilled, 346
   creamed, 347
   mock oysters, 347
   sautéed, 347
   soup, mock oyster, cream of, 311
   steamed, 346
   with tomatoes, 346

Pan-broiled meats, bacon, 37
   bear, 38
   beefsteak, 38; stuffed, 38
   big game, steaks, 38
   elk, 38
   ham, 38; and veal with sage, 38;
      steaks, 38
   hamburger steaks, 38
   lamb chops, patties, or steaks, 38
   mutton chops, 38
   pork chops, 37; sausage, 38, 114;
      steaks, 38

Pan-broiled meats (*cont'd*)
  veal and ham with sage, 38
  venison, 38
Pan-broiling, meat thermometer, use
    of, 36
  method, 35–36
  time and temperature tables, 32
Pancakes, apple, 200
  baking powder, 417
  buckwheat, 417, 420
  cheese-filled, 200
  corn-meal, 417
  crêpes suzette, 504
  filled, or blintzes, 199–200; with
    apples, 200; cheese, 200; spinach,
    200
  from mix, 429
  Pfannkuchen, 247
  soy, 417
  spinach-filled, 200
  Swedish, 247
  thin, 247, 418
  yeast, 418
Pancreas, how to prepare, 76–77
Panocha fudge, 533
Pantothenic acid, solubility of, 295
Papaya, appetizers, 255
Paprika, salads, 275–276; -cucumber,
    276; stuffed rings, 275–276
  value of, 275
Para-aminobenzoic acid, solubility of,
    295
Parsley, -anchovy omelet, 245
  and spinach with bacon, garlic, 360
  See also leafy vegetables
Parsnips, 347
  baked, 347–348; with cheese, 348
  broiled, 348
  chilled, 348
  fried, 348
  sautéed, 347
Pasha, or Russian cheesecake, 500–501
Patties, beef, ground, 111
  brain, 85
  fish, 168
  game, 111
  ham, 112
  heart, 93, 112
  kidney, 84–85
  lamb, 111, 112; broiled, 34; pan-
    broiled, 38
  liver, 85
  meat, broiled, 34
  mutton, 111
  soybean, 173
  veal, 111, 112
Patty shells, 381

Peach, appetizers, -black raspberry,
    255; frozen purée, 256
  juice or purée, directions for can-
    ning, 458–459; freezing, 454
  pie, 512, 518
  sauce, 473
  stuffing, 133
Peaches, "baked," 471
  directions for canning, 456–457;
    freezing, 453–454
  dried, cooked, 475
  glazed, 471
  loosening skins, 452–453, 469
  spiced, 464
  stuffed, 472
  with brandy, 475; custard sauce,
    471; crumbs, 472
Peanut brittle, 530–531
Peanut butter, biscuits, 425
  bread, 427
  candy, 537–538
  cookies, 520, 524
  non-hydrogenated, where to buy,
    542
  salad dressing, 290
Pear, appetizers, frozen purée, 256;
    -orange, 254; -persimmon, 255
  juice or purée, directions for can-
    ning, 458–459
  salad, 281
  sauce, 473
Pears, directions for canning, 456–457
  dried, cooked, 475
  glazed, 471
  spiced, 464
  stewed whole, 472
  with brandy, 475; crumbs, 472; cus-
    tard sauce, 471; orange sauce, 472
Peas, edible-pod, creamed, 339
  simmered in milk, 338
  steamed, 338
  with meat, 338
Peas, fresh, 348
  creamed, 349
  directions for freezing, 454–455
  simmered in milk, 348–349
  soufflé, 195, 349
  soup, cream of, 311
  steamed, 349
  with other vegetables, 349
Peas, split, creamed, 179
  effect of fat, 175; molasses, 175;
    salt, 175; soda, 175
  how to prepare, 175
  protein in, 171
  seasoned, with meat, 178–179
  soaking, 175

Peas, split *(cont'd)*
soup, I, 316; II, 316
soup, cream of, 311
with cheese, 179; chicken, 179; curry, 75
Pecan, fudge, 536
pie, 514
pralines, 536
roll, 532
Peelings of fruit and vegetables, contribution to flavor, 318
mineral concentration in, 318
value in preventing vitamin loss, 262, 319, 454; in soup making, 293, 295–296, 297
waste resulting from removal, 263, 318–319
Peppermint icing, 508
Pepper-pot, soup, 305
stew, 117
Pepper, aspic, 283
red bell, advantages of, 112
relish, 461
salads, 275–276; bell pepper-watercress, 276; stuffed rings, 275–276
Peppers, chili relleno, 192–193
creamed, 332
directions for canning, 457
how to stuff, 112
pickled, 462
sautéed, 332
simmered in milk, 332
stuffed, 112–113, 192–193, 215; with brains, 81; creamed chicken, ham, oysters, or shrimp, 113; ground beef, 112–113; ground beef and leftover meats, 113; heart, 94; leftover meats, 113; liver, 92; macaroni and cheese, 113; meat loaf, 113
stuffed rings, salad, 275–276
vitamin A in, 331
vitamin C in, 112, 275
Persimmon, appetizers, frozen, 256; -grapefruit, 254; -pear, 255
Persimmons, as dessert, 477
directions for freezing, 453–454
vitamin A in, 476
Pfannkuchen, 247
Pheasant, roast, 47
Phosphorus, in brewers' yeast, 446; fish, 147; meat, 21
Pickles, bread-and-butter, 463
cauliflower, 463
cucumber, 462–463
dill, 463
gherkins, 463

Pickles *(cont'd)*
onions, 463; small, 463
peppers, 462
watermelon rind, 464
Pickling, 460–464
cucumber pickles, 462
fruit, spiced, 464
method, 460
peppers, 462
relishes, 461
Picnic ham, definition of, 26
Pie crusts, advantages of freezing, 508; of using lard, 508
boiling water, 510
crisp, 510
crumb, 510–511
effect of stirring, 508
flaky, 509
how to handle, 508; to produce flakiness, 508
sogginess, how to prevent, 513
use of oil, 508; wheat germ, 508
Pie fillings, custard, 513–515, 518
eggnog, 497
fruit, 511–512, 518
gelatin chiffon, 495, 496, 497
meringue cream, 516–517
of prepared puddings, 491
Pies, almond, 517; -custard, 514
apple, 512; -custard, 514; open-top, 512
apricot, 512, 518
banana, 517; -custard, 514
beef and kidney, 71
berry, 512, 518
cherry, 512
chiffon-cream, 517; how to prepare, 515
coconut, 517; -custard, 514
custard, 513–514; variations of, 514–515
date-custard, 514; -nut, 517
eggnog, 497
fruit, 511–512; -cream, 517; fresh, 518
gelatin chiffon, 494–495, 496, 497, 517–518
grape, 512
heart, 96
lemon, 517; -custard, 514
maple-nut, 517
meringue for, 516; how to prepare, 515
meringue-cream, 516; how to prepare, 515
mince, 512
orange-custard, 514

Pies *(cont'd)*
  peach, 512, 518
  pecan, 515
  pineapple, 512; -custard, 514
  prune, 513
  pumpkin, 514–515
  raisin, 513; -nut, 515
  rhubarb, 512
  rice, 198
  shepherd's, 214
  spaghetti, 198
  squash, 514–515
  tamale, 197–198
Pig, roast suckling, 46–47
Pigs' feet, braised, 118–119
  calcium in, 21, 117
  pickled, 118
  stewed, 119
Pigs in blankets, 114
Pimento sauce, 137
Pimentos, salads, 275–276; stuffed
    rings, 275–276
  stuffed, 193
  value of, 275
Pineapple, aspic, -avocado, 285;
    -cranberry, 286; -cucumber, 286;
    -watercress, 284
  cookies, 520
  curry sauce, 144
  filled halves, 477–478
  gelatin, effect on, 282
  icing, 507
  kisses, 532
  -lime sponge, 495
  -nut bread, 427
  pie, 512; -custard, 514
  stuffing, 133
Pinto-bean soup, 316
Piquant sauce, 137–138
Pizza, 188–190
Plant sprays, effect on food, 10
Plate of beef, definition of, 24
Plum, juice or purée, directions for
    canning, 458–459
  pudding, 499
  sauce, 473
Plums, directions for canning, 456–
    457; freezing, 453–454
  spiced, 464
Poor man's rice pudding, 488
Popcorn, 530
  balls, 530
  cheese, 530
Pork, B vitamins in, 29
  backbones, pickled, 118; stewed,
    120–121
  barbecued, 51

Pork *(cont'd)*
  braised roast, 65
  chop suey, 201
  chops, broiled, 35; pan-broiled, 37;
    sautéed, 41; stuffed, 35, 37; with
    cabbage or sauerkraut, 37
  chow mein, 201
  cold roast, 222
  cuts of, 25–26
  danger of trichinae in, 29
  dressing for, 130
  gravy, 127
  ham, *see* ham
  head cheese, 121–122
  loaf, 110
  marinated, cold, 217
  overcooking, harm from, 29
  pig, suckling, roast, 46–47
  pigs' feet, braised, 118–119; pickled,
    118; stewed, 119
  pigs in blankets, 114
  roast leg, loin, shoulder, or tender-
    loin, 46; stuffed, 46
  salads, 233
  sausage, pan-broiled, 38; seasoned,
    114; with apples and sauerkraut,
    114; cabbage and yams, 114; liver
    loaf, 92
  scrapple, 122
  spareribs, 47, 119–120; braised, 120;
    pickled, 118; roast, 47; stewed,
    121; stuffed, 47; with apples, 120;
    sauerkraut, 47, 120
  steaks, broiled, 35; pan-broiled, 38;
    sautéed, 41
  tenderloin, sautéed, 41
  undercooking, danger from, 29
  with lentils, 213
  See also brains, ground meats, ham,
    heart, kidney, leftover meats,
    liver, tongue, tripe
Porterhouse steaks, definition of,
    24
Postum, 446
Potato substitutes, 389
  apples, 390
  bananas, 389–390
  barley, hulled, 391
  beans, red, Mexican style, 392
  buckwheat groats, 392–393
  corn, 393–396
  lentils, 396–397
  lima beans, 400
  millet, 391
  rice, 397–398
  soybeans, fresh, 400
  squash, winter, 401–402

Potato substitutes (*cont'd*)
wheat, unground, 196–197, 398–399
wild rice, 398
See also beans, macaroni, parsnips, rutabagas
Potatoes, white, baked, 376–377; new, 377; shredded, 387–388
broiled, 379
chips, 382
creamed, 380; with peas, 380; shredded, 388
French-fried, 382
fried, American, 380–381; leftover, 381; oven, 379; Spanish, 381; whole, 381
hash-browned, 378; quick, 387
iron in, 375
mashed, 382–383; patties, 383–384
oven "French fries," 379
pancakes, 388; with vegetables, 388
patties, 383–384
patty shells, 381
peeling of, 376
preparation of, 376
puffs, 384; fried, 384
soufflé, 196
soup, cream of, 311; with leeks, 310
stuffed, 377–378
stuffing, 131
salads, American, 386; German, 386–387
scalloped, 384
shepherd's pie, 214
steamed, 388; leftover, 388–389
to be served with a roast, 381
vitamin C in, 375; retention of, 376, 377–378, 384
Pot roast, beef, 63–64; with cherries, 65; sour cream, 65
heart, 65
Potted meats, *see* braised meats
Powdered milk recipes:
batter for French-fried foods, 158
biscuits, 424
brain patties, 85
brain sausage, 82
breads, 409; nut, 426; quick mix, 428–429; steamed brown, 425
broccoli with cream sauce, 365–366
brownies, 524–525
cakes, 505; cheese, 500–501
cake icings, 506–508
candies, 532–538
cereals, 436
cheese blintzes, 199–200
chews, 525–526
chicken with noodles, 73

Powdered milk recipes (*cont'd*)
chili relleno, 192, 193
cookies, 519–524
corn fritters, 395; patties, 396; pudding, 396
cornbread, 421, 422
corn-meal mush, 198
creamed lima beans, 177; lentils or split peas, 179
"creamed" rice, 397–398
croquettes, 206–207
custards, 484–486
fish loaf, 168
fish patties, 168
French toast, 247
fruit whips, 483
fruities, 529
gingerbread, 498–499
gravy made with thickening added to liquid, 126
hard sauce, 500
head cheese, 121–122
heart cutlets, 94
junket, 490
kidney patties, 84–85
lasagne with cheese, 182
liver casserole with rice, 88–89
liver patties, 85
macaroni, noodles, or spaghetti, 182–184
marshmallow cream, 489
meat loaf, 109; heart, 93; liver, 91
milk drinks, 443–450
mock liverwurst, 229
muffins, 423
Newburg, sea food, 167; shrimp, 167
New Zealand spinach sautéed in batter, 359
noodles, 186–188
omelets, 244–247
pancakes, 247, 417, 418
pies, custard, 514–515; fruit, 518; meringue-cream, 516
puddings, 486–488, 491, 492
rarebits, 249–250
reconstituted milk, 450
rice, 182–184
rolls, 412–415
sauces, 135–138
scrapple, 122
shepherd's pie, 214
soufflés, 194–196
soups, 297, 308, 309–310
sponges, 492, 494
stewed backbones, 121
stuffings, 129–131
tamale loaf, 198; pie, 197–198

Powdered milk recipes (cont'd)
  tiger's milk, 447
  tortes, 502–503
  trifle, 493
  waffles, 419, 420
  whips, 495–496
  yogurt, 449
  zucchini patties, 354
Prairie chicken, roast, 47
Pralines, pecan, 536
Pressed tongue, 227
Pressure cooker, use in soup making,
    294; vegetable cooking, 323, 365
Protein, effect of boiling on, 53; high
    temperature on, 14, 16–18, 20, 21,
    22, 236
  importance to health, 20
  in cheese, 235; dry beans, 171, 313–
    314; eggs, 235; fish, 145, 146, 147;
    gelatin, 282; glandular meats, 77;
    heart, 77; meat, 20; milk, 438;
    nuts, 502, 528; soybeans, 171;
    tiger's milk, 446; wheat germ,
    437
  use in cooking leafy vegetables, 356
Prune, aspic, with apricots, 286
  -nut bread, 427
  pie, 513
  salad, stuffed, 281
  stuffing, 133
Prunes, cooked, 475
Puddings, bread, 486; cottage-cheese,
    487; date-nut, 487
  chiffon-cream, 517
  date, 500
  flaming, 491
  fruit, 491
  meringue cream, 517
  plum, 499–500; hard sauce for, 500
  prepared, 491; cake filling, 491;
    flaming, 491; fruit, 491; pie
    filling, 491
  rice, 487; cream, 490; poor man's,
    487–488
  See also Bavarian creams, custards,
    junket, sponges
Puffed-wheat bars, 531
Puffs, cheese, 427–428
  cream, 428
Pumpkin pie, 514–515

Quick-bread mix, 428–429
Quick breads, 415–416
  biscuits, 424–425
  cornbread, 421–422
  flour for, 416
  mix, 428–429; for biscuits, 430;

Quick breads (cont'd)
  coffee cake, 432; cookies, 431;
    gingerbread, 499; muffins, 430;
    nut loaf, 432; pancakes, 429; spice
    cake, 433; waffles, 430
  muffins, 423–424
  nut breads, 426–427
  pancakes, 417–419
  soda, effect of, 415; substitute for,
    415–416
  steamed, 425
  waffles, 419–421
  yeast in, 416

Rabbit, braised, 61
  fried, 58
  roast, 46
  stewed, 73
Rack of lamb, definition of, 25
Radish tops, with kale and sour
    cream, 360–361
  See also leafy vegetables
Raisin pie, 513; -nut pie, 515
Raisins, cooked, 475
Rarebit, baked, 250
  mushroom, 250
  oyster, 250
  Swiss style, 250
  tomato, 250
  Welsh, 249–250
Raspberries, as dessert, 473–474
  directions for canning, 456–457;
    freezing, 453–454
  how to handle, 469; prepare, 473–
    474
Raspberry, appetizers, 255
  pie, 512, 518
  yogurt, 444–445
Recipes, changes, reasons for, 7–8
  creating and revising, 539–541
  explanation of, 4–5, 12–13
  four fundamental, 4
  meat, reasons for multiplicity of,
    51
Reconstituted milk, 450
Red beans, Mexican style, 392
Refrigerator cookies, 522, 523–524
Relishes, cabbage, 461
  cauliflower, 461
  celery-horseradish, 461
  corn, 461
  cucumber, 461
  pepper, 461
  tomato, green, 461
Rhubarb, directions for canning, 457;
    freezing, 454

Rhubarb (cont'd)
pie, 512
steamed, 478
Rhubarb chard, creamed, 357–358
See also leafy vegetables
Rib roast, definition of, 23
prime, 23; standing, 23
Rib steaks, beef, definition of, 24;
veal, 25
Riboflavin, *see* vitamin B₂
Rice, B vitamins in, 180; losses in
washing, 180
brown, 180
casserole with brains, 89; fish, 166;
kidneys, 89; liver, 88–89
converted, definition of, 180
cooked in milk, 181
cooked with tomatoes, 398
cream, 490
"creamed," 397–398
cooking water, amount to use, 181
fried, 191–192
how to cook, 181
how to store, 130; wash, 180
muffins, 424
omelet, 245
pie, 198
pudding, 487; poor-man's, 488
Spanish rice with meat, 190
stuffing, 131, 132
-tomato soup, 307
with beef, 184; cheese, 182; chicken,
183; clams, 183; fish, 183; ham,
183; lamb, 183; liver, 183; mushrooms, 183; oysters, 183; peas,
183; salmon, 183; seeds, 183;
shrimp, 184; veal, 183; vegetables,
184
Rice polish recipes:
biscuits, 424
breads, 426; steamed brown, 426
cookies, 519–524
cornbread, 422
gingerbread, 499
meat loaf, 109
muffins, 423
pancakes, 417
pie crust, 509
plum pudding, 499
rolls, 413
waffles, 419
Rigatoni, 186
Roasting meats, characteristics of individual roasts, effect on cooking
time, 43
cooking times and temperatures, 44
method, 41–43

Roasting meats (cont'd)
slow, 47–49
thermometer, need for, 42
Roasts, bear, 47
beef, less tender cuts, 45; tender
cuts, 45
big game, 47
buffalo, 47
chicken, 45–46
duck, 46; wild, 47
elk, 47
goose, 46
grouse, 47
ham, 46
lamb, 46
liver, 46
moose, 47
mutton, 46
pheasant, 47
pork, 46
prairie chicken, 47
rabbit, 46
spareribs, 47; barbecued or glazed,
47
squab, 47
suckling pig, 46–47
turkey, 47; wild, 47
veal, 47
venison, 47
wild duck, 47
wild turkey, 47
Roe, fish, baked, 155
broiled, 156
chilled, with capers and olives, 224;
egg sauce, 224; onion sauce, 224
fried with skate, 161
Rolls, almond, 413–414
butter, 414–415
butterhorns, 415
cinnamon, 414
directions for cutting, 413
orange, 414
wheat-germ, 412–413
Rose hips, extracting vitamin C
from, 465–466
nutritive value, 465
Round of beef, definition of, 24; of
veal, 25
Rump roast, definition of, 24
Russian beet soup, 307
Rutabagas, baked, 373
cooking methods, 365
leftover, 373
mashed, 373
simmered in milk, 372–373
steamed, 373
See also turnips

Rye, bread, 412
  muffins, 424
  waffles, 420

Salad dressings, cheese, 289, 290, 291
  cooked, 291–292
  cream, 289, 291, 292
  French, 288–289
  fruit, 292
  lemon juice for, 288
  low calorie, 290; cheese, 291;
    "cream," 291
  mayonnaise, 289
  nut, 289
  nutritive value, 260, 287
  oils for, 287–288
  peanut butter and banana, 290
  olive, 289
  seasoned vinegar for, 289
  sour cream, 291, 292
  Thousand Island, 290, 292
  tomato-soup, 289
  vinegar for, 288
  yogurt, 290–291
Salad greens, *see* greens
Salad ingredients, chilling, impor-
    tance of, 262, 263
  discoloration of, 263
  drying of, 260–261
  effect of cutting and peeling, 263;
    soaking, 262–263
  green leaves, value of, 261
  handling of, 260–263
  how to buy, 261; prepare, 261–
    263; store, 263
  losses during preparation, 262–263
  minerals in, 261
  nutritive importance, 260, 261
  sugar in, 262
  vitamins in, 261
  washing of, 260–261
  when to gather, 261
  See also tossed salads
Salad oils, 260, 264, 287–288
  See also vegetable oils
Salad-seasoned vinegar, 289
Salads, apple, 270; carrot, 273; car-
    rot and orange, 270
  as first course, advantages of, 260
  avocado, 271–272
  candle, 280
  carrot, 273; and apple, 273; apple
    and orange, 270
  cole slaw, 272–273
  cottage cheese, 278–279
  cucumber, 274–275

Salads (*cont'd*)
  finger, 267; combined with other
    foods, 269–270; with French
    dressing, 268
  fruit, 279–280; candle, 280; salad
    bowl, 280–281
  gelatin, 281–286
  grapefruit, 281
  melon, 281
  orange, 281
  pear, 281
  potato, American, 386; German,
    386–387
  prune, stuffed, 281
  tomato, platter, 276–277; sliced,
    280–281; stuffed, 277–278
  tossed, 266–267; importance of, 264–
    265
  See also gelatin salads, salads for
    entrées, tossed salads
Salads for entrées, aspic, 230–231
  beef, corned, 233
  brain, 81–82; with sour cream or
    yogurt, 82
  brains, 232
  cheese, 230
  chicken, 232
  cottage cheese, 232
  crab, 232
  egg, 230
  egg, American cheese, 232
  fish, 230, 232, 233
  ham, 233
  heart, 233
  how to prepare, 229–230
  kidney, 233
  lamb, 233–234
  liver, 233
  lobster, 232
  mayonnaise with cheese, egg, fish,
    or meat, 230
  meat, 230
  pork, roast, 233
  shrimp, 232–233
  sweetbreads, 233
  tongue, 234
  turkey, 232
  veal, 234
Salmon, with macaroni, noodles, rice,
    or spaghetti, 183
Salsify, *see* oyster plant
Salt, effect on meats, 19, 39, 53, 69;
    on fish, 147; dry beans, lentils,
    peas, 175; in fish, 147; meats, 19
  need for, 219–220
Salt pork, definition of, 26
Sandwich spreads, brain, 82

Sauces, almond, 143
  barbecue, 140; for canning, 460; spiced, 460
  brown, 136
  butter, garlic, 142; herb, 142; lemon, 142
  caper, 136
  caraway, 136
  celery, 136
  cheese, 136; -pimento, 136
  chili, 140; for canning, 459–460
  citron-cherry, 143
  cream, medium, 135; variations of, 135–138
  creole, 140; uncooked, 141
  curry, 137; pineapple, 144
  delicious, 137
  dill, 137
  egg, 137
  hard, 500
  Hollandaise, easy, 138–139; mock, 137
  horseradish, 137; mustard, 143–144
  how to prepare, 134–135, 138
  Italian, 140; for canning, 460
  lemon, 139, 143
  Mexican, 141; for canning, 460
  milk in, 135
  mint, 143
  Mornay, 137
  mushroom, 136
  mustard, 137; -horseradish, 143–144
  naming of, 134
  olive, 137
  onion, 137, 144
  pimento, 137
  piquant, 137–138
  sour cream, 143; variations of, 143–144
  Spanish, 141
  spiced, 142
  tartar, 144; hot, 137
  tomato, 140
  tomato catsup, for canning, 460
  vinegar, 139
  whole-wheat flour in, 135
  yogurt, 143; variations of, 143–144
Sauerkraut, -tomato juice appetizer, 252
  with apples, 373–374; cabbage, 368, 373; caraway seeds, 373; duck, 61; ham, 373; pineapple, 373; pork chops, 37; sausage and apples, 114; spareribs, 47, 120; tomatoes, 374; wieners, 107, 374

Sausage, brain, 82
  broiled liver sausage, 105
  liver-sausage crisps, 105
  mock liverwurst, 228–229
  pigs in blankets, 114
  pork, pan-broiled, 38
  pork, seasoned, 114
  pork, with apples and sauerkraut, 114; liver loaf, 92; soy beans, 174
  with baked eggs, 241; beans, 177; scrambled eggs, 238
Sautéed meats, bear, 40
  beef paprika, 40
  beef Stroganoff, 40
  brains with chives, 40; eggplant, 80; lemon sauce, 79; scrambled eggs, 80; sour cream, 80; tomatoes, 80; vegetables, 80; yogurt, 80
  heart, 95
  kidneys, 83
  lamb steaks, 40
  liver, 40–41; with bacon or onions, 41
  liver-sausage crisps, 105
  mock oysters, 80
  pork chops, steaks, or tenderloin, 41
  round steak, 40
  sweetbreads, 99; with ham, 99
  Swiss steak, quick, 41
  tripe, 117
  veal cutlets, 39–40; in batter, 40
Sautéing of meats, meat thermometer, use of, 39
  method, 39
  time and temperature tables, 32
Sautéing fish, 161
Sea food, *see* clams, crab, crawfish, fish, lobster, mussels, oysters, roe, scallops, shrimp
Scallops, broiled, 156
  French-fried, 160
  mock, 159
Scoring meats, 62–63
  effect of, 62
  methods, 62–63
Scrapple, 122
Searing meat, disadvantage of, 62
  effect of, 20
  method, 36
Seasonings, aromatic oils in, 5, 147
  how to use, 5; with meats, 19; fish, 147
Shanks, beef, definition of, 23; veal, 25

Shellfish, *see* clams, crab, crawfish, lobster, mussels, oysters, scallops, shrimp
Shepherd's pie, 214
Sherbets, frozen fruit purées, 256
frozen tomato appetizer, 256
fruit, 482, 497–498
orange, 497–498
tomato, 256
Short ribs of beef, braised, 67
definition of, 24
Shoulder of veal, definition of, 25
Shrimp, and avocado salad, 271–272
appetizer, 258; in grapefruit halves, 252–253
bisque, 313
broiled, 156
casserole with brains, 80
chilled, with mushrooms, 223
creamed with brains, 79; with dill, 164
curried, 75, 165
deviled, 169–170
egg foo yung, 202
flaked fish loaf, chilled, 226
French-fried, 159–160
how to clean, 151
Newburg, 167
salads, 232–233
soufflé, 195
steamed, 163
with creamed eggs, 243; fried rice, 192; macaroni, noodles, rice, or spaghetti, 184; noodles, 187–188
Shrinkage of meat, temperature effect on, 14–15, 17
Sirloin of beef, definition of, 24; veal, 25
Skewer cooking, flaming, 102
method, 102
Skewered, ham with broiled yams, 379
lamb, 103; with broiled yams, 379
meat with fruit, 103
oysters, 103
shish kebab, 103
shrimp, 103
top sirloin of beef, 103
veal, 103
Slow braising, 68–69
Slow roasting, 47–49
Smooth diets, vegetables for, 326
Smothered meats, *see* braised meats
Soaking foods, effect of, 21, 77, 146, 175, 262–263, 317–318, 364–365, 469, 540

Soda, effect on B vitamins, 175; vitamin C, 319; in making breads, 415
Soufflés, brains, 196
broccoli, 196
carrot, 195
cheese, 194
chicken, 195
corn, 195
crab, 195
fish, 195
ham, 195
liver, 195
lobster, 195
mushroom, 195
nutritive value, 193
pea, 195
potato, 196
preparation of, 193
shrimp, 195
Spanish, 196
spinach, 196
sweetbreads, 196
Soup garnishes and accompaniments, 298–299
Soup making, acids, use of, 294
bones and meat scraps in, 293–294
calcium in, 294, 296
cooking temperatures, 294
extracting gelatin for, 294; meat juices for, 294
leftovers in, 294
meat, when to add, 297
minerals in, 295
parings in, 293, 295
powdered milk in, 297
salt, when to add, 294
soy flour in, 297
stock, bones to buy for, 296; uses for, 296
vegetables for, 296–297; how to prepare, 296
vitamins in, 295
Soups, bean, black, 315; chili, 315; kidney, 315; leftover, 315; lima, 315; minestrone, 316; navy, 314–315; pinto, 316; without bones, 315
bisques, fish, 312; mushroom, 313; salmon, 313; shellfish, 313; tomato, 313
bouillon, beef, 302; chicken, 302; jellied, 302; with chicken, 302; tomato, 302
chowder, clam with milk, 319; tomatoes, 304; vegetables, 321; corn, 310; oyster, 311

Soups (*cont'd*)

consommé, beef, 301–302; jellied, 312; with egg, 302

cream, avocado, 310; chicken, 308, with cucumbers, 308, mushrooms, 309; leek and potato, 310–311; mixed vegetables, 311; mock oyster, 311; mushroom, 311; oyster, 311; pea, 311; potato, 311; split pea, 311; tomato, 311; turkey, 309; vegetable, 309–310; watercress, 312

lentil, 315

onion, 302

pureé, buckwheat-tomato, 306; mixed vegetable, 305–306; spinach, 306

split-pea, I, 316; II, 316

stock for, 300; beef, 300; chicken, 300; clear, 301; dark, 301; light, 301; of uncooked meat and fresh bones, 301; vegetable-cooking water, 301

vegetable, with meat, 303–305; chicken, 304; chicken gumbo, 304; ground meat, 303–304; heart, 304; Italian meat soup, 304–305; pepper-pot, 305; tongue, 304; turkey, 304; with meat balls, 305

vegetable, without meat, 306–307; borsch, or Russian beet soup, 307; corn, 307; okra, 307; rice-tomato, 307

Sour cream, biscuits, 425

salad dressing, 291, 292

sauce, 143

Soy, chews, 526

nuts, 531–532

pancakes, 417

Soybeans, amino acids in, 171

B vitamins in, 171

calcium in, 171

protein in, 171

soy grits, use of, 172

soy nuts, 531–532

starch, lack of, 171

Soybeans, dried, "baked," 173

chili, 173; with meat and beans, 179–180

Chinese, 173

cooked, 172–173

creamed, 173

how to prepare, 172

loaf, 173

patties, 173

savory, 173

Spanish style, 173

Soybeans, dried (*cont'd*)

with bacon, 174; beef, 174; chicken, 174; green onions, 174; ham, 174; sausage, 174; tomatoes, 174; wieners, 174, vegetables, 174

Soybeans, fresh, 400

chilled, 400

creamed, 400

simmered in milk, 400

steamed, 400

Soy flour, value of in breadmaking, 403; in soups, 297

Soy flour recipes:

biscuits, 424

breads, 426; steamed brown, 426

cookies, 519–524

cornbread, 422

gingerbread, 499

meat loaf, 109

muffins, 423

omelets, fluffy, 244–245

pancakes, 417

pie crusts, 509

plum pudding, 499

rolls, 413

soufflés, 194–195

soups, 304, 310, 313, 314

waffles, 419

Soy grits, advantages of using, 172

definition of, 172

how to prepare, 172, 174–175

Soy grits recipes:

almond-custard pie, 514

Bavarian cream, 497

breads, 409, 426; steamed brown, 426

brownies, 524–525

cereals, 436

chews, 525, 526

chili with meat and beans, 179–180

cookies, 519, 522, 524

cornbread, 422

corn-meal mush, 198

croquettes, 206–207

custards, 484, 486

marshmallow cream, 489

meat loaf, 109

muffins, 423

softened soy grits, 174–175

soufflés, 194–195

soups, 304, 306, 307, 310, 313, 314

soybeans, substitute for, 172–174

summer squash in batter, 351

tamale pie, 197–198

tortes, 503

zucchini, stuffed baked, 355

Spaghetti, *see* macaroni, noodles or spaghetti
Spaghetti pie, 198
Spanish, chicken, 72
  omelet, 246
  rice with meat, 190
  sauce, 141
  soufflé, 196
  -style chicken, 58
  -style eggs, 238
  -style soybeans, 173
  wieners, 106
Spareribs, definition of, 25
  barbecued, 47, 119–120; braised, 120; pickled, 118; roast, 47; stewed, 121; stuffed, 47; with apples, 120; sauerkraut, 47, 120
Spencer steaks, definition of, 24
Spice, brownies, 525
  cake, 432–433
  cookies, 431, 522, 524
Spiced, fruit, 464; stuffing, 133
  honey-nut bread, 427
  sauce, 142
Spinach, and parsley with bacon and garlic, 360
  directions for freezing, 454–455
  -filled pancakes, 200
  oxalic acid in, 356
  purée, soup, 306
  soufflé, 196
  See also leafy vegetables
Split peas, *see* peas, split
Sponges, banana, 494
  how to make, 494
  lemon, 495
  lime-pineapple, 495
  marshmallow, 492
  orange, 495
  strawberry, 494
  yogurt, 495
Squab, braised, 61
  roast, 47
Squash, crookneck, 354
  See also squash, summer
Squash, summer, baked, 350; with sauce, 350
  broiled, 350
  creamed, 350
  directions for freezing, 454–455
  fried in batter, 351; with crumbs, 351; tomatoes, 351
  sautéed, 350; with bacon, 350–351; other vegetables, 350
  steamed, 351
  with cheese, 349

Squash, winter, acorn, baked, 401
  browned, 401
  mashed, 402; leftover, 402
  pie, 514–515
  steamed, 402
  stuffed, 401
  varieties of, 401
Stainless-steel cooking utensils, 6–7
  disadvantages of, 6-7
Steaks, broiled, 33, 35
  chicken-fried, 40
  definition of, club, 24; filet mignon, 25; flank, 24; New York cut, 25; porterhouse, 24; rib, 24; round, 24–25; sirloin, 24; Spencer, 24; Swiss, 24; T-bone, 24
  marinated flank, 101
  pan-broiled, 38; stuffed, 38
  pounded, 35
  round, marinated, 101
  Swiss, 65; broiled, 35; quick, 41
  tenderized, 35
Steamed meats, *see* braised meats
Steaming fish, 162
Steel-cut oats, 435; value of, 435
Stewing, cuts to use, 69
  meat bones, use of, 69
  method, 69
  salt, use of, 69
Stews, beef, 70–71; with dumplings, 71–72; fruit, 71; wheat, 71
  beef and kidney pie, 71
  beef paprika, 71
  chicken, 72; with dumplings, 73; mushrooms and olives, 73; noodles, 73; paprika, 73; pineapple, 73; rice, 73; vegetables, 73
  chicken curry, 74–75; with tuna, 75
  chicken pie, 72
  heart, 71
  Hawaiian chicken, 75
  Hungarian goulash, 71
  kidney and beef, 208
  lamb, braised, 67–68
  liver, 90–91
  New England boiled dinner, 71
  pepper-pot, 117
  pigs' feet, 119
  rabbit, 73
  Spanish chicken, 72
  spareribs, 121
  veal, braised, 67–68
Stock for soup, *see* soups
Strawberries, how to handle, 469; prepare, 473–474
  served with stems, 473

Strawberry, appetizer, frozen purée, 256
  pie, 512, 518
  sponge, 495
String beans, *see* beans, green string
"Strong-flavored" vegetables, 364–365
  cooking methods, 365
  enzymes in, 364–365
  indigestion from, 364
  soaking, effect of, 364
  sulfur in, 364–365
  See also broccoli, Brussels sprouts, cabbage, cauliflower, onions, rutabagas, turnips
Stuffed, acorn squash, 401
  artichokes, 327
  beefsteak, 38
  braised flank of beef, 64–65
  braised pork shoulder, 65
  breast of lamb, 65; veal, 65
  celery, 269
  chili peppers, 192–193
  chilled baked fish ring, 223
  cold roast chicken, 222
  cucumbers, 269
  cucumbers, with brains, 81
  dried fruit, 528–529
  eggplant, 217
  eggs, hard-cooked, 244
  fish, baked, 152–153
  fish fillets, 153
  fried squid, 161
  heart, braised, 54–55
  leg of lamb, barbecued, 51
  meat loaf, 110
  mutton chops, 38
  onions, 372; with brains, 81
  paprika rings, salad, 275–276
  peaches, 472
  peppers, 112–113, 192–193, 215; with brains, 81; creamed chicken, ham, oysters, or shrimp, 113; ground beef, 112–113; ground beef and leftover meats, 113; heart, 94; leftover meats, 113; liver, 92; macaroni and cheese, 113; meat loaf, 113
  pepper rings, salad, 275–276
  pimentos, 193; rings, salad, 275–276
  pork chops, 35, 37
  potatoes, sweet, 377; white, 378
  prune, salad, 281
  rigatoni, 186
  roast meats, beef, 45; chicken, 45–46; duck, 46; goose, 46; grouse, 47; lamb, 46; liver, 46; pheasant,

Stuffed (*cont'd*)
  47; pork, 46; prairie chicken, 47; rabbit, 46; spareribs, 47; squab, 47; suckling pig, 46–47; turkey, 47; veal, 47; wild duck, 47; wild turkey, 47
  spareribs, 47
  tomatoes, baked, 354; salad, 277–278; with brains, 81
  tripe, 117
  wieners, 106
  zucchini, baked, 355; with brains, 81
Stuffings, apple, 133
  apricot, 133
  barley, hulled, 132
  buckwheat, 132
  celery, 131
  chestnut, 130
  chicken, 130
  cornbread, 130
  crumb, 129–130
  duck, 130
  eggplant, 131
  for fish, 131; beef, lamb, mutton, or pork, 130; poultry, 130
  how to lace roasts, 128–129; to pack stuffing, 128
  meats to stuff, 128; pockets in, 128
  millet, 132
  mushroom, 131
  onion, 131
  oyster, 131
  peach, 133
  pineapple, 133
  potato, 131
  preparation of, 129; vegetables for, 129
  prune, 133
  rice, 131, 132; wild, 132
  spiced-fruit, 133
  turkey, 130
  unground wheat, 132
  wild rice, 132
Sucrose, *see* sugar
Suckling pig, 46–47
Sugar, cookies, 519–520
  disadvantages of use, 527–528
  losses in cooking vegetables, 318; soaking, 262, 318; standing, 319
  relation to tooth decay, 527–528
Sulfur, effect of soaking, 364
  effect of heat on, 242, 364–365
  in "strong-flavored" vegetables, 364–365

Summer squash, *see* squash, summer
Swedish pancakes, 247
Sweet potatoes or yams, baked, 377, 379; glazed, 377; leftover, 378; stuffed, 377
    broiled, 379; on skewers, 379; with bananas, 379
    casserole, 385; with apples, 385
    chips, 382
    French-fried, 382
    fried, American, 381; with apple or pineapple, 381
    glazed, 378
    hash-browned, 378
    leftover baked, 378
    mashed, 383
    oven "French fries," 379
    patty shells, 381
    scalloped, 384–385
    steamed, 388
    stuffed, 378
    vitamin A in, 376
Sweet-sour, beans, green string, 343
    lamb tongues, 115
    lentils, 396–397
    purple cabbage, 368–369
    tongues, 115
Sweetbreads, appetizer, 259
    baked, 96–97; with other meats, 97
    braised, 99
    broiled, 35, 97
    creamed, 98
    creamed with brains, 79
    definition of, 77
    economy of, 96
    for salads, 96
    how to prepare, 96
    in bacon rings, 97
    Newburg, 167–168
    nutritional importance of, 76–77
    salads, 233
    sautéed, 99; with ham, 99
    soufflé, 196
Swiss steak, 65
    broiled, 35
    quick, 41
Swiss-style rarebit, 250

Tables of cooking times and temperatures for broiling, pan-broiling, sautéing meats, 32; roasting, barbecuing, 76
Taffy, molasses, 530
Tamale loaf, 198; pie, 197–198
Tartar sauce, 144; hot, 137
T-bone steaks, definition of, 24

Temperatures, effect on amino acids, 20; aromatic oils, 5; connective tissue of meat, 16–18, 22, 52–53; ground meat, 18; meat, 14–22; protein, 14, 16–18, 20–22, 52–53
    for braising, 52–53; for slow braising, 68; slow roasting, 47–49
    for broiling, 15
    for cooking eggs, 239; fish, 147–148, 151, 157–158; kidneys, 83; meat loaves, 108; soup, 294
    for meringues, 515
    for slow roasting, 48–49
    meat, internal, 17; when broiling, pan-broiling, sautéing, 32; roasting, barbecuing, 44; slow roasting, 48–49
    tables for broiling, pan-broiling, sautéing meats, 32; roasting, barbecuing, 44
    to destroy trichinae, 29
Tenderizing meats, by acids, 21, 53
    by pounding, 18
    by scoring, 62–63
Tenderloin of pork, definition of, 26
Tenderness of meat, how to judge, 22–23, 26–28; relation to fat content, 26
Thermometers, use in cooking meat, 14, 17, 19; barbecuing, 50; broiling, 31; chops or steaks, 35; meat loaves, 108; pan-broiling, 36; pork, 30; roasting, 42; sautéing, 39; slow braising, 68; slow roasting, 49
    use in cooking fish, 147–148, 152, 157
    use in making custards, 485
Thermostats, oven, inaccuracy of, 42
Thousand Island dressing, 290–292
Thymus, *see* sweetbreads
Tiger's milk, 447
    instant, where to buy, 447
    nutritive value, 446
Tiger's milk recipes:
    chili with meat and beans, 179–180
    deviled sea food, 170
    meat loaf, 109
    pizza, 190
    soups, 304–306
    spaghetti with beef, 185
    Spanish rice with meat, 190
    tomato sauce, 140
    yogurt popsicles, 449

Timetables, for broiling, pan-broiling, sautéing, 32
for roasting, barbecuing, 44
Toast, French, 247
Tomato, appetizer, frozen, 256
aspic, I, 283; II, 283; -cucumber, 285
bisque, 313
bouillon, jellied, 302
-buckwheat purée, soup of, 306
catsup, 460
gravy, 127
juice appetizers, 252; -grapefruit, 252; -sauerkraut, 252
juice and purée, directions for canning, 458; freezing, 454
omelet, 245
relish, 461
-rice soup, 307
salads, 276–278; platter, 276–277; stuffed, 277–278
sauces, 140–141; directions for canning, 459–460
sherbet, 256
soup, cream of, 311
-soup salad dressing, 289
Tomatoes, baked, 353; stuffed, 353
broiled, 352–353
directions for canning, cold-pack, 457; open-kettle, 459
loosening skins, 452–453, 469
paraffin on, 276
sautéed, 353; with brains, 80
stewed, 351–352; with corn, 352
stuffed, 354; salad, 277–278; with brains, 81
with green onions, 352; liver, 90
Tongue, beef or pork, rolled with bacon, 116; braised, 55
browned beef, pork, or veal, 115
creamed lamb, 55
how to prepare, 114
pork, cold, 222
pork, with apple rings, 116
pressed, 227
salads, 234
soup, 304
sweet-sour lamb, 115; beef or veal, 115
with soybeans, 174
See also leftover meats
Tooth decay, relation to sugar intake, 527–528
Top sirloin, definition of, 24
Tortes, almond, 503
walnut, 502–503

Tossed salads, directions for making, 264–265
oil, amount to use, 265; how to add, 264; purpose of, 264
purpose of tossing, 264–265
suggested variations, 266–268
Trichinae, danger of, 129
in pork, 29; pork sausage, 29; tenderized hams, 29
temperature at which destroyed, 29
Trichinosis, how spread, 29–30
prevalence of, 29
symptoms of, 29
Trifle, Americanized, 493
Tripe, creamed, 116
creole, 117
broiled, 116–117
pepper-pot soup, 305
pepper-pot stew, 117
sautéed, 117
stuffed, 117
Tuna, casseroles, 205–206; with brains, 80; potato chips, 165
creamed with brains, 79
curried with chicken, 75
deviled, 169–170
omelet, 245
patties, 169
with noodles, 187–188
Turkey, curried, 75
dressing, 130
fried, 58–59
gravy, 127
Hawaiian, 76
roast, 47; wild, 47
soup, 304, 309
with baked sweetbreads, 97
Turnips, 374
baked, 374
crisp shredded, 374
cooking methods, 365
creamed, 374
mashed, 374–375
sautéed, 375
scalloped, 375
steamed, 375
Turnip tops, steamed, 363–364; with vinegar sauce, 364
vitamin A in, 355
See also leafy vegetables

Uncooked candies, *see* candies
Utensils, *see* cooking utensils, kitchen equipment

Veal, and ham with sage, 38
braised rump or shoulder, 65

Veal (*cont'd*)
  breast, stuffed, 65
  chilled barbecued, 221
  croquettes, 207
  curried, 75, 105
  cutlets, broiled, 35; sautéed, 39–40; in batter, 40
  cuts of, 25
  goulash, 216
  gravy, 127
  Hawaiian, 76
  in blankets, 108
  loaf, chilled, 227
  patties, 112
  riblets, braised, 67
  roast breast, leg, loin, rib, or shoulder, 47; stuffed, 47
  salads, 234
  shanks, braised, 66
  skewered, 103; with fruit, 103
  steak, marinated, 101
  stew, 67–68
  with baked sweetbreads, 97; noodles, 187
  See also brains, ground meats, heart, kidney, leftover meats, liver, tongue, tripe
Vegetable-cooking water, definition of, 297
Vegetable marrow, 349, 354
  See also squash, summer
Vegetable oils, as seasoning for cooked vegetables, 326
  beaten into butter, 7–8
  in salad dressings, 260, 277–288
  kinds, 287
  rancidity, danger of, 288
  relation to cholesterol, 7, 11, 287
  storage of, 288
  unsaturated fatty acid content, 287
  use in cooking meat, 19; frying fish, 157
  use to prevent coronary disease, 7–8, 11
  vitamin E, need for, 8, 288
Vegetable parings, *see* peelings
Vegetable purées, *see* soups
Vegetables, chilling, importance of, 262, 263, 319, 320, 321, 322, 365, 376
  chopping, effect of, 263, 320, 365
  cooking water, use of, 321
  creaming, 326
  cream sauce for, 326
  flavor losses, 262, 318, 319, 320
  frozen, how to prepare, 320

Vegetables (*cont'd*)
  handling of, 260–263, 317, 364–365, 375–376
  how to buy, 261, 317; preserve vitamins, 319–320, 322, 376
  leafy, 355–357
  mineral losses, 263, 317–318
  peeling, 263, 318–319, 376
  potatoes, 375–376
  preparation of, 319–321, 364–365, 376
  preserving color of, 263, 320–321, 365
  reheating, 321, 376
  salt, when to add, 320
  seasoning, 326; use of mayonnaise, 326; sugar, 326; vegetable oils, 326
  shredding, 325
  soaking, 263, 317–318, 364–365, 375
  "strong-flavored," 364–365
  vitamin losses, 262–263, 317–321, 375
Vegetables, cooking methods, baking, 325; in casserole, 325
  boiling, 322; effect of, 317–318, 375–376
  broiling, 325
  double-boiler cooking, 323–324
  frying, 325
  ideal method, requirements of, 322
  pressure cooking, 323
  sautéing, 324
  simmering in milk, 324–325
  steaming, 323
  waterless method, 322–323
Vegetable salads, *see* salads
Vegetable soups, *see* soups
Venison, chicken-fried, 40
  meat loaf, 110
  pan-broiled, 38
  roast, 47
Vinegar, egg white, effect on, 238
  salad-seasoned, 289
  sauce, 139
  use in cooking meat, 21, 53; in cooking kidneys, 83; bony meats, 117–118
  use in dissolving calcium, 117–118, 294
  use in making soups, 294–295; 314
  use in retarding enzyme action, 460, 465
Vitamin A, destruction by heat, 319
  destruction by oxygen, 261; room temperature, 468
  in animal fat, 27–28; appetizers, 251; eggs, 235; green salads, 261;

Vitamin A (*cont'd*)
  in animal fat (*cont'd*)
    leafy vegetables, 355; peppers, 331; persimmons, 476; sweet potatoes and yams, 376
Vitamin B complex, in buckwheat, 392; cereal, 434; fish, 145–146; glandular meats, 77, 220; green salads, 261; heart, 77; liver paste, 228; meat, 21; milk, 439, 440; nuts, 502, 528; pork, 29; soybeans, 171; tiger's milk, 446; wheat germ, 437; yeast, 406; yogurt, 220
  losses during soaking, 21, 77, 175, 263, 317; in hot weather, 219
  solubility of, 76, 263, 317, 469
  storage of, 76
  synthesis by yogurt bacteria, 441–442
Vitamin B₁, destruction by high heat, 320
  solubility, 295
Vitamin B₂, cancer, relation to, 10–11
  destruction by light, 6, 236–237, 262, 319, 320; room temperature, 468
  in cheese, 235; eggs, 235; green salads, 261; milk, 438
  solubility of, 295
Vitamin C, destruction at room temperature, 468; by alkali, 319; by copper, 263, 319; iron, 319; by heat, 252, 295; by oxygen, 261, 319, 469
  extraction of, from rose hips, 465–466
  in appetizers, 251, 252; citrus fruits, 220, 252; guavas, 468, 476; green salads, 261; kohlrabi, 343; peppers, 112, 275, 331; pickles, 460; rose hips, 465; salads, 220, 260; tomatoes, 220; white potatoes, 375
  losses during cooking, 108, 112, 204, 317–318; in hot weather, 219–220; soaking, 263, 317–318, 540; thawing, 469
  preservation by heating, 108, 319
  preventing loss of, 453, 468–470
  ripening, effect on, 331, 468
  solubility of, 76, 263, 295, 317, 469
  storage of, 76
  trichinosis, relation to, 29
  variation with ripeness, 112
Vitamin D, relation to trichinosis, 29
Vitamin E, destruction by high heat, 157; oxygen, 261

Vitamin E (*cont'd*)
  in bread, 403, 404; cereal, 434; green salads, 261; salad oils, 260; wheat germ, 437
  need with vegetable oils, 8, 157
Vitamin K, in green salads, 261

Waffles, baking-powder, 419
  buckwheat, 420
  corn-meal, 420
  from mix, 430
  gingerbread, 420
  rye, 420
  yeast, 420
Walnut-date creams, 536
Washing foods, nutritive losses from, 77, 146, 180, 260, 263
Watercress, aspic, 283; and grapefruit, 286; -pineapple, 284
  soup, cream of, 312
  with mushroom sauce, 363
  See also leafy vegetables
Watermelon, bowl, 474–475
  pickles, 464
Welsh rarebit, 249
Wheat, cracked, 399–400
  simmered, 391, 399–400
  sweet-sour, 397
  with sour cream, 400
Wheat germ, and middlings, 436
  as cereal, 435
  fudge, 533
  how to introduce, 435; keep, 420
  nutritive value, 435, 437
  toasted, 437
  where to buy, 542–543
Wheat-germ-and-oatmeal cookies, 520–521
Wheat germ recipes:
  apple Betty, 488; crisp, 488; sauce, 473
  biscuits, 424
  brain croquettes, 80
  brains in casserole, 80
  brain sausage, 82
  breads, 412; nut, 426; quick mix, 428–429; steamed brown, 425–426
  brownies, 524–525
  candies, fudge, 533; pineapple kisses, 532
  casseroles, 205–206
  cereals, 436–437
  chews, 525–526
  cookies, 519–524
  corn, patties, 396; scalloped, 396
  cornbread, 421, 422

Wheat germ recipes (*cont'd*)
  croquettes, 206–207
  custards, 484, 486
  deviled sea food, 169, 170
  fish loaf, 168
  gingerbread, 498–499
  ground beef broiled on toast, 111
  ground beef in pepper rings, 111
  heart cutlets, 94
  junket, 490
  meat loaf, beef, 108–109; game, 110;
    ham, 109; heart, 110; Italian, 109;
    lamb, 109–110; pork, 110
  muffins, 423
  New Zealand spinach sautéed in
    batter, 359
  omelet, fluffy, 244–245
  pancakes, 417, 418
  patties, beef, 111; brain, 85; corn,
    396; fish, 168–169; game, 111;
    ham, 112; heart, 112; kidney, 84–
    85; lamb, 111–112; liver, 85; mut-
    ton, 111; veal, 111, 112
  pie crusts, 509–511
  plum pudding, 499
  rolls, 412–413
  scrapple, 122
  soufflés, 194–196
  stuffed eggplant, 217–218
  stuffed meat loaf, 110
  stuffings, celery, 131; chestnut, 130;
    cornbread, 130; crumb, 129–130;
    eggplant, 131; mushroom, 131;
    onion, 131; oyster, 131; potato,
    131; rice, 131
  summer squash in batter, 351
  tortes, 502–503
  waffles, 419, 420
  zucchini patties, 354
  zucchini, stuffed baked, 355
Wheat, whole or unground, as a
    cereal, 196–197
  cooked in tomato juice, 399
  cooked under pressure, 197
  creamed, 399
  serving suggestions, 196, 197
  steamed, 398
  stuffing, 132
  with braised beef brisket, 64
Whip, orange, 495–496
  other fruits, 496
Whole-wheat bread, 408–411
Whole-wheat bread mix, 406
Wieners, broiled, 35
  disadvantage of, 103
  French-fried, 106
  how to prepare, 105

Wieners (*cont'd*)
  in blankets, 106
  paprika, 106
  quality of meat in, 103
  Spanish, 106
  stuffed, 106
  with barbecue sauce, 106; cabbage,
    106–107; cheese, 106; eggs, 106;
    omelet or scrambled eggs, 107,
    238; sauerkraut, 107, 374; sour
    cream, 107; soy beans, 174
Wild duck, roast, 47
Wild greens, 359
Wild rice, 398
Wild-rice stuffing, 132
Wild turkey, roast, 47

Yams, *see* sweet potatoes
Yeast, muffins, 424
  pancakes, 418
  waffles, 421–422
Yeast, bakers', advantages of using,
    406–407, 416
  amounts to use, 407
  effect of chilling, 407; heating, 407
  how to buy, 406–407
  optimum temperature for, 407
Yeast, brewers', where to buy, 542–
    543
Yeast, brewers', recipes:
  breads, 426; steamed brown, 426
  chocolate brownies, 524
  cookies, 519, 522
  gingerbread, 449
  meat loaf, 109
  milk, malted, 444
  muffins, 423
  plum pudding, 499
  rolls, 413
  soufflés, 194–195
  tiger's milk, 447
  tomato-juice appetizer, 252
  waffles, 419
Yogurt, advantages of using, 441–442
  digestive value, 441
  electric yogurt maker, 448; where
    to buy, 448
  how to introduce, 442; use, 442
  importance of temperature for,
    447–448
  nutritive value, 441–442
  popsicles, 449
  preparation of, 441, 447–448, 449
  raspberry, 444–445
  salad dressing, 290–291
  sauce, 143; variations, 143–144
  sponge, 495

Yogurt (*cont'd*)
    where to buy, 542–543
    with antibiotics, value, 442
Youngberry, appetizer, frozen purée,
    256
    pie, 512, 518
Youngberries, as dessert, 473–474
    how to handle, 469

Youngberries (*cont'd*)
    how to prepare, 473–474

Zucchini, directions for freezing, 454
    patties, 354
    stuffed baked, 355
    stuffed with brains, 81
    See also squash, summer

Equivalents

a pinch = less than 1/8 teaspoon
3 teaspoons = 1 tablespoon
2 tablespoons = 1/8 cup
4 tablespoons = 1/4 cup
6 tablespoons = 1/3 cup
8 tablespoons = 1/2 cup
12 tablespoons = 3/4 cup
16 tablespoons = 1 cup
1 fluid ounce = 2 tablespoons
1/2 pint = 1 cup
1 pint = 2 cups
2 pints = 1 quart
4 cups = 1 quart
4 quarts = 1 gallon
1 gill = 1/2 cup
4 gills = 1 pint
8 quarts = 1 peck
4 pecks = 1 bushel
16 ounces = 1 pound
16 fluid ounces = 2 cups
28 grams = 1 ounce
454 grams = 1 pound
4 cups flour = 1 pound
2 cups granulated sugar = 1 pound
2 3/4 cups brown sugar = 1 pound